Anxiety Culture

Anxiety Culture

The New Global State of Human Affairs

Edited by
JOHN P. ALLEGRANTE, ULRICH HOINKES,
MICHAEL I. SCHAPIRA, AND KAREN STRUVE

With a foreword by
RENATA SALECL

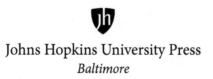

Johns Hopkins University Press
Baltimore

Johns Hopkins University Press
2715 North Charles Street
Baltimore, Maryland 21218
www.press.jhu.edu

Library of Congress Cataloging-in-Publication Data

Names: Allegrante, John P. (John Philip), 1952- editor. | Hoinkes, Ulrich,
editor. | Schapira, Michael I., 1983- editor. | Struve, Karen, editor.
Title: Anxiety culture : the new global state of human affairs / edited by
John P. Allegrante, Ulrich Hoinkes, Michael I. Schapira, Karen Struve,
Description: Baltimore, Maryland : Johns Hopkins University Press, [2024] |
Includes bibliographical references and index.
Identifiers: LCCN 2024021121 (print) | LCCN 2024021122 (ebook) |
ISBN 9781421450360 (hardcover) | ISBN 9781421450377 (epub)
Subjects: LCSH: Anxiety—Social aspects. | World health. |
Civilization, Modern. | Culture.
Classification: LCC BF575.A6 A77 2024 (print) | LCC BF575.A6 (ebook) |
DDC 152.4/6—dc23/eng/20240603
LC record available at https://lccn.loc.gov/2024021121
LC ebook record available at https://lccn.loc.gov/2024021122

A catalog record for this book is available from the British Library.

Special discounts are available for bulk purchases of this book.
For more information, please contact Special Sales at specialsales@jh.edu.

For Asher, Edda Marlie, Vera, and Jonna and Philipp

CONTENTS

Wherever one looks around the world, anxiety is on the rise. With devastating wars, climate change and economic inequality, we face existential concerns related to the survival of the planet and our species. Furthermore, capitalism's promotion of individualism and the ideology of choice has contributed to people's increased dread regarding their private lives. The internet has opened new avenues of anxiety with new types of manipulation, surveillance, and aggression. At the same time, social media encourages people to constantly engage in self-promotion, to try to stand out from the crowd and curate a perfect image of their lives. On the one hand, people are striving to get noticed and not be dismissed, but on the other hand they are not allowed to be ignored, which is why more and more people are experiencing surveillance anxiety.

The essays contained in this volume comprehensively explore how people's anxieties are affected by the multifarious changes we have experienced in the past decades. In an interdisciplinary way, the authors in this volume assess various social and psychological interpretations of anxiety—as well as the semantics of an appellation like "anxiety culture"—to show how broader cultural, economic, political, and social factors influence what is at a particular time for people anxiety-provoking.

From the era of Ronald Reagan and Margaret Thatcher—both of whom championed rugged individualism—people living in Western democracies have been hearing that there is no society, that it is the individual who is ultimately responsible for his or her well-being, and that their success and happiness are related to individual choices. When people are bombarded with the idea that everything in their lives is a matter of choice, that they are free to make out of themselves what they desire, and that there are limitless ways to find enjoyment in life, they often end up anxious that they did not make the right choices. Some might also be full of guilt or feel inadequate when they do not come close to the ideals of success that are culturally and economically propagated.

When people speak about anxiety today, they often invoke the idea that they are now asked to make choices concerning their sexuality, marriage, and reproductive health that once were not regarded as choices in the past. However, the more options there are, the more it can seem impossible to achieve an ideal result. This is the case not only for people who are continually changing their electricity provider in the hope of finding the better deal but also for those searching for their ideal love partner. That is why some claim that love is especially anxiety-provoking today.

The French psychoanalyst Jacques Lacan pointed out that, for people, the questions about their relationships and their standing in a broader social space, which Lacan names the "Big Other," is "anxiogenic."[1] Questions like "Who am I?" or "Who am I for the Other?" never get a satisfying answer. If on the one hand people are still concerned about the question of the desire of the Other (i.e., how others regard them and how they are viewed in society as a whole), on the other hand they are under pressure to choose their lives independently of social constraints. Psychoanalysts thus often encounter patients who come to analysis with the demand, "I need to decide what I want out of my life."

When people are struggling over their choices, they often search for an authority who might appease their anxiety.[2] With the demise of traditional cultural authorities, new leaders (from coaches to trendsetters on social media) are becoming points of reference and identification. Thus, someone today might encounter therapists who specialize in consumer and life-choice anxieties. Some are even taking fashion as anxiety-provoking[3] because it tempts the consumer with unique identities that shift with the season and express the fragmented moralities of cultural diversity and social uncertainty.[4]

As the editors and authors of this book rightly argue, public health has been dramatically affected by increased anxiety among the general population, especially among the young. Yet, the ideology that presents one's health as a matter of personal choice has also contributed to anxiety. When people fall ill, they are often reminded that their illness might be related to their unhealthy lifestyle. They are told they have not eaten the right food, exercised sufficiently, or successfully coped with stress. Even overcoming illness, as has been propagated by some self-help gurus, is viewed as a matter of choice. One often hears that one needs to choose to overcome illness, work hard to change bad habits, and embrace positive thoughts.

In this context, it is not surprising that anxiety and choice have played an essential role in the global public discourse about wearing masks, physical distancing, and vaccination at the time of the COVID-19 pandemic. People who constantly hear how important it is to make the right choices, especially when it comes to their bodies and their individual health, become overwhelmed with anxiety over the question of what to put into one's body and who to listen to for guidance about vaccination.

An analysis of the cultural aspects of anxiety opens the question of what role anxiety plays in upholding the dominant ideologies and economic systems and to what extent it influences social change. The anxiety culture in which we live today—the topical construct of this volume—is of great help to the dominant capitalist ideology that cherishes individual choices and the free market. This is because it often makes people feel responsible for everything happening in their lives. The cultural, economic, and political circumstances under which people live might offer them no possibilities to enhance their well-being. Guilt that they did not make the right choices might paralyze people and prevent them from cooperating and fighting for social change, whether it be in response to climate change, migration and immigration, or the fast pace of technological change.

Anxiety, however, can also be a mobilizing factor. Individually, anxiety can help make us reflect on our actions. Socially, anxiety might mobilize people to prevent future catastrophes that they dread. Years ago, I asked an American military colonel how he copes when his soldiers are under anxiety. He pointed out that he was most afraid of soldiers who do not have anxiety when they engage in the battle since they might end up being ruthless killers.[5]

The solution for our culture of anxiety is to channel this often-uncomfortable feeling into a direction of positive social action and not into something that allows dreaded catastrophes to happen. This book is an ambitious step forward in that direction.

Renata Salecl

NOTES

1. Jacques Lacan, *Anxiety: The Seminar of Jacques Lacan, Book X*, trans. A. R. Price (Cambridge, MA: Polity, 2016).

2. Renata Salecl, *The Tyranny of Choice* (London: Profile Books, 2011).

3. Alison Clarke and Daniel Miller, "Fashion and Anxiety," *Fashion Theory* 6, no. 2 (May 2002): 191–213.

4. Rebecca Arnold, *Fashion, Desire and Anxiety: Image and Morality in the Twentieth Century* (London: Rutgers University Press, 2001).

5. Renata Salecl, *On Anxiety* (London: Routledge, 2004).

This is a volume that aspires to a great scholarly ambition. The story behind that ambition and the basis for the collaboration is worth briefly recounting. Thus, an account of the origins of this book not only reveals the historical background and motivation behind writing it but also the hope that it might be instructive to the reader as they make their way through the various sections and to those scholar-researchers interested in formulating projects of an interdisciplinary nature that this book seeks to catalyze and inform.

The four editors come from different disciplinary backgrounds and occupy different ranks within the academy. Among our two senior scholars and cofounders of the Anxiety Culture Project, John P. Allegrante is a leading scholar in the behavioral health sciences whose research and scholarship focuses on public health and health promotion in the United States and Nordic contexts; Ulrich Hoinkes is a specialist in sociolinguistics and romance language studies who is a former head of the German Association for Catalan Studies. The two junior scholars are both humanities-focused, with Michael I. Schapira concentrating on the historical and philosophical underpinnings of the modern university and Karen Struve on 18th and 20th Century Francophone literature. Anxiety culture was never an articulated part of any aspect of our primary research interests nine years ago, when the acquaintances between the two senior members of our editorial team were first made at Columbia University in New York in March 2015 and then reified in Kiel, Germany, later that year, in June.

The occasion of the Kiel meeting was an informal conference that brought together delegations of education scholars from the Christian Albrechts University of Kiel, the IPN Leibniz Institute for Science and Mathematics Education (in Northern Germany), and Teachers College, Columbia University (in New York City). The modest goals of the conference were to share research, explore and elucidate some cross-cultural points of comparison, and open a dialogue about the possibilities for formal future collaboration around themes of mutual interest. One theme that emerged over the course of the three-day meeting was the prevalence of "threats and dangers in public education" in subfields as diverse as second-language literacy, teacher education (or what is often called "didactics" in Europe), health and science education, and educational policy studies. Despite bringing together scholars from two of the wealthiest advanced economies in the global north, both with long established and in many cases envied institutions of higher education, the meeting produced a clear sense of unease pervading the enterprise of public secondary education and the broader society.

Following the Kiel meeting, a number of conferences and symposia were convened, both in Germany and the United States, to further elucidate, understand, and better articulate the contours of this unease and its implications for public education.[1] As with any descriptive exercise of this nature, there were vigorous and heated debates during these intellectual salons about the appropriate terminology. Was "threats and dangers" adequate? Are we talking about "mere discourse" or "existential realities"? Should "public education" remain the orienting frame, and if so, should the emphasis lie with "public" or "education"? Such discussions not only brought us to anxiety culture as a workable construct but also gave shape to what the editors realized was a potentially exciting and important research program that stretched far beyond the bounds of discipline-based educational scholarship and the American-German contexts. Two main factors were behind this realization. The first was that anxiety culture presented not only a timely theoretical question for the academy but also a socially and culturally relevant question to be addressed in response to the cultural, political, and societal imperatives of the moment. And since it is omnipresent (both in terms of topics and geographical areas), examining the construct from interdisciplinary perspectives seemed warranted and necessary. The second was the ease with which participants from diverse fields of scholarship entered such interdisciplinary conversations about a wide-ranging semantic field of anxiety, from unease to panic, and the enthusiasm with which they exited them. This included both individual scholars from new applied fields such as climate change and technology studies to more established fields such as anthropology, philosophy, and political science. Also included were representatives from institutional partners such as the Council for European Studies and the Alliance Program at Columbia University, the IPN Leibniz Institute for Science and Mathematics Education at Kiel

University, and EUCOR, the five-university alliance across three European countries.

To preserve the interdisciplinary nature of the collaboration, we eventually established four basic research clusters, all representing pressing planetary challenges of the moment and each specific enough to delimit the aspect of anxiety culture under investigation but capacious enough to integrate different streams of research and methodologic approaches and generate a useful set of middle-range concepts. Three of these (climate change, population health, and technology) were present from the origins of our discussions, but the concern with migration, language, and culture arose later in light of the great wave of refugee migration to Europe in 2016 and what we have witnessed subsequently along the southern border of the United States and elsewhere.[2] And cross-cutting each of the areas, of course, the broader influences of the deeply divisive cultural and political polarization that have emerged in the last decade in the United States and across the post-World War II liberal democracies of Europe, most notably the Russian invasion of Ukraine in 2022 and the Israel-Hamas war that broke out in 2023.

We first sketched out our notion of the construct of anxiety culture in a 2018 paper published in *EuropeNow* that became the basis for this book.[3] Against this backdrop, work on the book began in 2019, a year before COVID-19 disrupted our lives, when the Johns Hopkins University Press accepted a proposal from the editors to produce this volume. Thus, much of the work on the book occurred during the course of an unfolding pandemic that would take the lives of over 6.8 million globally.[4] Despite the deprivations and dislocations the pandemic caused, we and especially our contributors—almost one third of whom had participated in one or more of the Anxiety Culture Project conferences and symposia—adapted and persevered with remarkable resilience. The resulting book contains an introduction by the editors and is followed by 22 chapters that have been organized across six parts: Part I—Disciplinary Perspectives on Anxiety; Part II—Climate Change and the Environment; Part III—Population Health and Social Well-Being; Part IV—Migration, Language, and Culture; Part V—Technology; and Part VI—a Coda. An introductory essay to each of the parts briefly explicates the rationale behind the specific cluster and provides an advanced organizer about what each of the chapters in the part contains and contributes. A cursory glance at the table of contents should also tell the reader how productive the clusters have been for gathering a diverse range of scholarly perspectives and integrating novel and important sets of interests such as migration (Part IV). For example, that part contains contributions which reinterrogate the fields of literary studies, bilingual education, and migration studies through the heuristic of the construct anxiety culture. Moreover, these contributions do not stand in isolation from one another but rather together help establish a set of middle range concepts (e.g., around stress and stage-affect theory, about crossing borders) that we believe can serve as a conceptual and practical bridge for interdisciplinary examination of different phenomena related to the movement of peoples.

We must acknowledge and thank the many individuals, colleagues, and collaborators who have contributed to the development of this book. In addition to the contributing authors who persevered during long periods of hardship associated with the social isolation and uncertainty imposed by the pandemic to write the compelling essays that appear in the volume, we owe a debt of gratitude in particular to the following individuals: Prof. Dr. Olaf Köller (IPN Leibniz Institute for Science and Mathematics Education), Dr. Emmanuel Kattan (Columbia University Alliance Program), Dr. Markus Lemmens (EUCOR), and Dr. Nicole Shea (then with the Council for European Studies) for the intellectual enthusiasm and generous administrative support they extended to the project from the outset; Prof. Thomas James (then Dean of Teachers College, Columbia University) and Prof. Jeffrey Sachs (Columbia University), for their enthusiastic encouragement of the book; Profs. Renata Salecl and John Baldacchino for contributing the illuminating essays that make up their respective Foreword and Afterword; and Robin Coleman, acquisitions editor at the Johns Hopkins University Press, whose early encouragement and confidence in the idea for this book made it possible. In addition we must acknowledge and thank the editorial staff at the Johns Hopkins University Press, including Diem Bloom, director of publishing operations; Marlee Brooks, editorial assistant; Sophia Franchi, acquisitions coordinator; Bea Jackson, book designer; Kris Lykke, marketing specialist; and Molly Seamans, art director, all of whom brought their formidable creative talents to this book. Thanks also to Angela Piliouras, Rebecca Faith, and the production team at Westchester Publishing Services for the superb copyediting and other aspects of the production process, and Devon Thomas of DevIndexing indexing service whose work will surely facilitate the reader in navigating this volume.

We also thank the Hamburg Foundation, the Alfred Toepfer Foundation and Gut Siggen Seminar Center, the Representation of Schleswig-Holstein in Berlin, the Consulate General of the Federal Republic of Germany in New York, and the New York University Center for European and Mediterranean Studies, all of which provided conference venue and travel support for the various meetings of the Anxiety Culture Project. We would be remiss if we did not also acknowledge the Centre on Humanities in Education at the Christian Albrechts University of Kiel, the IPN Leibniz Institute for Science and Mathematics Education, and Teachers College, Columbia University—all parties to a multiyear Memorandum of Understanding that grew out of the project and provided a cross-institutional framework that nurtured this collaboration. Each institutional entity invested in the project through various intramural funding, sabbatical leaves, and other forms of generous support at critical junctures that enabled us to devote unfettered attention to completing the work of curating this book.

Finally, there is the incalculable debt to be paid to our spouses, children, and other family members, whose devotion, support, and understanding have fueled and inspired us during the myriad tasks and challenges of completing a book of this nature.

J.P.A.   *New York, New York*
U.H.   *Kiel, Germany*
M.I.S.   *St Andrews, Scotland*
K.S.   *Bremen, Germany*

May 2024

NOTES

1. See Appendix for a listing of the Anxiety Culture Project conferences and symposia.

2. This strand developed most strongly in the summer of 2016, as Angela Merkel, then Chancellor of Germany, pursued the most generous (though not immune to serious critique) refugee policy among her European colleagues. As a bustling port due to its famous canal, Kiel had an abundance of cargo containers that were retrofitted into small family apartments, several of which were erected hundreds of yards from some of our project offices on the campus of Kiel University.

3. See Michael I. Schapira, Ulrich Hoinkes, and John P. Allegrante, "Anxiety Culture: The New Global State of Human Affairs?" *EuropeNow*, 2018, https://www.europenowjournal.org/2018/07/01/anxiety-culture-the-new-global-state-of-human-affairs/.

4. As of March 2023, when the Johns Hopkins University Coronavirus Resource Center suspended operations and stopped collecting data. See https://coronavirus.jhu.edu/map.html.

Introduction

Anxiety as a New Global Narrative

MICHAEL I. SCHAPIRA, KAREN STRUVE,
ULRICH HOINKES, AND JOHN P. ALLEGRANTE

Anecdotal evidence abounds that one of the defining features of contemporary existence, on the collective and the individual level, is the pervasiveness of anxiety. Concerns are proliferating around aspects of our living conditions that seem to be spinning out of control: climate change and its consequences on food systems, the ability to inhabit large areas of the world (e.g., coastlines, deserts, islands), and the stability of ecosystems; increasing prevalence of mental illness, addiction, and chronic medical conditions like obesity in populations; massive population migration and the ensuing disturbances in social and political orders, most recently seen in the Russia-Ukraine war that broke out in early 2022; drastic technological changes with regard to our forms of communication, commerce, and employment; spiraling inequalities within and between nations; a building legitimation crisis in democratic societies and the attendant rise of populism, nationalism, and militarism; terrorism, mass shootings, and the ubiquity of media accounts of mass violence; forms of indebtedness (student, medical, or consumer debt) that lead to chronic insecurity throughout the life cycle; and, to bury the lead and reference the conditions under which this Introduction was written, the as-yet-to-be-understood post-COVID-19 reality, with the global pandemic already having shown a powerful capacity to manifest and then fray the fragile social fabric of national and global culture. That this is by no means an exhaustive list, and that it cuts across cultures, underscores the axiomatic manner in which anxiety is now invoked as the characteristic mood of our age.

Empirical evidence shows that anxiety is a pervasive feature of modern life. Take the field of psychology, where, though long established as an issue of concern, anxiety has moved to the center of clinical concerns.[1] In 1980 the third edition of the American Psychological Association's *Diagnostic and Statistical Manual* (*DSM III*) devoted 15 pages to anxiety disorders. In 1987 the revised edition included 18 pages of such disorders, but by the *DSM IV*'s publication in 1994, the entries had increased to 51 pages, only to be eclipsed in the *DSM V* (2013) by 99 pages on anxiety and related conditions.[2] The National Institute of Mental Health in the United States estimates that 31% of adults will experience an anxiety disorder in their lifetime.[3] Given its prevalence at the clinical individual level, one would be fully warranted in following Ivan Illich's concept of cultural and social "iatrogenesis," and scaling up these individualized medical concerns to cultural and social phenomena.[4] Indeed, the blurring of diagnostic lines (between individual and society, or between descriptive and normative intentions) perfectly maps onto anxiety's uncanny effect of forcing emotional states and concepts to float without the consoling anchor of a well-defined referent.

Aside from its prevalence in professional and nontechnical everyday discourse, the many valences of anxiety throughout history, from its origins in the ancient world to its development as the underside of Western Enlightenment, naturally suggest it as an important keyword for our times. Etymologically, anxiety derives from *Angh*, an Indo-Germanic root referring to "narrowing, constricting, and tightening feelings, usually in the chest and throat," normally in response to fears, threats, and dangers.[5] The physiological dimension of anxiety is very much present in the diagnostic criteria of the *DSM*, but you can also see it in Aristotelian conceptions of moral education, which aim to develop virtuous dispositions that allow us to confront fear in a healthy manner (which, contra anxiety, involves learning how to attach different emotional states to their proper objects).[6] Freud brought anxiety into a modern psychological idiom by distinguishing fear, in which the affective dimension of threats and dangers can attach itself to an object, from anxiety, in which the affective dimension persists in a generalized state of uncertainty and insecurity.[7] Kierkegaard alighted on this feeling of dread, or Martin Heidegger on *Angst*, centering anxiety in the development of existentialism and the processes through which lives are given meaning against a backdrop of both radical freedom and radical insecurity. And today, much in the spirit of this historical trajectory, we see the proliferation of crises, the limits of which we struggle to define and the future toward which they move difficult to imagine.[8]

There are many consequences of living in this state of anxiety on an individual or collective level. Invoking crisis or danger tends to speed up our thinking and lend a sense of urgency to our actions, but might this come at the expense of a deeper understanding of the changing face of our societies? As educators (in addition to scholar-researchers), we are as keenly aware as the American philosopher John Dewey that learning possibilities follow from a slower, patient, and more reflective approach to confounding features of our environment.[9] In this volume we aim to develop the construct of "anxiety culture" as a fruitful heuristic for analyzing a variety or phenomena in our often bewildering times. In the Preface to *The Human Condition*, Hannah Arendt characterized her task as "nothing more than to think what we are doing."[10] We proceed in the same spirit but emphasize the affective dimension that structures our field of action or paralyzes us, Hamlet-like, in peculiar forms of incapacity. This does not mean that the affective dimension drives out fact-based discussions of these problems but notes the many ways that anxiety as a structuring construct can provide an important clue for understanding phenomena as diverse as literary production, political discourse, and changing conventions in public health.

As a heuristic, this construct of anxiety culture draws our attention to various mechanisms in social life related to public discourse and internal thought patterns. These different discursive spaces create their own special forms of anxiety that proliferate in the media and often show up as broad social moods. The challenge is to recognize this kind of anxiety as it is made by a curious admixture of public communication and social action. Anxiety culture is much more than fear about threatening developments and potentially dangerous incidents. It has become characteristic of our dealing—intellectually, cognitively and emotionally—with the increasing problems and undefined solutions in a rapidly changing world. If anxiety culture is about having fears, they are much more generated by feeling the pulse of contemporary life and struggling to conceive of the future than by a cold, analytic study of the present. In other words, an examination of anxiety culture is an attempt to resist the reductive leap toward solutions or definitive understandings and rather to develop a generative new set of conceptual tools for understanding and coping with the present moment. Thus, anxiety, as Kierkegaard put it, "is our best teacher."

To this end we have organized a volume of essays that takes up this theme of anxiety culture from a variety of disciplinary perspectives and interpretations. Before explaining some of the principles guiding our selection of topics and contributors, we would like to make some provisional methodological comments. We see the emerging research agenda around anxiety culture in the tradition of middle range theory (or generative of derivate middle range concepts) akin to the social theories of Zygmunt Bauman and Ulrich Beck, which combines the sociological and analytic project of concept formation with the empirical analyses of various disciplines.[11] As will become clear, we believe that this approach provides the appropriate framework for the interdisciplinary research agenda that we hope will result from our efforts in this volume. It is thus to questions of methodology that we now turn.

Anxiety Culture and Middle Range Theory

The designation of a particular historical juncture as being an anxiety culture is not specific to the present. In 1948, W. H. Auden was awarded the Pulitzer Prize for Poetry for his long verse poem *The Age of Anxiety*. Two years later, the psychologist Rollo May published *The Meaning of Anxiety*, which claimed, "The evidence is overwhelming that we live today in an 'age of anxiety' . . . The ordinary stresses and strains of life in the changing world of today are such that few if any escape the need to confront anxiety and deal with it in some manner."[12] Despite long stretches of affluence in the United States and Western Europe an anxious mood emerged out of World War II. Prior historical periods of war and social upheaval have also generated reflections on anxiety; therefore, it is incumbent on us to develop our understanding of anxiety culture as a useful heuristic for the contemporary moment without reducing it to a mere occurrence of a more general, transhistorical phenomenon.

We propose anxiety culture as an instance of *middle range theorizing*. The term derives from the sociologist Robert K. Merton, who contrasted it with *grand theory* to avoid the temptation to universalize our judgments about an epoch or social phenomenon.[13] As Anders Blok has recently insisted, middle range theorizing is concerned with the production of *concepts* that satisfy both empirical and theoretical ambitions.[14] Put another way, middle range theorizing aims to produce concepts with enough theoretical grounding to move past a purely descriptive enterprise, while at the same time retaining enough of an empirical grounding to resist the universalizing tendencies of social theory.

As will become evident in thematic subdivisions of this volume, anxiety culture brings a specific set of concerns about contemporary life to the fore, particularly those surrounding the experience or discussion of threats and dangers. Yet, it can be situated within a broader field of modern social theory that is motivated by overlapping interests.

The first such area is how to understand the role that *fear* plays in the contemporary world, both as a personal experience and as a social mood. The German sociologist Heinz Bude argues that an understanding of fear as a social mood must displace our tendency to reduce it to a biographical event or clinical diagnosis. "It is through concepts of fear," he writes in a recent book, "that society takes its own pulse."[15] The late Polish sociologist and philosopher Zygmunt Bauman calls fear "the most sinister of the demons nesting in the open societies of our time," warning that the insecurity and sense of impotence that it generates "won't be exorcized until we find (or more precisely *construct*)" the conceptual and practical tools to regain a sense of agency.[16] Such tools, the argument implies, are not currently available; thus, fear lends to the intimately related construct of anxiety.

For Bauman fear is one feature of what he has characterized as "liquid modernity." Another feature is *uncertainty*, or the experience of living through times of incessant change and conceptual upheaval. One important methodological consequence of studying an unstable object is the avoidance of grand theories and the application of middle range concepts to a diverse set of social phenomena. (Bauman has also written books on *Liquid Love*, *Liquid Fears*, and *Liquid Surveillance*.) To this end, the American sociologist Daniel Little has argued that the experience of chronic or structural uncertainty is "not well understood." Comprehensive theories like world systems theory, rational choice theory, or modernization theory have proven analytically deficient, leading Little to conclude that "it is a radical misunderstanding of the nature of the social to imagine that there might be such theories."[17] As a construct, anxiety culture is a further contribution to this understanding of uncertainty, which Bauman and Little recognize is serviced better by middle range concepts (informed by both theoretical and empirical concerns) than totalizing theories. Moreover, such middle range concepts have the potential to encourage interdisciplinary dialogue and research, as they are not the sole province of sociology, but rather can provide the "loose couplings" that have been proven to bring disciplinary units together.[18]

A final associated discourse worth mentioning is Ulrich Beck's conception of the "risk society." Before his untimely death in 2015, Beck produced a rich and suggestive body of work surrounding the reversals of our collective understanding of positive and negative externalities in different social formations (what he calls, disarmingly, "goods" and "bads"). Joshua Yates summarizes the general picture this way:

> Put simply, risk society signals a new phase of modernity in which what were once pursued and fought over as the "goods" of modern industrial societies, things like incomes, jobs, and social security, are today off-set by conflicts over what Beck calls the "bads." These include the very means by which many of the old goods were in fact attained. More pointedly, they involve the threatening and incalculable side effects and so-called "externalities" produced by nuclear and chemical power, genetic research, the extraction of fossil fuels, and the overall obsession with ensuring sustained economic growth.[19]

Nowhere is such a reversal felt more strongly, for example, than in the domain of climate change, where the high quality of life produced by industrialization is now seen as the primary agent in the endangerment of the very conditions sustaining life. Or, to turn again to the circumstances in which this Introduction was written, flourishing global networks of communication, commerce, and cultural exchange allowed the spread of a lethal pathogen that brought social and economic life as we have known it to a standstill. The imperative of anxiety culture is to understand how positive actions can undergo such a sudden reversal.

We view anxiety culture as participating in this cluster of middle range theories, making an important contribution by attending to the tangle of concepts and experiences that constitute our understanding of anxiety—fear, uncertainty, risk, threats and dangers, crisis, and the unsettling of our most basic claims to stability. While the origins of such an approach are grounded in the social sciences, we hope that this volume proves it is relevant also for conversations that cut across a wide range of disciplines and professional competencies.

The Shapes of Anxiety Culture

With these methodological commitments in mind, we have organized the contributions into four primary research clusters: *Climate Change and the Environment*; *Population Health and Social Well-Being*; *Migration, Language, and Culture*; and *Technology*. These clusters are preceded by a more theory-focused section on philosophical and disciplinary approaches to anxiety and followed by a more practically oriented section of selected essays on the implications of anxiety. We recognize that such a proliferation of perspectives may devolve into a cacophonous roar, drowning out the clear account that one would expect from an edited collection on a single theme. As practitioners of middle range theory, our goal is not to provide a definitive account of anxiety culture but rather to set out an ambitious research agenda that can transcend the reductive tendencies of a more restrictive disciplinary approach. The contributions are engaged in a process of concept formation that provides conduits between theoretical and practical registers. It is important that this range of concepts emerges out of and reworks specific contexts that are associated with anxiety so that a truly multidimensional understanding of anxiety culture can emerge.

Considering our methodological commitments, we have selected contributions that generally fit three categories—case studies with a strong disciplinary or geographical perspective, conceptual analyses that integrate disciplinary perspectives, and reflections tied to specific practice or policy domains.

As the earlier reference to the *DSM* suggests, anxiety tends to find its primary articulation as a medical or psychological idiom. Attempts to apply it to historical, political, or cultural phenomena are often viewed as analogical, lacking the analytic, diagnostic precision of medicine or psychology. There is much to be commended in the psychological and biomedical domains (e.g., as evidenced in the section on population health and social well-being). Clearly, we believe that such a restricted understanding of anxiety as a clinical manifestation forecloses its potential to serve as a fruitful heuristic for our times, because our interest is in tending to both "anxiety" and "culture." In fact, varying disciplinary perspectives beyond psychology and medicine have integrated their findings on anxiety into their own methodologies and theoretical lexicons. Take, for example, evolving understandings of climate change: Dominic Boyer deploys psychoanalytic resources to understand the development of petro-economies such as Houston, noting various destructive forms of mania and perversion; whereas Michel Bourban uses similar resources to map out sources of hope and constructive agency in the climate emergency.

Each research cluster includes demonstrations of anxiety taking up residence in different disciplines. While this is, in one sense, proof of concept that anxiety is a fruitful heuristic for understanding different aspects of culture, it would not alone fulfill the ambitions of this collection. We also aim to stake out an emergent research agenda, one that makes meaningful connections across disciplinary boundaries. Thus, we also included contributions that are more explicitly engaged in developing anxiety at a more conceptual register. The first section lays out a set of historical, philosophical, and literary coordinates to help locate the subsequent discussions that tread more familiar ground for a work on anxiety culture (e.g., behavioral health, areas of social and political threat, etc.). Behavioral neurobiologist and medical psychologist Frauke Nees builds on her work on the deep history of consciousness, showing how anxiety is a key lynchpin in the formation of human processes of learning and cognition, as well as the building block for human culture. In contrast to discussions of anxiety culture that bear an overly presentist focus, Nees argues that anxiety is part of an extended process of human beings defining their place in the natural world. Such extensions of the object of inquiry to deeper historical frames, and the conceptual armature that is built through this process, is but one instance of how we aim to provide useful frameworks for emerging research agendas on anxiety culture. Other instances are threaded through the sections centering on the four core clusters of research interest.

The final section of the book presents some additional, concluding perspectives that address the very question that an anxiety culture, with its thorny resistance to clearly defined domains of action, makes it so hard to pose: What is to be done? Definitive, univocal answers would violate the spirit and the findings of the book, but we nevertheless think that incorporating some of the broader challenges and potential solutions rounds out the emerging research agenda that this book stakes out. If anxiety culture is a useful heuristic for understanding our new global condition, then policy-related and other considerations would benefit tremendously from a discussion of how to formulate and carry out policy and practice against background conditions created by the growing threats to democracy both in the United States and elsewhere, the singular existential threat posed by climate change, and the limits of conventional therapeutic culture. (In a loose way, this tracks the ideal vs. non-ideal theory debate in political philosophy.)

Consider how the COVID-19 pandemic both disrupted and foregrounded questions of education—from the practical issue of how it is to be delivered without undermining public health concerns, to more holistic questions of whether the disruption is a convenient time to radically reconfigure educational paradigms. Do we limit such concerns to their immediate context at this inflective moment? We believe that discussions of education policy and practice and other action must widen their aperture and ultimately reckon with the deeper currents of social change explored in this book (e.g., how rapid developments in climate change, migration, and technology inevitably inform the discussion of pandemic and post-pandemic era education).

An Emergent Research Agenda

This volume is neither meant to be a polemic, nor a jeremiad for a more self-assured cultural formation, nor a bit of academic opportunism to push a pre-set package of interests. It is rather a contribution toward what we hope is an emerging research agenda around what we believe is a valuable, but under-examined, heuristic through which to understand the global state of human affairs at this historical conjuncture.

We began with a direct question: What is anxiety culture? This short narrative about the purpose of the book demonstrates that we did not enter this project with a clear definition or answer to this question, nor do we expect the reader to leave with just one answer. In fact, we had no clear-cut expectation of who would make meaningful contributions to this unfolding conversation. Thus, we hope this volume sharpens our understanding while at the same time pushing us toward new areas of thought and insight. Coming to grips with a phenomenon as immediately felt, but as beguiling to conceive as what we call anxiety culture, was a process and valuable intellectual enterprise that brought a great deal of perspective, reinforcing the oft-forgotten lesson, to invoke John Dewey once more, that knowledge can only result from collective effort.[20]

NOTES

1. Handbooks on the assessment, diagnosis, and treatment of clinical anxiety abound. See Martin M. Antony and Murray B. Stein, eds., *Oxford Handbook of Anxiety and Related Disorders* (Oxford: Oxford University Press, 2008); Robert Blanchard, Guy Greibel, and David Nutt, eds., *Handbook of Anxiety and Fear* (Amsterdam: Elsevier, 2008); Bunmi O. Olatunji, ed., *The Cambridge Handbook of Anxiety and Related Disorders* (Cambridge: Cambridge University Press, 2019); and Eric Bui, Meredith E. Charney, and Amanda W. Baker, eds., *Clinical Handbook of Anxiety Disorders* (London: Springer Nature Switzerland AG, 2020). All of these treatments of the topic are clinically oriented and focus almost exclusively on the biology of anxiety and the chemical or psychopharmacologic treatment of anxiety. None of these books share this volume's interdisciplinary focus on the culture of anxiety, cross-cultural perspectives, and social context.

2. See Allan Horowitz, *Anxiety: A Short History* (Baltimore: Johns Hopkins University Press, 2013), 143–161.

3. National Institute of Mental Health, "Any Anxiety Disorder," accessed April 30, 2024, https://www.nimh.nih.gov/health/statistics/any-anxiety-disorder.

4. Ivan Illich, *Medical Nemesis: The Expropriation of Health* (New York: Pantheon, 1982).

5. Horowitz, *Anxiety*, 5.

6. See also Martha Nussbaum, *Political Emotions* (Cambridge, MA: Harvard University Press, 2015) for an account of emotional states and their relationship with politics, in particular Section III: Public Emotions. Nussbaum has extended this analysis to the present political context (i.e., post-Brexit, post-Trump election) in *The Monarchy of Fear: A Philosopher Looks at our Political Crisis* (New York: Simon and Schuster, 2018).

7. Freud wrote in his *Introductory Lectures on Psychoanalysis* that "The problem of anxiety is a nodal point at which the most various and important questions converge, a riddle whose solution would be bound to throw a flood of light on our whole mental existence." His views on anxiety changed throughout his career, with earlier conceptions adopting a physiological model of undischarged libido, and later conceptions turning around the psychic dynamics of the ego and its defensive mechanisms against threats and dangers. For a useful gloss of these changes, see Charles Shepherdson's foreword to Roberto Harari, *Lacan's Seminar on Anxiety: An Introduction* (New York: Other Press, 2001), ix–xii.

8. See Janet Roitman, *Anti-Crisis* (Durham, NC: Duke University Press, 2014) and Zygmunt Bauman and Carlo Bordoni, *State of Crisis* (Cambridge, UK: Polity Press, 2014).

9. John Dewey, *Democracy and Education* (New York: Columbia University Press, 2024).

10. Hannah Arendt, *The Human Condition* (Chicago: University of Chicago Press, 1998), 5.

11. Peter Hedström and Lars Udehn, "Analytical Sociology and Theories of the Middle Range," in *The Oxford Handbook of Analytical Sociology, Oxford Handbooks*, eds. Peter Bearman and Peter Hedström (Oxford: Oxford Academic, 2017).

12. Rollo May, *The Meaning of Anxiety* (New York: W. W. Norton, 1977), ix.

13. The skepticism toward grand narratives is also, of course, a hallmark of postmodern, post-colonial, and post-structuralist critique. By invoking "middle range theory," we do not want to delimit our focus to a purely sociological lens. We also think the aforementioned perspectives from literary studies and historiography can help produce fruitful concepts that elucidate aspects of anxiety culture.

14. Anders Blok, "Towards Cosmopolitan Middle-Range Theorizing: A Metamorphosis in the Practice of Social Theory?" *Current Sociology* 63, no. 1 (January 2015): 110–114.

15. Heinz Bude, *Society of Fear* (Cambridge, UK: Polity, 2017).

16. Zygmunt Bauman, *Liquid Modernity* (Cambridge, UK: Polity, 2007), 26.

17. Daniel Little, *New Directions in the Philosophy of Social Science* (London: Rowan and Littlefield, 2016), xiv.

18. Tony Becher and Paul R. Trowler, *Academic Tribes and Territories: Intellectual Enquiry and the Cultures of Discipline* (Buckingham, UK: SRHE and Open University Press, 2001).

19. Joshua Yates, quoted in Ulrich Beck, *The Metamorphosis of the World* (Cambridge, UK: Polity Press, 2016), 66–67.

20. John Dewey, *America's Public Philosopher: Essays on Social Justice, Economics, Education, and the Future of Democracy*, ed. Eric Thomas Weber (New York: Columbia University Press, 2021).

PART ONE

DISCIPLINARY PERSPECTIVES ON ANXIETY

Introduction

MICHAEL I. SCHAPIRA

In the 19th and early 20th centuries, two disciplines could lay claim to anxiety as an object of inquiry—philosophy and psychology. The Danish philosopher Søren Kierkegaard set anxiety in an existential idiom, describing the dizziness that attends free beings with undetermined futures. As with many of Kierkegaard's concepts, anxiety was taken up by Martin Heidegger, who understood the richness of this countermovement to modernity's emphasis on individual agency and its capacity to increasingly enlarge the sphere of freedom once the shackles of superstition, dogma, and the like were set aside. It is through the concept of anxiety that strains in 20th century philosophy—existentialism, phenomenology—were able to flourish and bequeath a lasting influence on the discipline, particularly in the dialectical imaginary that could think of capacity and incapacity in their irreducible relationship.

Freud had a similar deflationary ambition in introducing anxiety into a psychoanalytic framework for understanding the human psyche. By deflationary I refer not to his ambitions—"There is no question that the problem of anxiety is a nodal point at which the most various and important questions converge, a riddle whose solution would cast a flood of light upon our whole mental existence" he wrote in his *General Introduction to Psychoanalysis*[1]—but rather to his own sense of the limits of agency and freedom. Anxiety posed its own set of challenges to both the analyst and the patient, as it furiously resisted determination in this or that object (unlike the easier to understand experience of fear).

In the 21st century the picture looks quite different. Developments in technology have fundamentally altered the conceptual and practical aspects of psychology, especially with the introduction of neuroimaging and experimental designs that rendered obsolete many of Freud's insights. Similarly, the consolidation of philosophy (at least in the Anglo-American scene) around analytic methods, and the development of the social sciences that are more catholic in their influence, have scattered the originary theories of Kierkegaard and Heidegger in the arts and led to their being discarded by those with a more analytical bent. Anxiety, as with many objects of inquiry, has not been unscathed by the disciplinary reorganization of the academy.

In this section we capture the nature of this changing landscape. Ulrich Hoinkes and Michael Schapira provide an exploration of anxiety in philosophy and the human sciences, beginning with Kierkegaard and moving through 21st century social theory and the emerging area of post-humanism. With this broad, historically informed framework in mind, we reflect on two further areas in which anxiety has spurred a great deal of scholarly development.

Liya Yu approaches our topic from a neuropolitical perspective, fusing the insights of neuroscience with anxieties about the future of liberal democratic politics. She points to two important challenges that must be addressed to ensure conditions amenable to democratic life—the threat of cognitive closure and the dehumanized perception of others.

Frauke Nees brings us up to date on neuroscientific research on anxiety—both as it relates to cognitive development and how people learn from and adapt to changing environments. Nees suggests that anxiety culture may be registering particular effects on the brain, which advances in this field are now beginning to understand with greater clarity.

Underlying both Nees and Yu's contributions is the necessity of *learning* as a way to cope with the effects of anxiety—whether for healthy brain development or the maintenance of a healthy political order. It was Kierkegaard who described anxiety as a kind of school, and whether it is at the forefront of cognitive science or in the more interpretative human and social sciences, developments in disciplinary research about anxiety have much to teach us about a world that seems increasingly harder to firmly grasp.

NOTES

1. Sigmund Freud, *A General Introduction to Psychoanalysis* (New York: Liverlight, 1920), 340.

CHAPTER ONE

Vulnerable Political Brains
in Anxiety Cultures

LIYA YU

Maintaining a liberal and inclusionary brain is one of the most difficult cognitive feats of our time. This is because liberal cognitive capacities such as embracing randomness, diversity, and ambiguity do not come easily to us; our brains are overwhelmed by the dizzying speed in which our modern world has developed and unsure how to cope with the hyperdiverse and hyper-mobile societies that we live in today. We need to confront the possibility that upholding liberal cognitive capacities might feel neither most comfortable nor most natural to us, and it might require a lifetime's effort to maintain these capacities at the brain level—even if we wholeheartedly profess liberal and inclusionary values and ideals.

There exists a troubling explanatory chasm between how "anxiety cultures" are consciously experienced and enacted by individuals on the one hand, and how they are unconsciously processed at the neurocognitive level on the other hand. An indicator of this chasm is the way in which political analysts and intellectuals have been taken by surprise by various recent election and referendum results in Western democracies, as well as by the troubling and ongoing rise of sociopolitical movements countering liberal norms and institutions.

Political theorists from Aristotle, Hobbes, and Bentham, to Rousseau and Marx have made various claims about the political animal and its natural tendencies toward freedom and toleration. Likewise, post-war liberal political theories about the foundations of cooperation, toleration, and diversity are usually based on highly speculative and subjective theories about human nature.[1] The majority of these political theories are unable to verify the validity of their speculative claims against the actual realities of the political brain and are often unaware of the neurocognitive limitations faced by individuals within liberal democratic societies.

A neuropolitical perspective, based on careful political theorizing of social and political neuroscience insights, challenges us with uncomfortable truths about our cognitive dispositions, forcing us to reconsider the racial, classist, gender, and cultural biases inherent in many speculative theories about human nature that are currently used to analyze our political world. It prevents us from engaging in moral self-righteousness and the common assumption that noble liberal beliefs and values can automatically protect us from dehumanizing others.

This chapter's contribution contends that the first step toward overcoming the chasm between political reality and brain reality is to acknowledge that our brains are vulnerable and that this vulnerability might in some respects be irresolvable. We need to examine the political brain in the context of hyperdiverse, hypermobile, and uncertain societies, especially the challenges our socially evolved brains face in these environments. What are the cognitive conditions necessary for citizens to cooperate peacefully in this setting, and which cognitive limitations are potentially most disruptive? How can we begin to devise a neuropolitical theory that outlines the cognitive conditions under which individuals in anxiety culture societies operate?

In essence, I argue that our brains—irrespective of whether we identify as liberals, democrats, libertarians, or conservatives—are all susceptible to various neurocognitive tendencies that can potentially undermine the conditions necessary for cooperation, toleration, and diversity in liberal democratic society. In fact, of all political orientations, liberalism might be the least neurocognitively comfortable and satisfying one, requiring us to overcome our exclusionary and closed-minded political brain tendencies. This can be exacerbated by conditions of threat, anxiety, and loss of personal control.

Not only are our brains ill-equipped to handle the sociopolitical realities that accompany liberal democratic procedures, but we might never be able to completely overcome our brains' biases and dehumanizing abilities, nor can we prevent people from preferring cognitive closure over openness toward ambiguity, uncertainty, and risk. Nevertheless, a neuropolitical approach can bring about a paradigm shift in our understanding of anxiety cultures and the illiberal politics that often accompany them. In addition, social neuroscience research is beginning to offer meaningful strategies for overcoming some of our cognitive biases. In turn, this has practical implications for the setting of norms and standards of political discourse, institutional design, and deliberative procedures that need to be explored.

This chapter singles out two core cognitive limitations that deserve special attention: the need for *cognitive closure* and *dehumanized perception* of others, both of which, in different ways, run counter to the openness and creative adaptability required of citizens in liberal democracies.

The Need for Cognitive Closure

Neuropolitical insights present a rather worrying picture of how cognitive pressures can quickly lead to preferences for hierarchical rather than egalitarian systems, and how liberalism, unlike conservatism, requires us to devote more cognitive effort and engagement into making judgments about the world. In addition, conservatives are self-reportedly happier than liberals.[2] To put it bluntly, our brains need to work harder to be liberal, open, and inclusive.

One of our core vulnerabilities is the desire for cognitive closure. This is particularly relevant for anxiety cultures, because the possibility of achieving cognitive closure is constantly thwarted by the ambiguous, uncertain, and indefinite conditions that prevail in such cultures. Political psychologists and neuroscientists have begun to explore the relationship between partisanship and political beliefs on the one hand and neurocognitive and behavioral functioning on the other.

The groundwork for the study of personality differences between conservatives and liberals (and leftists) was laid in the aftermath of WWII by researchers such as German-Jewish émigré Theodor W. Adorno, Gordon Allport, and others. Since then, research on partisan differences along behavioral, psychological, physiological, neurocognitive, and even genetic lines has expanded considerably.[3]

Even though some of the claims, especially those purporting genetically verifiable differences, are controversial and contested, it is possible to argue that a preliminary picture of the conservative versus the liberal brain has begun to emerge: conservatives seem to be more sensitive to threats and disgust, more resistant to change, and less accepting of new information. Conservatives also prefer to justify rather than question the status quo, and they choose order and adherence to rules in preference to uncertainty and moral ambiguity.

Liberals, on the other hand, are less sensitive to threats and can tolerate more repulsive stimuli due to a higher disgust threshold. They more readily question existing social inequality and authority; in addition, they are also more open to new experiences and willing to embrace ambiguity and uncertainty. The conservative brain has been characterized by John R. Hibbing and his colleagues as exhibiting a "negativity bias."[4] According to this characterization, the world, for the conservative brain, is foremost a place of danger; rules and deference to authority-based systems help to keep this danger at bay.

It is important not to disparage the conservative brain for characteristics that not long ago might have served vital evolutionary purposes—constantly looking out for potential danger and maintaining the hard-won survival of the status quo made sense for human beings in a world that until recently was filled with predators, unpredictable natural disasters, and fatal illnesses. Instead, we should ask anew which cognitive conditions are necessary now for us to thrive together in hyperdiverse and uncertain societies.

Studies have shown the political brain to be highly suggestible. For example, consider that simply exposing people to disgusting odors can decrease their approval of LGBTQI+ people, that sitting in a messy room or on a hard and uncomfortable chair can lead to harsher moral judgments, and that staging a polling place in a religious place (e.g., a church) versus a more neutral place (e.g., a school) increases the chance of people voting for right-of-center candidates.[5] A study in Iceland shows that if politicians were exposed to higher levels of threat (to the self, group, and system), they would score higher in political conservatism and closed-mindedness.[6]

The suggestibility of our political brains in general, and the ill-adaptation of the conservative brain in particular within the context of anxiety cultures, is one of the most concerning insights to emerge from these studies. It is crucial to pay attention to how anxiety cultures are viscerally experienced by individuals, especially in the form of loss of agency and control, and what consequences this has on political orientation. Studies on the relationship between exposure to existential threats and coping strategies for fear and anxiety show an increase in system justification and right-wing orientation with an increase of threats.[7] Support for religious and authoritarian systems has been observed to increase with a lowered perception of personal control.[8]

Ironically, anxiety cultures can thus get trapped in a vicious circle of causing closed-minded and conservative reactions to anxiety, which in turn create further anxiety-based narratives and models of problem solving. Sadly, the persistence of anxiety cultures also becomes a self-fulfilling prophecy for those whose brains tend to seek the most negative and anxiety-filled interpretations of our world.

This perspective of our political brains as being especially susceptible to conditioning by threat and fear can help explain, for example, why experiences of war, poverty, exclusion, and catastrophe can lead to an increase in conservatism, as in the case of various immigrant groups that supported President Donald Trump during the 2016 and 2020 elections. Likewise, it might help explain why a swath of hitherto liberal society turned fascist, as during Germany's transformation from liberal Weimar Republic to the Nazi's Third Reich.

Cognitive Vulnerabilities During the Pandemic

In the context of the COVID-19 pandemic, our vulnerable brains exhibited exclusionary and epistemological biases in terms of the increased hate and racism directed against people from Asian diaspora communities and the perplexing rise of conspiracy theories and the anti-vaccination movement.

In Germany, for example, this cognitive failure to correctly assess the pandemic threat in regard to one's own self-interest also occurred at the highest political and media levels: in January and February 2020, that is, when COVID-19 first broke out in the city of Wuhan, major German news outlets ran predominantly dehumanizing images of Chinese people and disgust-inducing, civilization-shaming stories about Asian wet markets—making the virus seem endemic to China and "dirty, civilizationary inferior, and distant Asia."

This led to political misjudgments and missed chances to prepare for the pandemic. It seemed unimaginable to political decision-makers, including Germany's health minister Jens Spahn, that the virus could eventually reach Germany, so no precautions were taken. Indeed, when Spahn and his ministry of health were contacted in early February by a German mask and personal protective equipment (PPE) manufacturer who voiced his concern about the big shipments going to China at the time, asking if the German government would like the manufacturer to save some for Germany's own mask and PPE stock, the ministry of health ignored them.

As a result, Germany, like many other Western countries at the time, suffered from severe mask and PPE shortages at the beginning of the pandemic. In hindsight, shortages could have been avoided if the government and the media had assessed the pandemic threat correctly instead of perceiving COVID-19 to be endemic to China and Chinese society's civilizational-inferior eating habits.

In another instance of the vulnerability of our brains during the pandemic, conspiracy theories often presented a challenge as perplexing as the virus itself. Traditional liberal persuasive strategies often proved inadequate to tackle these cognitive failures or to shake the tenacious conviction with which people held onto conspiracy theories and false beliefs. Appeals to liberal values and rational consensus, shaming people for endangering others with their actions, or providing ever more scientific information and data to counter erroneous beliefs did not yield the desired effects.

In fact, as Crystal Lee and her colleagues discovered, COVID-19 skeptics, who are commonly perceived as irrational and anti-science, use an ample amount of orthodox data visualization to make their point on social media, even if that point is to subvert what they deem the "wrong" science.[9] Anti-mask Twitter users therefore do not need more data to be convinced; rather, we might have to develop counterintuitive strategies that can reach these users at a deeper epistemic level.

Others contemplated that if we had axed the pillars of liberal democracy— free speech and individual civil liberties—and implemented authoritarian measures such as suppression of free speech and coercion, the problem could have been overcome. Yet it is highly questionable whether oppressive measures would have in fact been effective at quelling conspiracy theories in the long run, because they still would have failed to address our underlying vulnerabilities in accurately gauging reality and social threat. In fact, studies show that authoritarian societies are just as (if not more) susceptible to conspiracy theories and rumors.[10]

By taking a cognitive perspective, I am not minimizing any of the abhorrent contents of conspiracy theories or the political damage they cause. Rather, I am trying to highlight the ease with which we can derail from a shared political reality and how this is linked to the way that we naturally make sense of the world. For example, some argue that instead of interpreting conspiracy theories as rooted merely in an emotion such as fear and anger, or primarily as the product of a certain personality trait or socioeconomic status, we should recognize the central role of cognitive function at play, such as hyperactive agency detection and illusory pattern processing.

In addition, one study showed that belief in conspiracy theories is correlated with higher levels of dopamine, a hormone involved in decision-making.[11] In other words, people who believe in conspiracy theories might be doing so not only because they feel anxious or angry about their political circumstances and their governments or merely because they are socioeconomically disenfranchised. Independent of those reasons, they might be overthinking the world around them: over-ascribing agency to powerful actors, overseeing connections and secret plots that in fact do not exist, and feeling an intense need to actively determine the outcome of their lives.

By allowing freedom of speech and diverse opinions to flourish and by not imposing one defining worldview on their citizens, liberal democracies specifically embrace the uncertainty and randomness of life. To deal with this uncertainty and randomness, we need to exercise cognitive restraint by refraining from over-ascribing agency or patterns to the world around us. The COVID-19 pandemic exposed the shocking number of citizens who do not necessarily possess this cognitive restraint and maturity, and too little attention has been devoted to this cognitive vulnerability toward conspiracy theories.

As counterintuitive as it might sound, the cognitive perspective allows us to see the origin of conspiracy theories not simply as a deficit of intellect or lack of educational skills, but as a much more fundamental, potentially destabilizing neuropolitical capacity that many citizens within liberal democracies succumb to across different gender, ethnic, racial, and socioeconomic identities across the whole political spectrum. It is up to us to address and attempt to overcome this tendency, but for that to happen, we must change our perspective.

Why Dehumanization Matters

In addition, I argue that our brains need to be able to perceive others as full human beings (i.e., able to include them in our sense of humanness) for genuine and stable inclusion to take place. I consider inclusion one of the most foundational pillars of liberal democratic societies, and one that is decisive in helping us to overcome today's deep divisions and polarization. Without humanization of the other, no lasting cooperation or meaningful solidarity can take place.[12]

I deliberately choose the criterion of dehumanization because it encompasses other forms of exclusion such as racism, sexism, homophobia, and classism (in the sense that these more commonly recognized categories of exclusion always entail some form of dehumanization of another group or individual). I argue that dehumanization is such a basic and universal exclusionary neurocognitive ability that any social contract theory aimed at inclusionary cooperation must take it into account to be persuasive and viable.

The term *dehumanized perception* refers to our brain's ability to rapidly and spontaneously deny humanity to other humans, especially those belonging to a perceived out-group. The picture that is emerging on dehumanization and its relation to social cognition is that dehumanizing other humans is an everyday, often subtle, phenomenon that we all engage in as part of how we function socially.

Although dehumanization has been studied by social psychology at the behavioral level for several decades, exploring the neural underpinnings of dehumanization is a relatively novel endeavor. I argue that the recent psychological and neuroscience data on dehumanization is highly relevant for theorizing about politics in hyperdiverse societies, to the point that any minimal theory of social cooperation needs to be aware of it.

Lasana T. Harris treats our in-built dehumanized perception of others as part of what he calls our "flexible social cognition" system—namely, our ability to imagine and infer the mental states, beliefs, and feelings of other individuals. Thus, the fundamental neurocognitive aspect of dehumanization is the inability to infer someone else's mental state.[13] This inability can be directly observed in fMRI studies as an absence of neural activity in brain regions that are responsible for empathic concern.

The neurocognitive mechanisms underlying dehumanization have been linked to troubling sociopolitical outcomes: intergroup aggression, torture, and mass atrocities; the neglect of vulnerable out-groups; rejection of refugees; support for stronger retributive punishment in legal contexts; hostility toward social welfare programs; and the denial of adequate pain medication in medical settings.[14]

In addition, the tendency to apply dehumanizing categories is also of concern, such as categorizing certain human groups into animals (e.g., stereotype of the coarse and uneducated Mexican immigrant), or machines (e.g., stereotypes of overachieving and ruthless Asians or Jews), or perceiving them as barbaric (e.g., Arabs and Muslims) and less developed on an evolutionary civilization scale.[15] These dehumanizing categories, often perpetuated in the media and in the language of US foreign policy since the 9/11 attacks, have led to the intensification of intergroup violence by those groups who feel dehumanized as well as a reduction in the willingness to pursue peaceful means to overcome conflict.[16]

Further, when testing the willingness of Italians to help Haitian and Japanese earthquake victims, a study found that Italians animalistically dehumanized Haitians and mechanistically dehumanized Japanese—both of which led to decreased willingness to help either group of earthquake victims.[17] In another study, explicit dehumanization between Palestinians and Jewish Israelis predicted preference for punitive over restorative forms of justice.[18]

The preexisting dehumanization of Asians during the COVID-19 pandemic was exacerbated by the association of all Asians with a threatening and impersonal virus. In addition, researchers in the United States proved that blatant dehumanization of Asians in general and Chinese people in particular increased during the pandemic, especially among those people who deemed the COVID-19 virus less risky to human health and believed in conspiracy theories. The blatant dehumanizing belief in the evolutionary inferiority of Asian and Chinese people combined with subtly denying Asians human warmth and complex emotions all contributed to the disinhibition of aggressive acts toward them abroad as they were collectively scapegoated for having caused a global pandemic.

In a different instance of animalistic dehumanization, social psychologist Philip Atiba Goff and his colleagues exposed its devastating consequences for Black children. Black boys are seen as less childlike than white boys, which is exacerbated when Black boys are dehumanized by being implicitly associated with apes. As a consequence, Black boys are more easily made targets of police violence and are seen as more responsible for their actions, even though they deserve as much presumption of innocence and protection as other children.[19]

A Novel Form of Persuasion

Encouraging studies also show how to partially overcome these tendencies, even though we might not be able to eradicate completely the dehumanizing tendencies of our brains. For example, a mental exercise as seemingly banal as imagining someone's vegetable preferences can help in inferring someone's mind and helping to humanize them. Paying attention to language by choosing relevant verbs to describe someone's mental state and ascribing a complex emotional inner life to individuals can also increase the likelihood of humanizing them.[20] Emphasizing similarities and shared universal characteristics between disparate social, cultural, and national groups can also help prevent cognitive dehumanization. On the international stage, rhetoric about civilizational clashes as put forward by Samuel Huntington or pitting the civilized West against the barbaric non-West can lead to toxic dehumanization outcomes and should therefore be avoided.

These strategies should not be confused with merely trying to increase empathy in people's brains but should be understood as a distinctive targeting of our brain's core dehumanization vulnerabilities. In fact, asking people to *excessively* humanize routinely dehumanized groups such as the homeless can actually lead to the reverse effect: people will avoid humanizing the most dehumanized individuals in society because they fear emotional exhaustion.[21] Although it might be relatively easy for people to affirm values around universal humanization, such as the right to dignity in the international human rights debate, realizing those abstract values in our concrete and contingent brains is potentially a far bigger challenge, as studies on how human rights education affects incidents of police brutality show.[22]

Going forward, researchers across disciplinary divides need to lay aside their ideological differences and embrace a neuropolitical paradigm shift through a truly interdisciplinary breakthrough in how to make sense of our political world. Otherwise, intellectual and political elites will continue to be left surprised and clueless about the ongoing shift toward illiberalism, authoritarianism, and right-wing conservatism across the globe. Researchers need to realize that brain insights into the distinct mechanisms of dehumanization, exclusion, and illiberalism can serve as a complementary analytical tool (in addition to more established modes of analysis in the social sciences) for making sense of political developments that defy traditional, ideology-based explanations. This also helps to demystify and humanize those people with whom we disagree politically. The ultimate aim is to access the neurocognitive underpinnings of everyone who lives in anxiety cultures, because it is the only way we stand a chance to address people across partisan divides.

Moreover, by approaching anxiety cultures through the lens of the political brain, we are beginning to bridge the epistemological chasm between the sciences and humanities, drawing a more bioholistic, comprehensive, and neurocognitively vulnerable picture of human beings in the realm of politics. Although highlighting our cognitive vulnerabilities in terms of our need for closure and our tendency to dehumanize others might lead to pessimism about our abilities to overcome today's anxiety cultures, this should not be a foregone conclusion. Rather, we should treat these insights as empowering knowledge that can help us understand what goes on in the brain of those who exclude others, which in turn allows us to come up with practical strategies that can more effectively address the exclusionary and illiberal cognitive tendencies of those people.

That the political artifice of liberal democracy based on inclusion, toleration, and equality has once been conceived and has at times even been partially realized in human history—despite the predicament of our vulnerable social brains—is a magnificent achievement and should in fact give us reason for cautious optimism. We need to stop presuming that anyone, including ourselves, is naturally made for the liberal life. Only then can we appreciate that the radical artificialness on which liberal democracies are built require an equally radical form of persuasion to survive.

NOTES

1. These include John Rawls, *A Theory of Justice* (Cambridge, MA: Belknap Press, 1971); Francis Fukuyama, *The End of History and the Last Man* (New York: Free Press, 1992); Will Kymlicka, *Multicultural Citizenship: A Liberal Theory of Minority Rights* (Oxford: Clarendon Press, 1995); Nancy Fraser, "Rethinking Recognition," *New Left Review* 3 (May/June 2000): 107–120; Martha Nussbaum, *Gender Justice, Development, and Rights* (Oxford: Oxford University Press, 2002); and Michael Walzer, *Politics and Passion: Towards a More Egalitarian Liberalism* (New Haven, CT: Yale University Press, 2004).

2. See Laura Van Berkel, Christian S Crandall, Scott Eidelman, and John C Blanchar, "Hierarchy, Dominance, and Deliberation: Egalitarian Values Require Mental Effort," *Personality and Social Psychology Bulletin* 41, no. 9 (2015): 1207–1222; Scott Eidelman, Christian S Crandall, Jeffrey A Goodman, and John C Blanchar, "Low-effort Thought Promotes Political Conservatism," *Personality and Social Psychology Bulletin* 38, no. 6 (2012): 808–820; and Becky Choma, Michael A. Busseri, and Stanley W. Sadava, "Liberal and Conservative Political Ideologies: Different Routes to Happiness?" *Journal of Research in Personality* 43, no. 3 (2009): 502–505.

3. See John Jost et al., "Political Neuroscience: The Beginning of a Beautiful Friendship," *Advances in Political Psychology* 35, no. 1 (2014): 3–42.

4. John Hibbing, Kevin B Smith, and John R Alford, "Differences in Negativity Bias Underlie Variations in Political Ideology," *Behavioral and Brain Sciences* 37, no. 3 (2014): 297–307.

5. Yoel Inbar, David Pizarro, and Paul Bloom, "Disgusting Smells Cause Decreased Liking of Gay Men," *Emotion* 12, no. 1 (2012): 23–37; Simone Schnall et al., "Disgust as Embodied Moral Judgment," *Personality and Social Psychology Bulletin* 34, no. 8 (2008): 1096–1099; Joshua Ackerman et al., "Incidental Haptic Sensations Influence Social Judgments and Decisions," *Science* 5986, no. 328 (2010): 1712–1715; and Abraham Rutchick, "Dues ex Machina: The Influence of Polling Place on Voting Behavior," *Political Psychology* 31, no. 2 (April 2010): 209–225.

6. Hulda Thorisdottir and John Jost, "Motivated Closed-mindedness Mediates the Effect of Threat on Political Conservatism," *Political Psychology* 32, no. 5 (2011): 785–811.

7. Brian Burke, Spee Kosloff, and Mark J. Landau, "Death Goes to the Polls: A Meta-analysis of Mortality Salience Effects on Political Attitudes," *Political Psychology* 34, no. 2 (2013): 183–200.

8. Aaron Kay et al., "God and the Government: Testing a Compensatory Control Mechanism for the Support of External Systems," *Journal of Personality and Social Psychology* 95, no. 1 (2008): 18–35.

9. Crystal Lee et al., "Viral Visualizations: How Coronavirus Skeptics use Orthodox Data Practices to Promote Unorthodox Science Online," *Proceedings of the 2021 CHI Conference on Human Factors in Computing Systems. Association for Computing Machinery* (2021): 1–18.

10. Haifeng Huang, "A War of (Mis)information: The Political Effects of Rumors and Rumor Rebuttals in an Authoritarian Country," *British Journal of Political Science* 47, no. 2 (2017): 283–311.

11. Katherina Schmack et al., "Linking Unfounded Beliefs to Genetic Dopamine Availability," *Frontiers in Human Neuroscience* 9 (2015): 521.

12. David Livingstone Smith, *On Inhumanity: Dehumanization and How to Resist it* (Oxford: Oxford University Press, 2020).

13. Lasana T. Harris, *Invisible Mind: Flexible Social Cognition and Dehumanization* (Cambridge, MA: MIT Press, 2017).

14. Lasana Harris and Susan T. Fisk, "Dehumanizing the Lowest of the Low: Neuroimaging Responses to Extreme Out-Groups," *Psychological Science* 17, no. 10 (2006): 847–853; Amy Cuddy et al., "The BIAS Map: Behaviors from Intergroup Affect and Stereotypes," *Journal of Personality and Social Psychology* 92, no. 4 (2007): 631–648; and Beatrice Capestany and Lasana Harris, "Disgust and Biological Descriptions Bias Logical Reasoning During Legal Decision-making," *Social Neuroscience* 9, no. 3 (2007): 265–277.

15. Nick Haslam, "Dehumanization: An Integrative Review," *Personality and Social Psychology Review* 10, no. 3 (2006): 252–264.

16. Nour Kteily et al., "They See us as Less than Human: Metadehumanization Predicts Intergroup Conflict via Reciprocal Dehumanization," *Journal of Personality and Social Psychology* 110, no. 3 (2016): 343–370.

17. Luca Andrighetto et al., "Human-itarian Aid? Two forms of Dehumanization and Willingness to Help After Natural Disasters," *British Journal of Social Psychology* 53, no. 3 (2014): 573–584.

18. Bernhard Leidner, Emanuele Castano, and Jeremy Ginges, "Dehumanization, Retributive and Restorative Justice, and Aggressive Versus Diplomatic Intergroup Conflict Resolution Strategies," *Personality and Social Psychology Bulletin* 39, no. 2 (2013): 181–192.

19. Philip Goff et al., "The Essence of Innocence: Consequences of Dehumanizing Black Children," *Journal of Personality and Social Psychology* 106, no. 4 (2014): 526–545.

20. Gün R. Semin and Klaus Fiedler, "The Cognitive Functions of Linguistic Categories in Describing Persons: Social Cognition and Language," *Journal of Personality and Social Psychology* 54, no. 4 (1988): 558–568.

21. C. Daryl Cameron, Lasana T. Harris, and B. Keith Payne, "The Emotional Cost of Humanity: Anticipated Exhaustion Motivates Dehumanization of Stigmatized Targets," *Social Psychological and Personality Science* 7, no. 2 (2016): 105–112.

22. Liya Yu, *Vulnerable Minds: The Neuropolitics of Divided Societies* (New York: Columbia University Press, 2022).

CHAPTER TWO

The Cognitive Neuroscience of Anxiety

Changing Environment, Changing Brain, Changing Self?

FRAUKE NEES

If the human brain were so simple that we could understand it, we would be so simple that we couldn't.

Emerson H. Pugh

That individuals vary in their anxiety levels is common wisdom. We all know a colleague or friend who is more tightly wound than others or who marvels at others' ability to just go with the flow. Anxiety has become a kind of cultural condition of modern society, of which we all reflect to varying degrees.

Highly anxious individuals have an attentional bias toward threat-related stimuli and a negative interpretation of emotionally ambiguous stimuli. These dysfunctional processes relate to the cognitive control of emotional processes and behaviors and are associated with altered neural functions in specific brain regions that build a circuit, previously referred to as "fear network."[1] Those processes can even determine mental health and disease, with fear and avoidance of specific triggering cues as a common behavior prevalent in many anxiety disorders.

In our research group at the Institute of Medical Psychology and Medical Sociology, University Medical Center, Kiel University, we are working on the neurobiological mechanisms of learning and memory as well as related information processing in the brain. We are also studying cognitive, affective, and somatic dimensions, both in critical life periods as well as over the life span to develop and empirically evaluate related prevention and intervention programs.[2] In terms of learning, for example, the process of fear conditioning is an important mechanism for adaptive behavior that has also been implicated in the development of an anxious psychopathology. Through processes of fear conditioning, previously neutral (so-called conditioned) stimuli acquire a negative value when occurring together with a negative (unconditioned) stimulus, and can, in the future, provoke responses like emotional distress, vigilance, hyperarousal, or avoidance behavior that had only been specific to negative (unconditioned) stimuli.[3]

This also relates to the co-occurrence of pathologies like chronic pain or depression. Overwhelming evidence suggests that chronic pain, anxiety, and depression promote the development of each other and negatively impact the treatment success of each pathology. In the European Union, it is estimated that during the life span 27% of the population will suffer from a disorder like anxiety or depression and 20% from chronic pain, and these are the most significant risk factors for suicide.[4]

Therefore, research is needed to better disentangle antecedents and consequences of high anxiety levels and related consequences and also identify respective vulnerability and resilience factors. Findings on the role of stress and stressful experiences, including traumatic stress, and their impacts on brain circuits important for learning and emotional processing go in this direction. In this context the state of attention and self-awareness during stress and emotional processing is essential and useful for regulating emotional (brain) responsivity in negative states like high anxiety.

Fear versus Anxiety: Learning and Dynamic Interplay Between the Individual and the Environment

Anxiety represents a complex emotion that manifests in our thoughts and affects our behavior and brain responses including mutual changes in subcortical and cortical brain regions.[5] In *Physiologie des Passions* (1878), Charles Letourneau defined emotions like anxiety as "passions of a short duration." He was contemporary with the French neuroanatomist Paul Broca, who said that emotions are "intimately linked with organic life" and this causes an "abnormal excitation of the nervous network," reflected in heart rate changes and changes in secretions, or in an interruption of "the normal relationship between the peripheral nervous system and the brain." Despite the limited knowledge on brain physiology and anatomy available at the end of the 19th century, the views and assumptions of Letourneau were premonitory: motivational, cognitive, and behavioral development entails co-constructive interactions between social and environmental influences on the one hand and the neurobiological inheritance of the individual on the other.

Without aiming to make a point on differences between perceived and actual societal states, just looking at our current society, it seems that a broad and uncontrollable feeling of anxiety is increasingly produced, which is reflected, for example, in a negative feeling over an uncertain future. Such a feeling of anxiety is different from a concrete immediate feeling of fear, which is often perceived as being more controllable and manageable. Although, from a neuroscience perspective, feelings of fear and anxiety partially overlap, sharing common pathways, they are still treated as two conceptually distinct constructs, even when such conceptual frameworks do not totally meet the considerably more complex circuitry. This framework provides a useful heuristic for achieving a more nuanced understanding of the role of brain mechanisms for feelings of fear and anxiety, and whether they are in the healthy or pathological range.

Whether we have a feeling of fear or anxiety also determines how we integrate current and past experiences into our thoughts and behaviors, and thus how we learn from experiences. Single stimuli (so-called conditioned cues) may evoke phasic fear responses, whereas broader contexts lead to sustained anxiety responses.[6] In particular, while responses to a cue quickly subside after its offset, contexts produce a more unpredictable feeling due to the absence of such a clear stimulus signal. Indeed multisensory, diffuse, and continuously present internal or external environments do not signal an exact time of onset or of non-occurrence of a threatening event. These contexts do not only cover environmental characteristics but also cultural and social settings, cognitive sets, and internal states. Moreover, learning is a dynamic process, not a steady state phenomenon, that varies as a function of the contingency between our made experiences and the stimuli that affect us. This learning process provides a basis to adapt to any changing environment, including an anxiety culture. In this vein, the way we learn reflects the cumulative reciprocal interactions between our individual neurobiological predispositions and responses, including genetic background and brain change, as well as social and cultural influences and our volitional choices and actions.[7]

Brain Correlates of Anxiety (Disorders)

Studies of patients with anxiety disorders and post-traumatic stress disorder (PTSD) provide a foundation for our understanding of the neural underpinnings of anxiety in humans. Figure 2.1 provides an overview on brain correlates of PTSD.

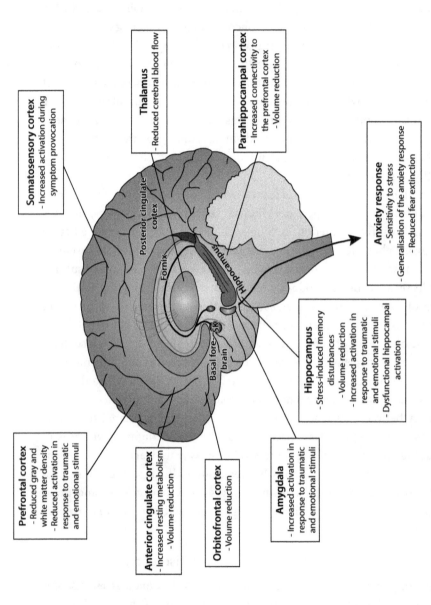

Figure 2.1. Post-traumatic stress disorder related brain regions identified from functional and structural magnetic resonance imaging. Adapted from Frauke Nees et al., "Neurogenic Approaches to Stress and Fear in Humans as Pathophysiological Mechanisms for Posttraumatic Stress Disorder," *Biological Psychology* 83, no. 10 (2018): 810–820.

Dysregulation in limbic brain regions like the amygdala, a region involved in the processing of emotionally salient stimuli and respective behavioral defensive responsivity, together with frontal brain for inhibitory top-down control of emotional-processing structures, have been found as core areas of anxiety models.[8] Among the limbic areas, the hippocampus plays a role in memory and stress sensitivity processes. In frontal areas, the prefrontal cortex (PFC) carries out executive functions such as decision-making, planning, social behavior, and predicting consequences for behaviors and processing of rewards, and the orbitofrontal cortex (OFC) controls impulses and regulates mood. The involvement of this brain circuitry demonstrates that the overwhelming feeling of anxiety integrates the whole personal system with sensory, affective, and cognitive components and covers also internal bodily states.

Few people today would dispute that chronic stress causes changes in those neuro-modulatory systems that in turn induce anxiety. The stronger emotional effort in daily life and the role of anxiety-specific connections in estimating the value and probability of uncertain threats may result in a more and more stressed population, where the sensitivity in detecting salient changes in the environment is increased. Amygdala and dorsal anterior cingulate cortex abnormalities, for example, are found in response to negative emotional stimuli in adults with childhood maltreatment and seem to represent predisposing factors, whereas dysfunctions in hippocampus-vmPFC connectivity may serve as acquired factors that become evident after the development of PTSD, and thus might be indicative of PTSD susceptibility (Fig. 2.2). Specifically, a

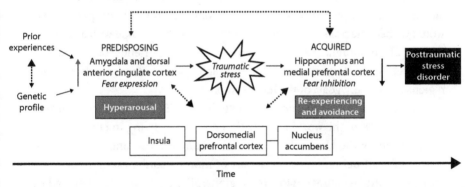

Figure 2.2. Supposed model of predisposing qualities quantified by the experience of a traumatic event and psychological and brain changes and correlates. Adapted from Frauke Nees et al., "Neurogenic Approaches to Stress and Fear in Humans as Pathophysiological Mechanisms for Posttraumatic Stress Disorder," *Biological Psychology* 83, no. 10 (2018): 810–820.

greater engagement of lateral and medial PFC for successful down-regulation of negative emotions, and thus more effort to regulate emotions in daily life, was characteristic for individuals with higher levels of anxiety.[9]

Effects of Environmental Challenges, Including Lifestyle and Living Environment, on the Brain

We, as living organisms, enact the world in which *we* exist: we actively constitute our environment and are simultaneously constituted by it. This means that there is not a pregiven world that *we* match or represent by means of our states in the central nervous system, but we rather shape and structure the environment. This occurs not only for ourselves but also for subsequent generations, for example, by building "nests," social networks, and homes. Accordingly, there is a coevolution of interrelated systems, where *we* adapt constantly to survive. This results from continuous bottom-up and top-down processes, including changes in the brain, to allow for developing and stabilizing new learning strategies and flexible behavior—a process that is often seen as a process of enculturation.

Today's society is faced with multiple challenges, such as climate change, pandemics, high levels of mental illness, rapid changes in technology, or migration. These impact our social, private, and working lives, our individual freedoms, and our political systems. In the context of anxiety, if this has swelled into our (social) daily life, and an anxiety culture has induced a process of enculturation, where and how would *we,* the individual and the society, end up? Many people experience the current world as a place of increased insecurity. Those factors impact the structure of our brain. From a neurobiological perspective, would we become prefrontal overactive individuals able to cope with anxiety, or would we be more anticipation-oriented and less action-oriented due to a strong fear of future negative events, with an overactivation of emotion-related brain regions like the amygdala or the hippocampus?

For example, our living environments have shifted from rural to urban areas, with 68% of the world's population potentially living in cities by 2050, as predicted by the United Nations, and this might also affect our mental states and well-being.[10] Indeed, anxiety or mood disorders seem to be more frequent in urban compared to rural regions. Higher stress-related amygdala activity is associated with currently living in a city, whereas exposure to urban environments in the first 15 years of life resulted in stronger anterior cingulate activity in the face of stress. Urban upbringings were further associated with reduced gray matter volume and thickness in the dorsolateral and medial PFC, the anterior cingulate cortex, inferior parietal lobe, and the parahippocampal cortex. Moreover, a stronger amount of forest or green around the home address was associated with amygdala integrity. If adolescents have spent their entire life in rural areas they also had bigger hippocampi compared to those adolescents who spent their entire life in cities, and this was additionally associated with stronger cognitive (spatial) skills.[11]

These regions also change in response to anxiety or as a result of an anxiety disorder, and they have been highlighted in learning and memory processes, including the processing of contexts. Here, contexts not only entail the external (environmental and social) but also the internal (cognitive and hormonal) backdrop. They shape the perception of past memories and experiences, enabling the flexible representation and retrieval of information, and have a central role in resolving ambiguity. This might also be important when it comes to anxiety, as an important moderator of whether and how people unlearn aversive contextual experiences, triggered in the brain, for example, through the hippocampus.

Anxiety may also interrupt positive routines and habits, which normally result in automatic actions that favor specific decision-making processes to receive (further) positive experiences. If these habits are interrupted, we may fall into a lost stage of uncertainty and helplessness, losing the automatic positive focus, which is common for states of anxiety.

Cultural Neuroscience, (Brain) Development, and Generations

Modern humans live in an immersive culturally constructed niche of artifacts, skills, structures, practices, beliefs, and artificial landscapes, which exert profound influences on their lives across evolutionary, developmental, and behavioral scales. In terms of the brain, in a rather provocative essay, Terrence Deacon stated that brain evolution should be impossible. "How could random mutational changes to such a complex integrated system be anything other than catastrophic?"[12] Brain development, however, is of remarkable adaptability and flexibility and thus an evolutionary process in itself. Even in the face of critical and large environmental perturbation, functional system plasticity can be produced by developmental selection and can bias patterning mechanisms, which may contribute to developmental neural programs. This further relates to the multilevel interaction between developmental mechanisms, genes, and environment, with a critical contribution of the social world—a cumulative culture that may be constructed by these dynamics.

In a world on the move like our present one, a sequela of acculturation might be triggered. If this sequela of acculturation is evaluated as threat, it may become biologically embedded via changes in the stress system and related to changes in the brain, including responses through hippocampal, amygdala, and prefrontal activation.[13] Moreover, a prolonged activation of this system results in a (chronic) dysregulation and thereby enhances the development of physical and mental disorders. This can be moderated by a range of beneficial or adverse effects of health-related behaviors including sleep, alcohol, smoking, physical activity, or dietary practices, which can also represent consequences of acculturation.

So, because of the substantial amount of plasticity in the brain, during development and by providing systematically different sets of experiences, culture can have a persistent influence on our behavioral patterns. Neural correlates of behaviors typical for a culture that are repeatedly activated lead to culturally specific neural structures and activity.

Variation within groups is likely considerable, depending on the particular subculture or socioecological niche we inhabit, and therefore also in the type of experiences we are exposed to. Subsequent various learning strategies, including copying familiar others, may impact the way individuals adopt their behavior. This means that two individuals inhabiting the same geographical space may also acquire only partially overlapping subsets of cultural experiences.[14] Moreover, a set of traits characteristic for a group is not necessarily coherent when looking at the individual level. For example, even cross-cultural differences in cognitive styles and social orientation have been widely documented. When looking at the individual level, there is sometimes still little relationship among the measures used. This variability may be attributed to interactions between the individual and different aspects of its culture and can result in cross-temporally stable behavioral profiles emphasizing different aspects of cognitive style and social orientation.

Likewise, inferences about how a typical individual in a society would have acquired the same set of experiences that is typical in that society cannot just be made because this set of experiences is meant to be typical for the society. This can also be transferred to the neuroscientific perspective, in that two neural indicators of some cultural variation do not necessarily correlate when looking at them within individuals. Finally, behaviors that are typical for a group of individuals may be shaped by features of social and physical ecology in that individuals flexibly adapt to the respective requisites of the immediate surroundings, and those influences do not necessarily align with cultural prescriptions.

Such interactions and influences are powerful and may be critical, particularly during the early years of life, when individuals are much more sensitive and vulnerable to external influences because central developmental (brain) processes are still occurring (figure 2.3). Indeed, the experience of adverse life events early in life result in more negative outcomes compared to the experience of similar events during adulthood. Adolescence is known as a transition period, marked by physical and behavioral changes due to the acquisition and refinement of social, cognitive, and emotional skills to support successful passage into adulthood.

On a neural level, brain areas like the anterior cingulate cortex, ventral pallidum, ventral striatum (including the nucleus accumbens, OFC, amygdala, hippocampus, thalamus, and prefrontal cortex are critical components) play a role, and an imbalance between the prefrontal cortex and nucleus accumbens development occurs.[15] This imbalance might result in riskier behaviors, and can also determine the development of a range of mental disorders, including those related to anxiety. Brain circuits related to emotional learning and emotion expression like the amygdala are involved in blunted emotional reactivity in early development, which could trigger fear-associated memories emerging later in adolescence. Experiences during childhood and adolescence are therefore associated with important outcomes later in life, including challenges to physical and mental health as well as educational attainment and earnings.

Among adverse early life experiences, socioeconomic status (SES) is one of the strongest predictors for variation in measures of brain structure and function during adulthood. This involves the pace of brain development with a reduced protraction of structural network development and a reduced prolongation of functional network segregation associated with lower childhood SES, and thus less efficient cortical networks during adulthood.[16] Such effects might stem from the often-found stronger perception of stress under circumstances of low SES, which accelerates brain maturation. Moreover, in children, lower compared to higher SES environments were shown to result in a thinner cortex already in the first postnatal year, particularly in the frontal lobe. Later in life, between 3 and 20 years, SES served as a moderator for the negative relationship between age and cortical thickness, with a steeper curvilinear decrease in cortical thickness in younger children with lower SES background compared to children with higher SES background. During adolescence, from 12 to 18 years, this effect was particularly present in females.[17]

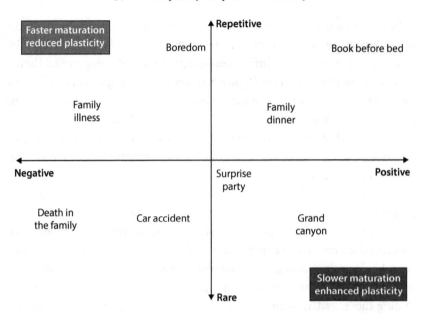

Figure 2.3. Overview on the effects of experiences early in life that affect the brain developmental processes. Adapted from Ursula Tooley et al., "Environmental Influences on the Pace of Brain Development," *Nature Reviews: Neuroscience* 22, no. 6 (2021): 372–384.

Chronic stress could initiate a faster aging process of the entire body through an increase in glucocorticoid levels and allostatic load and increased activation of the inflammation system. It may favor the use of stress regulation strategies and detection circuits in the brain, such as of the medial prefrontal cortex and the amygdala, which could result in a faster maturation of these areas. If the stress caused by SES is seen as a threat, it may be treated as an overall signal of lack of support, and protection and development would then proceed more quickly, triggering adaptive top-down processes. Indeed, children with low SES backgrounds, who perceive stronger levels of threat, entered puberty earlier.

Potential Consequences for Our Future Society and Ourselves

Given the context of an anxiety culture, the question is: Are we assembling a society of individuals who are more anxious, less able to successfully adapt to challenging situations, and stuck in a less flexible world that is also less hungry for experiences? Such questions are interesting on the one hand and challenging on the other hand, because from an evolutionary perspective, anxiety is a meaningful response mechanism to help the organism to survive and fight or flee critical, negative situations. Such meaningfulness also depends on the level or amount of anxiety. Our response capability when confronted with anxiety or threats lies in the so-called Yerkes-Dodson law. This law reflects a relationship between pressure and performance: performance generally increases with an increase in mental or physiological arousal, but this increase often occurs only up to a specific point. When the arousal becomes too high, which is particularly the case for very difficult or more complex tasks, it can turn into too much pressure to cope with the task and performance likely decreases.

Based on this law, scientists often talk about an inverted U-shape when speaking about potential negative effects of arousal (or stress) on cognitive processes that could affect our attention (e.g., tunnel vision), memory, and problem-solving. Such a relationship may also apply for contexts of increased anxiety. Neuropharmacological studies, for example, showed that anxiety is reduced following the augmentation of dopamine, a neurotransmitter that plays a major role in the motivational component of reward behavior signaling the perceived motivational prominence (i.e., aversiveness or desirability), but anxiety is only reduced until a tipping point is reached, after which higher levels then result in an elevation of anxiety.

If we then ask how all this would determine our own concepts and views as an individual, as a society, and as the world, the feeling of volition might be a critical issue. Volition means that events in our life are to some extent generated by our self and relates to the feeling of agency. Volition may become more and more lost when we are exposed to an anxiety culture.

From a neuroscientific perspective, various cues contribute to this sense of agency. Cues can be internal sensorimotor to external situational cues and they encompass the full spectrum including brain, body, and environment. Environment also refers to social factors, which largely determine human agency. Inferred over some aggregate of past experiences, agency might reflect an estimate of the controllability of important environmental events and stimuli—are they predominantly controllable (high agency) or are they consistently outside of our control (low agency)—and again, learning comes into play. Learned relationships between actions and contingent outcomes can then be triggered by these repeated experiences and result in either a direct enhancement of fitness or an indirect fitness benefit. In this vein, agency allows for adaptive behaviors, which can be challenged in the context of an anxiety culture when anxiety means a higher level of uncontrollability.

Interesting work has been conducted on the neuroscience of self and self-regulation, including the role of social distances. In *The Spaces Between Us*,

Michael Graziano elegantly describes how our personal space, the way of interacting with others, and the environment lead to a sense of self.[18] This personal space is also determined by continuous under-the-surface calculations of threat and negative emotions like anxiety. It further relates to the fundamental need of humans to belong, which encourages behaviors like being a good member of a group and requires the capacity of self-regulation. Self-regulation allows individuals to overcome or change emotions, thoughts, or behaviors in specific circumstances predisposed by culture, physiology, and learning. Although there is an impressive capacity of self-regulation, failures are common and individuals lose behavioral control in various circumstances. Self-regulation includes a specific amount of and need for inhibition, because group preferences do not always overlap or match the preferences (or enjoyment) for an individual. Such inhibition processes include stopping, interruption, or adjustment to changed feelings, thoughts, and actions for realizing personal goals or maintaining current standards. Inhibitions are critical for harmonious social relationships. From an evolutionary perspective, those who control undesirable impulses are undoubtedly favored.

But how does this relate to anxiety? Would it then be important, under social circumstances, to inhibit feelings of anxiety to protect the social group? Could this then potentially also help the individual to be less anxious? On the other hand, if a culture of anxiety is present within a group, should we consider anxiety as facilitating a group sharing a common feeling of a stronger group connection? How would such effects be represented in the brain?

The detection of threat relates to monitoring the environment for any negative cues, and several studies have shown that the amygdala plays a critical role when individuals respond to threatening stimuli.[19] This affective processing in the amygdala evolved during evolution as an adaptive process developed to protect animals from danger. It is also found in humans through responses to primary biologically relevant stimuli such as tastes, odors, or faces—even when those stimuli are below the level of an individual's awareness. Such threat detection also becomes relevant in social contexts, where it could, for example, include possible group exclusions. Feeling socially anxious or being worried about potential rejection may result in higher social sensitivity, which might also increase empathic responses, affect the ability to decode social information, and influence memory for social information. In situations in which social norms are violated, the amygdala is robustly activated.

Such factors are also relevant to the self, and evaluations of the self inevitably result in emotional responses that direct our actions and thoughts. Focusing too much on the self, however, can result in negative consequences for mental health. This is seen, for example, in patients with depression who are making negative self-attributions and ruminating about negative information. This goes along with several abnormalities in both cortical and subcortical regions in the brain, including the medial prefrontal cortex and ventral anterior cingulate cortex. Some research shows that brain stimulation of these areas helps alleviate depression in patients who were otherwise treatment resistant.[20]

Outlook

Applied cognitive neuroscience can help study how environment may change behaviors and attitudes. Through the combination of behavioral, self-reporting, and neural measures, in conjunction with carefully designed experiments, neuroscientific tools can be helpful for researchers from different fields including business, economy, or philosophy. It can be important for theory building and testing and to link areas and mechanisms hypothesized in those fields to cognitive processes and consequential behaviors and how they affect society. Finally, research and discussions should not only target the negative vulnerable side but should also increase insights into the neurosocial basis of resilience. The perception of and response to stress differs considerably between individuals, and these individuals can be divided into those who easily succumb to stress and those who are resilient, enabling them to show positive adaptation in an intensely challenging anxiety context.

NOTES

1. Christina Sehlmeyer et al., "Human Fear Conditioning and Extinction in Neuroimaging: A Systematic Review," *PLoS One* 4, no. 6 (2009): e5865.

2. See, for example, Frauke Nees et al., "Prediction Along a Developmental Perspective in Psychiatry: How far might we go?" *Frontiers in Systems Neuroscience* 15 (July 2021); Frauke Nees et al., "Neurogenic Approaches to Stress and Fear in Humans as Pathophysiological Mechanisms for Posttraumatic Stress Disorder," *Biological Psychology* 83, no. 10 (2018): 810–820; and Sebastien Siehl et al., "Structural White and Gray Matter Differences in a Large Sample of Patients with Posttraumatic Stress Disorder and a Healthy and Trauma-Exposed Control Group: Diffusion Tensor Imaging and Region-based Morphometry," *NeuroImage: Clinical* 28 (2020).

3. Shmuel Lissek et al., "Classical Fear Conditioning in the Anxiety Disorders: A Meta-analysis," *Behaviour Research and Therapy* 43, no. 11 (2005): 1391–1424.

4. Vladimir Valetic and Charles Raison, "Neurobiology of Depression, Fibromyalgia and Neuropathic Pain," *Frontiers in Bioscience (Landmark Edition)* 14, no. 14 (2009): 5291–5338; and Harald Breivik et al., "Survey of Chronic Pain in Europe: Prevalence, Impact of Daily Life, and Treatment," *European Journal of Pain* 10 no. 4 (2006): 287–333.

5. Jie Xu et al., "Anxious Brain Networks: A Coordinate-based Activation Likelihood Estimation Meta-analysis of Resting-state Functional Connectivity Studies in Anxiety," *Neuroscience and Biobehavioral Reviews* 96 (2019): 21–30.

6. I. M. Marks, "Behavioral Aspects of Panic Disorder," *The American Journal of Psychiatry* 144, no. 9 (1987): 1160–1165.

7. Thomas Goschke, "Volition und Kognative Kontrolle," in *Allgemeine Psychologie*, ed. J. Müsseler and M. Rieger (Heidelberg: Springer, 2017), 251–315; and Christian Grillon, "Associative Learning Deficits Increase Symptoms of Anxiety in Humans," *Biological Psychiatry* 51, no. 11 (2002): 851–858.

8. See Frauke Nees and Herta Flor, "Neuroanatomy and Neuroimaging," in *The Wiley Handbook of Anxiety Disorders*, eds. P. Emmelkamp and T. Ehring (London: Wiley, 2014), 233–253; and Gregory Fonzo and Amit Etkin, "Affective Neuroimaging in Generalized Anxiety Disorder: An Integrated Review," *Dialogues in Clinical Neuroscience* 19, no. 2 (2017): 169–179.

9. Laura Campbell-Sills et al., "Functioning of Neural Systems Supporting Emotion Regulation in Anxiety-prone Individuals," *NeuroImage* 54, no. 1 (2011): 689–696.

10. United Nations, "68% of the World Population Projected to Live in Urban Areas by 2050, says UN," May 16, 2018, www.un.org/development.desa/en/news/population/2018-revision-of-world-urbanization-prospects.html.

11. Simone Kühn et al., "In Search of Features that Constitute an 'Enriched Environment' in Humans: Associations Between Geographical Properties and Brain Structures," *Scientific Reports* 7, no. 1 (2017); and Bianca Besteher et al., "Associations Between Urban Upbringing and Cortical Thickness and Gyrification," *Journal of Psychiatric Research* 95 (2017): 114–120.

12. Terrence Deacon, *The Symbolic Species: The Co-evolution of Language and the Brain* (New York: W. W. Norton, 1987).

13. Bruce McEwen, "Physiology and Neurobiology of Stress and Adaptation: Central Role of the Brain," *Physiological Reviews* 87, no. 3 (2007): 873–904.

14. Luke Rendell et al., "Cognitive Culture: Theoretical and Empirical Insights into Social Learning Strategies," *Trends in Cognitive Sciences* 15, no. 2 (2011): 68–76.

15. Della Fuhrmann et al., "Adolescence as a Sensitive Period of Brain Development," *Trends in Cognitive Sciences* 19, no. 10 (2015): 558–566.

16. Martha Farah, "The Neuroscience of Socioeconomic Status: Correlates, Causes, and Consequences," *Neuron* 96, no. 1 (2017): 56–71; and Ursula Tooley et al., "Environmental Influences on the Pace of Brain Development," *Nature Reviews: Neuroscience* 22, no. 6 (2021): 372–384.

17. Shaili Jha et al., "Environmental Influences on Infant Cortical Thickness and Surface Area," *Cerebral Cortex* 29 no. 3 (2019): 1139–1149; Nadine Parker et. al, "Income Inequality, Gene Expression, and Brain Maturation During Adolescence," *Scientific Reports* 7, no. 1 (2017): 7397.

18. Michael Graziano, *The Spaces Between Us: A Story of Neuroscience, Evaluation, and Human Nature* (Oxford: Oxford University Press, 2018).

19. Joseph LeDoux, *The Emotional Brain: The Mysterious Underpinnings of Emotional Life* (New York: Simon and Schuster, 1996).

20. Helen Mayberg et al., "Deep Brain Stimulation for Treatment-Resistant Depression," *Neuron* 45, no. 5 (2005): 651–660.

CHAPTER THREE

Anxiety Culture as Social Reality and Object of Philosophical Consideration

ULRICH HOINKES AND
MICHAEL I. SCHAPIRA

The connection between the concepts of anxiety and culture raises fundamental definitional questions about the subject of our research project of the same name, especially because anxiety and fear are usually understood as natural rather than cultural emotional states. However, this also requires interpretation of the anthropological understanding of our time, which the French philosopher Corine Pelluchon has called the "age of the living."[1] As an expression of aliveness and the will to survive, anxiety is a central emotional state in our world, where a machine ethic is displacing animal and plant ethics, and where our future seems so technologized, automated, and determined by artificial intelligence that we as humans are struggling to find our place and meaning in it. If it is true that the Anthropocene threatens to marginalize humans themselves, that is, that we have long since entered a phase of transhumanism or posthumanism, then addressing the multiple realities of anxiety in our society is indicative of the place and function of the living in our cosmos, the individual as well as the universal. This raises the question of the dynamic potential of anxiety and eclipses its traditionally negative view as a provocateur of paralysis and irrationality. One might indeed consider these two undesirable consequences of fear to be avoidable in the context of a new ethics of anxiety culture.

Given the complex structure of our concept of anxiety culture, we must take its definitional approach very broadly. But then, what exactly is our object of inquiry? This is a notoriously complicated question, partially because we have already struck reductive (but quite useful and quite prevalent) biomedical definitions of anxiety (see the Introduction), and partially because of ongoing debates about method when it comes to a topic like culture. While we are not going to alight on a firm definition, our understanding of the concept will gain clarity within a matrix of sense-making frameworks that could plausibly be deployed when exploring a topic like anxiety culture.

If we accept that the epochal definitional task is the right approach, then we might be naturally drawn to the discipline of history. For example, following Eric Hobsbawm, we may intend anxiety culture as the name of some historical conjuncture, perhaps even in reference to some sort of structuring events that require the naming and policing of a boundary (as Hobsbawm does with the "long 19th century"). Or, if we want to take a slightly looser historical approach, we could follow 20th century developments in Marxist cultural analysis and attempt to put our arms around what Raymond Williams called a "structure of feeling."[2] We have in mind appellations like "The Society of the Spectacle," which names both a specific stage in capitalist development and its affective correlates as we interact with society's major instructions (politics, the legal system, the education system, and most importantly, various cultural and technological mediations of experience).[3] In either case anxiety culture is located temporally.

The confrontation with Marxist ideology in Europe led very early to a philosophical reference to the significance of feelings. No one else has expressed this as clearly as Ágnes Heller in *A Theory of Feelings*, in which she already proves to be a mastermind of sociocultural developments that bring value orientation, social action, and individual feelings into a close relationship.[4] Away from the emotional world of the bourgeois and toward the emotional world of the *citoyen* is her motto, which seems more topical than ever in today's anxiety culture.

What if we abandoned definition altogether and embraced the anthropological practice of thick description? We could examine patterns of social organization and social relation, or the systems by which meaning and value are produced in specific settings, and call this type of cultural form an anxiety culture. Though rooted in the specificity of ethnographic research and the subjective experiences of the researcher, this approach would mark a turn toward language and the symbolic register of value. Indeed, one of the virtues of the interpretive turn in the human sciences is that it took what were once interior, psychological categories and showed their public, culturally embedded character. This would be a salutary gesture for the study of anxiety, which traditional psychology has tried to contain within the (clinically examined) individual and pop social psychology has subjected to its dubious methodologies. Moreover, it may productively shift the understanding of anxiety from temporal to spatial terms.

Many other approaches are possible, from literary studies ("anxiety culture" as a metaphor generative of a set of associations), to media studies (tracking the prevalence of anxiety in various news and entertainment programs), to linguistics (anxiety is a notoriously difficult term to translate).[5] Indeed, the impetus for organizing this book is to give space for a fuller elaboration of these various approaches. The approach we will take in this chapter comes from the discipline of philosophy, with significant input from the human sciences.

Thereby, our guiding philosophical lights have two important sources: First, Ludwig Wittgenstein and his definitional approach of pointing to family resemblances instead of strict reference. On the other hand, we tie in with investigations of existential phenomenology of *Stimmung*, or "mood." In recent years, several public intellectuals have tried to analyze the social imprints and effects of fears with reference to our times, and scholars from a variety of disciplines are becoming increasingly aware that anxiety culture is the new global state of human affairs. Our aim in this chapter is to give some shape and language to this increasing awareness, and by not drawing a firm boundary around our object of inquiry and loosening our working definition we hope to capture specific aspects of our present anxiety culture in an experiential and reality-based way. In doing so, we want to highlight in this chapter that our anxiety culture has developed a problematic relationship with traditional truth claims, such that public discussions of anxiety are often focused, but not factual.

Fear and Angst

In *General Introduction to Psychoanalysis*, Sigmund Freud posited a key difference between fear and anxiety: "I think that anxiety is used in connection with a condition regardless of any objective, while fear is essentially directed toward an object."[6] This decoupling of a subjective experience from an objective correlate in reality has done much to push anxiety into the interior realm of the psyche. (In fact, Freud makes this distinction in the context of developing a "General Theory of the Neuroses.") However important this distinction has been, it has not fully expunged earlier understandings of anxiety that retained descriptions of fear and intended to describe more than the interior life of the neurotic. It also has not prevented fear and anxiety from finding new ways to intermix.

In questions of fear, theology was the leading discipline in European thought until the end of the 19th century. Even before psychoanalysis appeared on the scene in the 20th century and gave fear a completely new dimension of scientific consideration, it was the philosopher and theologian Søren Kierkegaard who, in his treatise *The Concept of Anxiety* (1844), proposed an interpretation of fear that further developed the traditional ideas of Christianity and made possible new ways of a philosophical-anthropological classification of fear.[7] In doing so, anxiety is placed in relation to the fundamentally givenness of human freedom, and a causal dependence between the two is postulated. Man is fearful because his path is not predestined and thus all essential decisions are demanded of him. This fundamental fear of man is qualitatively different from the fear of something concrete, such as a particular threat or danger. It is an indeterminate, diffuse fear that can be constructively directed through reflection and through faith-based closeness to God.

Philosophical existentialism was largely inspired by Kierkegaard and developed into a formative paradigm of human philosophical self-determination in the 20th century. In this context, both the basic element of a diffuse existential anxiety and the close interweaving of anxiety and freedom continued to prove to be the decisive parameters of anthropology and humanism. Our invocation of *Stimmung*, a key aspect of Heidegger's development of Kierkegaard's existentialism, notes this legacy. In the late 20th and early 21st century, however, we witnessed a profound shift in the way we think, interpret, and act about fears and their impact in the public sphere.

As early as the 1980s, public discourse took a new turn with the perception of an ethic and obligation to act in the face of dangers and threats that directly affect each individual as a member of modern society. The philosophical stance on this was now determined by a certain pragmatism, which ideologically referred to the foundations of postwar society with different emphases. Human rights and constitutional rights, democracy, political stability, capitalist economy, and ecological consequences were important signposts and admonitions for the parameters of governance and the steering of human action. Fear in its relevant dimension shifted away from the individual to a sociopsychological view and was presented as a phenomenon to be fundamentally overcome. The yardstick for overcoming fears was the calculated risk, which appears to be unavoidable but can be contained according to rational standards and thus in principle kept free of danger or free of the most debilitating consequences.

This shift in the understanding of fear and its relationship to freedom and anxiety is worth exploring in more detail. One key figure in this shift is Ulrich Beck. His "Risk Society" is a sociologist's comprehensive and formative attempt to ground and sustain this public belief in risk control.[8] In the theory of the risk society, fear is at best a warning signal that calls reason into action as a pragmatic decision maker and thus is itself not permanent.

If one reads Ulrich Beck's last book, posthumously published in 2016 under the title *The Metamorphosis of the World*, one realizes that even Beck recognized that the parameters of the risk society no longer apply and that we have to adapt to a completely changed world whose development forecasts now ultimately do reveal concrete dangers and will force us to make various changes of direction in our behavior (a primary object of his book is climate change).[9]

However, Beck's faith in reason did not yet allow him to recognize, even in this last work, the increasing and changing significance of fears in our contemporary world. In the public discourses of the present, on the other hand, critical and reflective voices that deal with the significance of fear in our present society are multiplying worldwide. In the following section we want to explore three representative publications that capture this new mood of fear, what we are characterizing as "focused, but not factual." Although this is similar to Freud's original definition of anxiety, we believe that it points to something quite different from an account of neurosis. We will return to this point in the final section of this chapter. But first, there is a growing public discourse around the family of fear, freedom, anxiety, and human action.

The Mood of the World

Beck's theory of a world in metamorphosis starts from the perception that the so-called side effects of our modern social systems, which can essentially be described as risks and longer-term dangers for all of us—such as nuclear contamination, refugee migrations, plastic pollution, or the autocratization of democratic states—must become the fundamental benchmarks of a new order of this world. At the same time, he emphasizes that this "concept of the world" has not yet been found.

> The reflexivity of second modernity is a result of the fact that societies are now confronted with the undesirable side effects of their own modernizing dynamics which they have often consciously accepted as collateral damage. It is not

poverty, but wealth, not crisis, but economic growth, coupled with the suppression of side effects, which are driving the side-effects metamorphosis of modern society. This is not abolished, but, rather, accelerated through inaction. It does not come from the centers of politics, but from the laboratories of technology, science, and business.[10]

Beck points out that the unintended side effects are shaking our modern civilization in its basic structures. We are not prepared for this in the Western industrialized world. We have no old or new ideology for this present reality; we can no longer rely on science, because it is itself the culprit; and in this situation, we are destabilizing the basis of our community in the sense of a loss of solidarity, which is the basis of democracy and which at the same time should be the guiding idea for cosmopolitanization. Several thinkers have stepped into this breach to generate a language and conceptual apparatus to describe and engage this emerging global state of affairs. Three such attempts emerged from within those technologically advanced, wealthy societies that were supposed to serve as advertisements for modernity's greatest achievements.[11]

Heinz Bude has pointed out that the basis for the social mediation of fears can be traced back to a phenomenon that the Germans describe with the difficult-to-translate word *Stimmung*. In English it roughly corresponds to "mood," but also "state of mind." There has been a long philosophical reflection in Germany on the phenomenon of *Stimmung* stretching back to Martin Heidegger:

> For Heidegger, mood (*Stimmung*) determines "how one is, and how one is faring"; how reality becomes accessible to us; what feelings, memories and thoughts suggest themselves and what are excluded from the outset; what kinds of behavior are deemed appropriate and what are rejected as inappropriate; and, above all, how the world represents itself to us as a whole.[12]

The mood is, as it were, the mirror of the external living conditions in the form of a collectively felt sensitivity of social subjects, who feel connected to each other through this mood. This is the essential difference to the personal mood of the individual. Bude defines the social character of mood beyond its psychological explanation as follows:

> What is crucial for mood, however, is how I am affected by a situation that is defined socially, spatially, historically and biographically, one that requires me to participate and play a role. In the mood of the situation, the self-generating

self experiences itself as a self that is already generated by the demands, sugges-
tions and syntheses of others. Every space of experienced presence has a mood
to which, without much conscious effort, I seamlessly adjust, and which I perceive either consciously by way of social contrast or which I succumb to without inward resistance.[13]

This approach to the difficult-to-analyze phenomenon of social anxieties via
the concept of moods may be a tradition particular to German thinkers. It offers the advantage of grounding anxieties in lived social relations rather than
from the unfounded and heavily mediated scaremongering of politicians and
the media. Politicians and the media reinforce general moods in the population by amplifying the emotions associated with them—primarily fear, but occasionally other affects that accompany it. For their part, however, they do
not generate the underlying moods that are due to the living conditions themselves. Understanding this is an essential step in understanding the anxiety
culture of our time.

Martha Nussbaum's book titled *Monarchy of Fear* is a very interesting exploration of this theme.[14] It is not, as one would expect from the author, a
strictly philosophical treatise, but rather a profound biographically motivated
reflection on the complex intermingling of personal experience, social mood,
and political reality. Nussbaum focuses on the function of feelings and emotions in public discourses about the current political situation of the time,
especially in the United States. In particular, she draws connections from
fear to other affects, such as anger and disgust.[15]

Anxiety in our society currently triggers emotions in many people who
then express personal fears, anger, or even disgust. But we must distinguish
this observation from the social relevance of anxiety, which is a much deeper
and solid form of critical perception of our living conditions. Nussbaum remains attached to an individual and personal concept of fear when she writes:

> But you don't need society to have fear; you need only yourself and a threaten-
> ing world. Fear, indeed, is intensely narcissistic. It drives out all thoughts of
> others, even if those thoughts have taken root in some form. An infant's fear is
> entirely focused on its own body. Even when, later on, we become capable of
> concern for others, fear often drives that concern away, returning us to infan-
> tile solipsism.[16]

This concept of individual fear does not really fit with the concept of anxiety
culture as we understand it. It stigmatizes fear and anxiety as self-centered and

as something bad in our society, because it proves to be antisocial when combined with other emotions. Pointing out such aberrations in social behavior patterns is an important contribution to upholding ethical principles that should govern our coexistence. But social anxiety as a reaction to the factually disturbing developments in our world—nationally as well as globally—is an equally important contribution to shaping all our actions into a social dynamic that enables us to have a good future.

This final point is underscored by Frank Biess, who in *German Angst: Fear and Democracy in the Federal Republic of Germany* underscores the complex dialectic between fear, anxiety, and democracy.[17] Biess, as a historian, is less concerned with the normative project of expunging or neutralizing fear and more concerned with describing how democracy emerged out of the fragile postwar situation. (We could call it *Germany: Year Zero* in homage to Rossellini's great depiction of this period.) Biess notes that fear and anxiety are quite useful analytic tools for the historian because they resist the temptation to sketch linear histories of development. This is particularly salient in the case of Germany, which like many other advanced, supposedly entrenched democracies, is facing a renewed challenge from right-wing anti-democratic political movements. Anxiety, as Biess understands it (harkening back to Kierkegaard in some sense), is often the ground for human actions and collective projects (he focuses on the Peace and Environmental movements in his book), but these are not wholly produced by the anxious psyche. Rather, returning to Bude, they are often reflective of concrete, lived realities (or the experience of crises, in Biess's understanding). Thus, understanding fear and anxiety becomes a key political task because they are not to be cast aside as irrational or socially destructive emotional states. Rather, they become a ground for political action that understanding may be able to bring into a more positive relationship with rational, collective action.

Anxiety Culture: Focused, but not Factual

In the foregoing discussion we highlighted how a number of thinkers have tried to deploy anxiety and fear to grapple with our current reality—whether that is democratic backsliding or contending with climate change. The main target of inquiry in all cases, we have argued, is something like a social mood but one that is related to concrete changes in people's lived realities and social conditions. This has allowed us to investigate a family of concepts (fear, anxiety, freedom, collective action, political organization) to sketch out some key features of what we are describing as anxiety culture, a new global state of affairs.

We posit that anxiety culture underwrites an orientation toward truth that is "focused, but not factual." What form of fear is at stake in our contemporary postmodern society? How might we describe the mood of anxiety culture? Five key characteristics of anxieties currently define us and are emerging with the perception of the major problem areas in our world today:

1. The anxieties of our time **are triggered by a loss of confidence in the future**, which in Western industrial societies relates to a triple concern: securing personal well-being, maintaining socioeconomic prosperity, and the increasing destruction of our natural environment.

2. The fears **focus on definable problem areas**, which can be marked with buzzwords such as *terrorism, political instability, artificial intelligence, migration, climate change, public health*, to name a few. These problem areas cannot be viewed in isolation from one another but rather reveal their complex interconnectedness.

3. Fears are **often expressed in society as general moods** (*Stimmungen*), that is, as affective patterns of action or emotional forms of evaluation, the starting point of which is usually an experience of crisis in which confidence in overcoming or solving this crisis is dwindling in public discourse.

4. Fears are focused within the respective prevailing public crisis discourses, that is, **their naming and recognition are an essential part of the discourse itself** and significantly shape it (e.g., as fear of Islam, fear of migrants, fear of environmental destruction, fear of viral epidemics, etc.).

5. The omnipresence of fears and the interdependence of their location in different problem areas **make it largely impossible to concretize the respective focuses as real and avertible dangers and threats**. Many fear scenarios are thus the focus of current debates, without their factual verification being the standard of judgment.

This is where the social experience of fear meets a bizarre development of our time, which has been called a post-factual mediated society. In our view, the now clearly recognized and widely exemplified phenomenon of a world "explained" on the basis of post-truths has not yet been convincingly analyzed. Most reason-oriented commentators are content with not understanding the other part of society and dismiss post-truth-led people as "poor misfits." Nevertheless, they now constitute a relevant voter profile for political parties. It is insufficient to dismiss the increased and politically relevant emergence of "irrational" ways of thinking and interpreting as aberrations of individuals or manipulated groups. Rather, it seems to find its justification in the new form of fear, which we can call a "focused, but not factually mediated fear" within the anxiety culture of our time.

This phenomenon is difficult to discern from the vantage point of public discourse, yet political leaders—with some significant exceptions!—and many dedicated public intellectuals strive to uphold the flag of reason in addressing our most pressing problem areas and future issues. For example, seemingly reasonable public voices encourage migrant phobia, downplay climate change impacts, or oppose protective measures against viral contagions. But truths and facts no longer reach many people in terms of their fundamentally fear-driven behavior. Thus, we all constantly contradict our own fears with our actions. Each of us has examples of this, whether on the topics of environmental protection, health protection, or data protection. At other times, our fears take precedence over the facts we know, for example, in racist behavior or religious prejudice—attitudes often detected even among our friends. It is therefore a socially relevant task of the humanities to analyze more closely the new form of fear that is characterized as "focused, but not factual."

As a finding of these observations, an urgent methodological postulate emerges: Anxiety culture must be defined and interpreted in such a way that it leaves room for a rational consideration and classification of things and develops a logic of action that remains reason oriented. The omnipresence of today's anxiety culture teaches us again and again that there is no indissoluble contradiction between fear and reason, even if this is a popular and recurring motif in the crisis discussions of democratic societies. In an anxiety culture like the present one, however, existential fears cannot be dispelled by arguments of reason. On topics such as climate change, migration, or pandemics, there is sufficient recourse to factual knowledge and rational judgments, at least in Western democracies, but the general fears and uncertainties do not diminish as a result. Rather, it seems as if—in opposition to the Enlightenment—rationality is no longer the yardstick of our public awareness and action but is rather a form of affective dealing with the threats and dangers that deeply define us. This image has in many cases become an emblem of our anxiety culture, but at the same time it is probably not as new as it might appear.

The history of the philosophy of emotions goes back to ancient Greece (Plato, Aristotle). This interest was suspended during the European Enlightenment (Kant declared feelings to be the "opponent of reason") and has only reentered mainstream philosophical thought since the 1960s. The Jewish/ Hungarian philosopher Ágnes Heller astonished many followers of the Hungarian school of her teacher György Lukács with the strong emphasis on feelings as part of a more developed Marxist philosophy of the present. In her article "From Utopia to Dystopia" she became very concrete in this regard and appears all the more modern in her thinking.[18] Heller explains that utopian concepts of social orders (e.g., communism, among others) tend to slow down social dynamics in times of crisis, while dystopias seem suited to frighten people, quite rationally, in a way that drives them to permanently change their lives and the destructive orders that determine them. This may sound idealistic, but in Heller's theory it is based on the concrete conviction that social change can only occur from the observation and awareness of everyday life. With this approach to everyday life, Heller exhibits a close affinity to modern social theories, which are always concerned with placing the individual or subject in a larger interpersonal context to facilitate a community-based ethic of action.

A condition of this concept is that rationality catches on with each individual subject if it is not to be imposed by the state. This is perhaps one of the greatest and most difficult challenges that Western democracies are currently facing. We are firmly convinced that it can only succeed if anxiety culture is recognized and taken seriously as the basic tone of our collective experience of reality. In the way our western states have been reacting to the coronavirus pandemic, the dilemma is evident in public discourse. In Germany, since the outbreak of the pandemic, the sociologist Heinz Bude, quoted earlier, and the philosopher Julian Nida-Rümelin have been advising the German government. Bude follows his reflections on the "society of fear" and "mood of the world" with a simple plea for "solidarity," without establishing an inner logic between anxiety culture, general uncertainty, and the ideal of solidarity. Nida-Rümelin adheres to a modern form of rational risk ethics that is essentially in the same tradition of trust in political rational decisions that Ulrich Beck joined for decades before he himself came to doubt it.[19]

The major task then is to explain the form of fear we all face: a focused fear that manifests itself in public discourses on several levels but that remains diffuse for many people because in their psyche the feeling of fear is not adequately connected with the correlating facts. Bringing together fears and facts is a task of prudent politics in our time. Such work will require the scientific backing from interdisciplinary analyses, hence our opening canvas of possible paths toward sense-making and our widened aperture by focusing on feeling and mood. There are of course more specific, traditionally scientific approaches to this topic. For example, Joseph Ledoux's *Anxious: The Modern Mind in the Age of Anxiety* is a magisterial neuroscientific analysis of fear, characterizing it as a fundamental principle of our social behavior and assigning it an essential function in human evolutionary development.[20] However, neuroscientific research often finds its way into public discourse of media and politics in the form of simplistic advice on overcoming fear. In the social classification of the problem, we often witness a relapse into the pragmatism of the late 20th century, which presents the risks of our time as controllable and attributes the actual problem to a form of wrong (i.e., too negative) thinking.

Our current anxiety culture, however, is neither pessimistic nor unfounded, and certainly it is not an aberration of human communities in Western democracies. Certainly, populism, conspiracy theories, and radical denial of facts are aberrations. When these proliferate, it is above all a sign of the mishandling of our anxiety culture, which always has the inherent potential to bring the Enlightenment into the age of the living (to again invoke Corine Pelluchon). Can we better achieve this goal in a still humanistic or in an already post-humanistic optic?

NOTES

1. Corine Pelluchon, *Les Lumières à l'âge du vivant* (Paris: Seuil, 2021).

2. Raymond Williams, *The Long Revolution* (New York: Columbia University Press, 1961), 63.

3. A masterful example of this with a less catchy name is Stuart Hall's "Great Moving Right Show," which unfolds the logic of Thatcherism through a renewed focus on "law and order" and educational policy. See Stuart Hall, *Selected Political Writings: The Great Moving Right Show and Other Essays* (Durham: Duke University Press, 2017), 172–186.

4. Agnes Heller, *A Theory of Feelings*, 2nd ed. (Lanham, MD: Lexington Books, 2009).

5. *Anxiety* and *fear*, for example, as a lexical opposition in everyday semantics of the English language, can hardly be translated into German with the opposing "Angst" and "Furcht," even if this has become common in the philosophical tradition after Kierkegaard. The lexical divisions of the semantic field of anxiety are not the same in different languages. This is also true with respect to central terms such as *angoisse* as opposed to *anxiété* and *peur* in French. In Spanish, too, the conceptual field is very complex even at its semantic core: *miedo, temor, ansiedad, pavor, angustia*, etc.

6. Sigmund Freud, *A General Introduction to Psychoanalysis* (New York: Liverlight, 1920), 340.

7. Søren Kierkegaard, *The Concept of Anxiety: A Simple Psychologically Orienting Deliberation on the Dogmatic Issue of Hereditary Sin* (Princeton: Princeton University Press, 1981).

8. Ulrich Beck, *Risk Society: Towards a New Modernity* (London: Sage Publications, 1992).

9. Ulrich Beck, *The Metamorphosis of the World* (Cambridge: Polity Press, 2016).

10. Beck, *The Metamorphosis of the World*, 48.

11. This understanding of modern development of course was premised on many unsustainably ideological commitments, pointed out from within these societies by groups like the Frankfurt School and from outside by innumerable postcolonial critics.

12. Heinz Bude, *The Mood of the World* (Cambridge: Polity, 2018), 10.

13. Bude, 27–28.

14. Martha Nussbaum, *The Monarchy of Fear* (New York: Simon and Schuster, 2019).

15. Here she is connecting with prior philosophical work on "Political Emotions." See Martha Nussbaum, *Political Emotions: Why Love Matters for Justice* (Cambridge, MA: Harvard University Press, 2015).

16. Nussbaum, *The Monarchy of Fear*, 21.

17. Frank Biess, *German Angst: Fear and Democracy in the Federal Republic of Germany* (Oxford: Oxford University Press, 2020).

18. Ágnes Heller, "From Utopia to Dystopia: A Story of Historical Imagination," *Graduate Faculty Philosophy Journal* 37, no. 2 (2016): 289–302.

19. Julian Nida-Rümelin, *Die gefährdete Rationalität der Demokratie: Ein politischer Trakta* (Hamburg: Edition Körber, 2020).

20. Joseph Ledoux, *Anxious: The Modern Mind in the Age of Anxiety* (London: OneWorld Publications, 2015).

PART TWO

CLIMATE CHANGE AND THE ENVIRONMENT

Introduction

MICHAEL I. SCHAPIRA

In exploring the many valences of anxiety culture, we are often moving between the micro and the macro, teasing out the implications of a prevailing mood on both daily practices and our ability to understand broad historical currents. Nowhere is this felt more acutely than around the topic of climate change. For example, a recent *New York Times* article began thus: "It would hit Alina Black in the snack aisle at Trader Joe's, a wave of guilt and shame that made her skin crawl. Something as simple as nuts. They came wrapped in plastic, often in layers of it, that she imagined leaving her house and traveling to a landfill, where it would remain through her lifetime and the lifetime of her children." The article, titled "Climate Change Enters the Therapy Room," tracks the once marginal but now influential field of ecopsychology, and in particular the work of psychologists Thomas J. Doherty and Susan Clayton on the phenomenon of "climate anxiety."[1] Such causal chains assembled by Black have required novel approaches from therapists trying to untie these emotional and intellectual knots.

This is but one instance of the reversals described, via Ulrich Beck, in the Introduction to this volume. Reason's post-Enlightenment refinement, once a source of liberation, now leads one straight to total paralysis. However, as Doherty and Clayton aim to prove, these conditions also point to novel perspectives on human psychology and unexplored paths forward.

Michel Bourban begins this section with an exploration of "eco-anxiety," both in its proximate causes in the Anthropocene and the ways that hope and confidence can be cultivated out of such a condition. Crucially, for Bourban, an important task for the climate-anxious modern subject is to cultivate suitable modes of communication, whether from climate scientists to the general public (e.g., in reports from the Intergovernmental Panel on Climate Change) or among citizens feeling acute disempowerment.

Many areas of the world do not seem particularly anxious about the effects of climate change. Take Houston, for example, whose growth is inextricably linked with the development of a fossil-fuel-driven petro-economy. Dominic Boyer reads Houston as a site of "petro-neuroses," "petromania," and "petro-perversions," all of which are expressive of an underlying death drive, first identified by Freud, but central to the working of petroculture. In yet another reversal, this death drive is in some senses a welcome phenomenon. As Boyer writes, "Mania is often the neurotic condition that immediately precedes either implosion and self-destruction or breakthrough and acceptance. In this respect, it is a healthy sign that petromania abounds today."

The final two contributions to this section bring us closer to the micro level of analysis, focusing on the effects of climate anxiety on concrete processes of learning and development. Kelsey Hudson and Eric Lewandowski describe the lived conditions of youth in the ongoing climate emergency, both in its harmful dimensions and the possibilities it opens for reestablishing meaningful connections to the natural world and to struggles for justice. Christian Martin and Kristina Allgoewer explore a different dimension of learning—namely, how machine learning can help us better understand the influence of anxiety on political affiliation. As they note, "climate anxiety is a politically cross-cutting issue that is not easily associated with traditional political preferences," and thus, as with the case of today's youth, will require a radical reimagining of the future.

NOTES

1. Ellen Barry, "Climate Change Enters the Therapy Room," *New York Times*, February 6, 2022.

Eco-Anxiety

A Philosophical Approach

MICHEL BOURBAN

*So that man, which looks too far before him, in the care of future
time, hath his heart all the day long, gnawed on by feare of death,
poverty, or other calamity; and has no repose, nor pause of his anxiety, but in sleep.*
　　　　　　Thomas Hobbes, Leviathan, *Chap. XII, "Of Religion"*

*Do not go gentle into that good night,
Old age should burn and rave at close of day;
Rage, rage against the dying of the light.*
　　　　Dylan Thomas, *"Do Not Go Gentle into that Good Night"*

Our shattering entry into the Anthropocene was marked by the crossing of
four planetary boundaries: the climate system, biodiversity, the nitrogen and
phosphorus cycles, and land use.[1] Climate change, accelerated loss of biodiversity, interference with the nitrogen and phosphorus cycles, and deforestation
have taken us out of the stable environmental conditions of the Holocene, into
an unknown geological epoch. If these transgressions persist, the entire planet
will likely be pushed into a new state that would be much less hospitable for
human societies, not to mention other species. The Anthropocene is a rupture
in Earth history, an irreversible ecological disruption, a geological bifurcation
with no foreseeable return to the normality of the Holocene.[2] Crossing the
planetary threshold of 2°C above preindustrial levels could even lead the entire Earth system into a "Hothouse Earth" trajectory, in which global warming may be substantially accelerated by a cascade of tipping points in the

climate system.[3] Earth system scientists warn us that "the evidence from tip-ping points alone suggests that we are in a state of planetary emergency: both the risk and urgency of the situation are acute." Indeed, "the intervention time left to prevent tipping could already have shrunk towards zero, whereas the reaction time to achieve net zero emissions is 30 years at best."[4]

Given this picture, it is very difficult not to feel anxious about the future of the planet, especially the future of the species and the sentient individuals Earth hosts. Environmental scientists have been warning us for decades that economic activities are pushing against and even crossing natural limits. Half a century ago, Donella Meadows and colleagues had already highlighted the (natural) limits to (economic) growth.[5] Back then, the tone was already quite alarmist, and the sense of urgency was rather pronounced. But as we entered the 21st century, the planetary boundary framework changed the game. This framework emphasizes nine planetary boundaries in the Earth system,[6] stresses the existence of tipping points,[7] and quantifies both the boundaries and their tipping points. Over the last decade, Earth system scientists have developed three key insights: (1) the Anthropocene probably started in the mid-1950s due to the exponential increase of material and energy flows under-lying our economic activities; (2) the Anthropocene is functionally and stratigraphically distinct from the Holocene, a remarkably stable epoch that lasted for more than 10,000 years, allowing our complex societies to develop; and (3) Earth's tipping points are too close for comfort and too risky to bet against. Now that we more accurately know the scale of what we are up against, feeling anxiety is close to unavoidable.[8] When scientists write that "we are in a state of *planetary emergency*" in the journal *Nature*,[9] when they explain that "The scale of recent changes across the climate system as a whole and the pre-sent state of many aspects of the climate system are *unprecedented* over many centuries to many thousands of years" and that "Many changes due to past and future greenhouse gas emissions are *irreversible* for centuries to millennia" in the latest IPCC Assessment Report, there are good reasons to feel not only alarmed but also anxious about the state of the planet in the near and distant future.[10]

In response to these more and more numerous, accurate, and accessible empirical data on the rapidly degrading state of the planet, there is a corre-sponding increase in pessimistic perceptions of the future through the lens of fictional narratives. The notion of "scenario," ubiquitous in IPCC reports and scientific articles on climate change, usually refers to a reasoned effort of anticipation in a film or a novel. Scenarios are fictions depicting possible worlds. They illustrate what kind of future might result from current trends, such as the continued use of fossil fuels to supply global energy demand. In the genre of eco-fiction and the subgenre of climate fiction ("cli-fi," for short), more and more novels and films explore apocalyptic and/or postapocalyptic scenarios in which anthropogenic ecological disaster completely changes the world as we know it.[11] Even if these "Anthropocene fictions" draw more or less accurately on scientific knowledge, they contribute to influencing popular perceptions of the near and distant future. Anthropocene fictions link numbers, graphs, and figures with our daily lives. They make the notion of the Anthropocene more tangible.

Scientific knowledge and Anthropocene fictions therefore contribute to making anxiety a defining feature of our time. Just as John Rawls perceived the "fact of reasonable pluralism" as a permanent feature of democratic public culture,[12] it makes sense to consider the "fact of anxiety" as a pervasive characteristic of life in the Anthropocene.[13] Global environmental changes such as anthropogenic mass extinction, climate change, and ozone depletion arguably give rise to a specific form of anxiety: eco-anxiety.[14] This chapter draws the contours of the notion of eco-anxiety and suggests possible remedies. In the spirit of the volume, the objective is to identify elements of anxiety culture without pretending to give definitive answers or trying to excessively restrict the understanding of anxiety. This is a contribution to an emergent research agenda on anxiety conceived as a new global state of human affairs.

What Is Eco-Anxiety?

Let us start with the following working definition:

> *Eco-anxiety* is a subjective trait, state, or disposition turned toward a possible objective state of the planet in the near or distant future. Its object is severe ecological risks that are not yet here (in space) or present (in time), but which might happen in the more or less distant future. It is a fear resulting from an acute awareness of the risks raised by global ecological issues. Eco-anxiety can lead to a generalized feeling of discouragement; taken to too high a degree, it can also become pathological, a fear of a fear, or an exaggeration of the probabilities of environmental dangers.[15]

There are three main elements of this definition. First, like any form of anxiety, eco-anxiety is *future oriented*. The envisioned future can be more or less determinate and more or less near, but it is both (a) threatening and (b) uncertain. Regarding (a), the main object of eco-anxiety is *ecological risks*, such as sea-level rise, mega-fires, and extreme climate events such as hurricanes, droughts, heat waves, and floods. Its object can also be the consequences of these phenomena on human and/or non-human beings, such as animal suffering, ecosystem degradation, species extinction, the disruption of agricultural systems and food supply chains, economic shocks, sociopolitical instability, as well as starvation, mass migration, conflict, and even societal collapse.[16] Regarding (b), risks and uncertainty are intrinsically linked. Risks are the product of magnitude and probability: the magnitude is a measure of the seriousness of the loss and damage at stake; the probability is a measure of the likelihood of such loss and damage occurring. That something is uncertain means that it currently has no calculable probability; it does not mean that its objective probability, if known, would be small.[17] Questions of probability can however become less relevant if the magnitude of the possible loss and damage is massive, such as the triggering of a Hothouse Earth pathway. In such cases, it is possible to replace the category of risk with that of danger. A cascade of tipping points in the climate system, such as rapid permafrost thawing, the weakening of terrestrial and oceanic carbon sinks, and the Amazon Forest dieback would represent positive global feedback loops over which no one would have any control. We can conceive these carbon cycle feedbacks as transcendental dangers, that is, dangers that threaten the very condition of human existence on the planet, or at least the conditions of a flourishing human life.[18]

Second, eco-anxiety is not only a state of uncertainty, but also of *fear* and *insecurity* in the face of ecological risks and transcendental dangers. Eco-anxiety is an emotion that reaches deep, a gut feeling that most, if not all, future scenarios are insecure. It is a constant or structural fear that we are contributing, with our individual and collective lifestyles, to creating a more dangerous world for young people and future generations. This feeling of fear and insecurity does not require the direct experience or observation of a dangerous anthropogenic ecological event to exist; imagining a risk or danger is sufficient to trigger it.[19] Eco-fictions, such as Kevin Reynolds's *Waterworld*, Roland Emmerich's *The Day After Tomorrow*, or Bong Joon-ho's *Snowpiercer* provide a visual representation of the dark side of the Anthropocene. These movies set in motion images that are the interpretative representation of a crucial concept in the Anthropocene: that of ecological disaster. Films allow us to apprehend concepts through imagination and emotions rather than through reason alone. Eco-fiction (and climate fiction) films seek above all to portray the notion of disaster, especially in the eco-apocalyptic and post-eco-apocalyptic subgenres, which trace the end of the world as we know it back to current environmental problems (and sometimes to the potentially catastrophic side effects of the technologies we might use to face them, such as geoengineering in the case of *Snowpiercer*).

The ecological disaster confronts us, whether we are actors or spectators, victims, or observers, with the unthinkable, the inconceivable, the impossible. The word that best corresponds to our direct or indirect exposure to disaster is stupefaction, which entails suspension of the movement of thought and action. The disaster lays bare a world in which reason has difficulty finding its bearings. Words resist, and a key objective of eco-fiction movies is to express the disaster through images rather than through concepts. Anthropocene fictions do not necessarily depict a world structured by a punctual and final disaster: the adverse effects of climate change and other environmental issues are gradual, widespread, and diverse. The ecological disaster is not simply a major, highly dramatic, and particularly destructive hazard; it is mostly a recurring, multifaceted phenomenon, occurring at various levels, and experienced in many ways.[20]

Third, eco-anxiety usually leads to a form of *paralysis*, or suspension of action. Fear can sometimes be motivating, for instance when it pushes us to avoid its object or its source, but it can also be paralyzing.[21] Eco-fictions can incite us to avoid the disaster they depict by changing our behaviors and reforming existing institutions, but they can just as easily block our individual actions by showing up the futility of our efforts. Likewise, learning about the existence of the nine planetary boundaries, the crossing of four of them, and the possibility of a Hothouse Earth pathway can be discouraging: what can I do as an individual in the face of such gigantic forces? Eco-anxiety can lead to a generalized feeling of discouragement regarding the future and what we can do about it, both individually and collectively.

This third feature shows how easily eco-anxiety can become difficult to live with. Neither eco-fiction film directors nor Earth system scientists wish to convey the message that individual action is futile. Quite the contrary: their films and publications are usually a call to action, both at the individual and the collective level. To take a recent example, Johan Rockström's and Owen Gaffney's book *Breaking Boundaries*, which has been adapted for the screen as a documentary, discusses individual and collective solutions to current ecological problems as much as the problems themselves.[22] At the same time, given the scale and the gravity of the problems they discuss and what is at stake (what Rockström and colleagues have called "the world's biggest gamble"[23]), one can understandably feel overwhelmed. Doom-and-gloom narratives can cause despair, which in turn can demotivate people in ways that could exacerbate ecological problems. When eco-anxiety gives way to despair, it becomes a fear of a fear, an exaggeration of the probabilities of transcendental dangers. At that point, there is little chance that eco-anxiety will leave space for possible solutions to avoid the realization of the darkest scenarios.[24]

How widespread is the phenomenon of eco-anxiety? Although degrees of eco-anxiety vary according to factors such as age, profession, and location, the (limited) available data indicate that it is spreading very fast. Two categories of people seem to be particularly affected by eco-anxiety: climate scientists, and children and young people. A first survey has found that many IPCC authors are suffering from eco-anxiety, with more than 60% of the respondents saying that they experience anxiety, grief, or other distress because of concerns over climate change. Eighty-two percent of the respondents report that they think they will see catastrophic impacts of climate change in their lifetime, and six in ten expect the world to warm by at least 3°C above preindustrial levels by 2100.[25] A second survey, the largest to date, has found that a huge and growing number of children and young people from a diverse range of countries with a diverse range of income and exposure to climate impacts are suffering from eco-anxiety.[26] While 59% say that they feel very or extremely worried about climate change, 45% say that their feelings about climate change negatively affect their daily lives. Seventy-five percent find the future frightening, 56% believe that humanity is doomed, 55% think that they will have fewer opportunities than their parents, 52% believe that their family's security will be threatened, and 39% are hesitant to have children. More than 50% say that they feel afraid, sad, anxious, angry, powerless, helpless, and/or guilty.

The psychological state of children and young people is not only affected by climate impacts but also by their perception of governments' failure to respond to climate change, which leads to feelings of betrayal and abandonment by adults. The study highlights that all these stressors will have "considerable, long-lasting and incremental negative implications for the mental health of children and young people." It also frames government failure as a "failure of ethical responsibility to care" and a source of "moral injury," understood as "the distressing psychological aftermath experienced when one perpetrates or witnesses actions that violate moral or core beliefs."[27] In other words, adults and governments hold a moral responsibility in the two major senses of this concept: they are responsible for the outcome of their lack of action on the psychological state of children and young people, and they are responsible for remedying this outcome by helping those who suffer from eco-anxiety.[28]

What Can Be Done About Eco-Anxiety?

Now that we know more about the meaning of eco-anxiety, we can ask what can be done about it. Since eco-anxiety is a distinctive feature of the Anthropocene, a key component of the fact of anxiety, it is in some sense unavoidable. The point is therefore not so much to try to escape this state as to mitigate it as far as possible to avoid its undesirable side effects such as paralysis and its pathological effects such as despair. We must live with eco-anxiety, but this does not mean that we cannot fight some of its most worrying manifestations.

Cultivating Hope and Confidence

A first intuitive counterpower that comes to mind when we wonder how to face eco-anxiety is of course *hope*. Some climate justice scholars have recently emphasized the value of hope in the climate change discourse by promoting "climate hope."[29] Hope applies to an object that is (1) desired, (2) believed to be possible but that remains uncertain, and (3) characterized by a certain mental emphasis that makes the desire and the belief of the person who hopes significant and stable. The mental emphasis is on the possibility of a positive outcome, but at the same time, hope and pessimism can coexist. As Dominic Roser explains, "I can believe X to have a low probability (condition 2) but can still desire X (condition 1) and psychologically rally around X (condition 3)."[30] He illustrates this with the case of the 1.5°C climate target: even if there is a low probability that we will keep the temperature increase below 1.5°C, this goal remains possible and desirable and can therefore be an object of hope. Roser adds that it is not only justifiable to hope to achieve the 1.5°C target but that also good reasons exist for cultivating hope of achieving this goal, since the advantages of hoping for this specific object (motivational and hedonic benefits) outweigh its disadvantages (temptation of wishful thinking, disappointment, and distraction). The motivational benefit of hope is especially relevant in discussions on eco-anxiety: one crucial reason why cultivating hope is so important is that hope can contribute to increasing the probability of achieving the hoped-for outcome. While anxiety can lead to overwhelm, discouragement, and even paralysis, hope can work as a remedy thanks to its instrumental value; a hopeful disposition can represent a source of personal motivation to overcome collective action problems. This point is also highlighted by Catriona

McKinnon: "Hope can increase the probability that a person's agency achieves its purpose, and so can galvanize the person's will as it aims at this purpose."[31]

Hope, however, is an ambiguous state, a double-edged sword. It is not necessarily energizing; quite the contrary, as Roser recognizes, "Dwelling on the imagined achievement instead of working towards it, hinders rather than spurs action."[32] In that sense, hope can also be a hindrance to successfully taking action that achieves the hoped-for object.[33] The main reason for this is that hope is not, contrary to a commonly shared conception, the opposite of anxiety.[34] Hope is a desire for an object we do not have or that does not exist, a desire whose fulfillment remains uncertain. This is why, as Spinoza famously observed, "there is no hope without fear nor fear without hope."[35] Hope and anxiety are both based on doubt, on uncertainty. To hope is to fear disappointment; to fear is to hope for reassurance.[36] Spinoza adds, "*Hope is* simply *an inconstant joy arising from the image of something in the future or in the past about whose outcome we are in doubt*."[37] This does not mean that one should stop hoping, which is neither possible nor desirable. This rather means that, in addition to cultivating hope, one should find other ways to mitigate eco-anxiety.

If hope is not the opposite of anxiety, what is? *Serenity* would be a more accurate candidate. Serenity is an inner peace, an absence of disorder, close to the Greek ideal of *ataraxia*. The problem with serenity is that it is a state proper to the wise, an ideal toward which one can only strive without ever fully reaching it. A more relevant (because easier to achieve) state to cultivate would be *confidence*. Confidence is less about the future than about the present, less about what we do not know than about what we do know, less about what does not depend on us than about what does.[38] There are surely many ways to cultivate confidence to reduce eco-anxiety, but here I would like to focus on the promotion of personal action against global environmental changes. Even if global and massive problems such as climate change and biodiversity loss can seem beyond our control, we can focus on what we can do here and now, on what we know about our individual carbon footprint and how we can reduce it, in short, on what depends on us.

There are two major categories of individual action that can be taken to face climate change with more confidence and less anxiety. The first is actions that directly reduce one's personal emissions. A recent review of the literature shows that there are five major high-impact actions that allow individuals in developed countries to substantially reduce their annual greenhouse gas (GHG) emissions:[39]

1. Adopting a plant-based diet (0.8 tCO_2e saved per year)
2. Buying green energy (1.5 tCO_2e saved per year)
3. Avoiding airplane travel (1.6 tCO_2e saved per roundtrip transatlantic flight)
4. Living car-free (2.4 tCO_2e saved per year)
5. Having one less child (58.6 tCO_2e saved per year)

All these actions need to be critically discussed, but they are representative of what needs to be done to seriously tackle high-emitting lifestyles of individuals in developed countries. In addition, some high-impact actions to reduce GHG emissions come with substantial ecological co-benefits. For instance, moving from currently dominant diets to diets that exclude animal products at a global level would not only reduce the GHG emissions of food by 49%; it would also reduce land use for food by 76%, eutrophication by 49%, and freshwater use by 19%.[40] Taking part in this kind of collective shift in habits can give confidence that the worst scenarios such as the Hothouse Earth pathway can still be avoided.

A second and related category of individual actions is to promote and support collective action against climate change. Individuals can do so by two means: by helping to design institutions better adapted to tackling climate change; and by participating in changing and creating social norms.[41] In the case of institutional reform, individuals have a wide range of possibilities at their disposal, from voting green to civil disobedience in response to government failure and pushing for more ambitious climate policies.[42] People can also write blogs and articles, petition their local government, email their representatives or executives, organize and/or attend demonstrations, and donate to or join NGOs.[43] In the case of social norm transformation and creation, individuals can for instance adapt their lifestyles and develop communication strategies to amplify the effects of their green behaviors. They can also frame greener lifestyles as appealing to influence other people to reduce their own carbon footprint. Abandoning the rhetoric of self-sacrifice and explaining the different ways in which more environmentally friendly lifestyles can be self-rewarding and contribute to happiness and well-being is a powerful tool to push other people to go green.[44] Here again, these actions can help build a climate of confidence that can work as a remedy to eco-anxiety and its manifestations.

The Power of Communication

One could object that, just like hope, confidence can remain wishful thinking in the face of experienced, observed, or imagined ecological disasters. When we feel high degrees of eco-anxiety, fear can lead to discouragement, which can lead to paralysis. How can this vicious circle be broken?

A key solution here is *adequate communication*. When they communicate the results of their empirical research, climate scientists should insist both on the urgency of the situation and on the available means to avoid dangerous climate change. Emotional appeals to fear to create a sense of urgency can backfire when they lead to paralysis or other psychological defense mechanisms, such as denial. For this reason, Susanne Moser explains that "fear appeals must be coupled with constructive information and support to reduce the danger."[45] IPCC authors have already to a certain extent taken this into account in their communication strategy, but there is still a bias toward technology fixes in most IPCC scenarios, which leads to an overestimation of the effectiveness of technological solutions and an underestimation of the effectiveness of changes in economies, societies, and especially lifestyles.[46] To combat eco-anxiety, they could and should say more about the environmental benefits of high-impact actions such as the aforementioned ones.

Likewise, when they communicate the results of their normative research, climate justice scholars should articulate abstract duties of global and intergenerational justice with concrete courses of action that would allow individual and collective agents to fulfill their duties. To reduce individuals' unwillingness to make lifestyle changes, so far philosophers have first and foremost promoted moral education and awareness through theories of environmental ethics, climate justice, or ecological citizenship to bring people to see environmental issues as moral problems and persuade them that they ought to take personal action against these issues. The task of urging moral agents to fulfill their ecological responsibilities remains incomplete however as long as philosophers do not also propose concrete courses of action. Regarding individual agents, philosophers should articulate the values, attitudes, and virtues they promote with behaviors that would allow people to reduce their overall environmental footprint. Regarding collective agents such as cities, states, or international organizations such as the UN or the EU, philosophers should explain how these agents can comply with their duties of justice by proposing feasible institutional reforms to existing municipal, national, and international environmental policies. So far, climate justice scholarship has mostly focused on the first, more abstract task of defining and justifying principles of climate justice at the individual and collective level. The time has come to link climate justice with climate action more systematically by proposing concrete and feasible courses of action.[47] This can play a part in replacing the vicious circle of

anxiety, fear, and paralysis with a virtuous circle of environmental awareness, confidence, and motivation. The challenge is tremendous, but we can at
least partially meet it with more adequate communication.

Finally, in addition to researchers, policymakers—both government officials
and citizens—also have a key role to play in combating eco-anxiety. As stressed
earlier, policymakers are not only responsible for the state of the planet, which
could definitely have been improved had they taken more ambitious action
sooner; they are also responsible for rising levels of eco-anxiety among children
and young people. This double outcome responsibility gives rise to a remedial
responsibility that policymakers can partially fulfill by way of two major steps.
The first step would be to officially recognize the feelings of young people by
hearing and respecting them. All too often, negative feelings caused by climate
anxiety have been dismissed, ignored, disavowed, rationalized, and negated by
those in positions of political power, and this is where things need to change
first. Here again, communication is key—when they communicate regarding
climate change, policymakers should directly address the legitimate concerns of
young people. The second step would be to act upon the negative feelings of
young people by taking ambitious environmental action. Once they have seriously acknowledged the negative feelings of young people, government officials
and citizens ought to act accordingly. This means placing environmental protection not only at the top of the political agenda but also at the center of policymaking. Otherwise, we will end up in the same situation as today, with discourses that seem to validate the worries of young people that are not followed
by corresponding actions. This is a question of integrity. Policymakers should
integrate their discourses and actions into a coherent whole, by designing
and implementing policies that correspond to the degree of emergency of
the situation. Otherwise, they will keep doing too little, too late.[48]

Conclusion

Eco-anxiety is a defining feature of the Anthropocene. It is a state of mind oriented toward an uncertain future characterized by ecological risks and
transcendental dangers. It is also a state of fear and insecurity in the face of an
observable or imaginable anthropogenic ecological disaster that can lead to
discouragement and even paralysis. It can be triggered by scientific data about
the state and the future of the world or by scenarios depicted in eco-fiction
novels and films, or both.

Although eco-anxiety has become somewhat unavoidable, it is possible to
mitigate its undesirable side effects such as paralysis and its pathological

effects such as despair. A first possible way to combat eco-anxiety is to culti-vate hope, in particular hope to limit global temperature rise below 1.5°C and therefore to avoid a Hothouse Earth pathway by the end of the century. Hope can be galvanizing and energizing, but it can also lead back to a key component of anxiety: fear. For the opposite of anxiety is not hope, but rather confidence. In addition to cultivating hope, climate change scholars should cultivate con-fidence by linking climate science and climate justice more systematically with climate action. This can play a part in replacing the vicious circle of anx-iety, fear, and paralysis with a virtuous circle of environmental awareness, confidence, and motivation. Adequate communication is key: appeals to fear, which are difficult to avoid in a state of planetary emergency, should be complemented by appeals to concrete courses of action that individuals can take to escape the psychological traps of paralysis and despair. Finally, ad-equate action by policymakers is probably the most effective remedy for eco-anxiety. Government officials and citizens should not only seriously ac-knowledge the negative feelings of children and young people in the face of global environmental changes, but they should also act accordingly by im-plementing long overdue ambitious environmental policies.

NOTES

1. Johann Rockström et al., "A Safe Operating Space for Humanity," *Nature* 461, no. 7263 (2009): 472–475; Will Steffen et al., "Planetary Boundaries: Guiding Human Development on a Changing Planet," *Science* 347, no. 6223 (2015).

2. Clive Hamilton, "The Anthropocene as Rupture," *The Anthropocene Review* 3, no. 2 (2016): 93–106.

3. Will Steffen et al., "Trajectories of the Earth System in the Anthropocene," *Proceedings of the National Academy of Sciences* 115, no. 33 (2018): 8252–8259.

4. Timothy Lenton et al., "Climate Tipping Points—Too Risky to Bet Against," *Nature* 575 (2019): 592–595.

5. Donella Meadows et al., *The Limits to Growth* (New York: Universe Books, 1972).

6. These nine boundaries are the following: the big three—the climate system, the ozone layer, and the ocean; the four biosphere boundaries—biodiversity, land, fresh water, and nutri-ents; and the two aliens—novel entities and aerosols.

7. The nine major active tipping points are the two ice sheets in Greenland and West Ant-arctica, Arctic and East Antarctic Sea ice, the boreal forest and the Amazon rainforest, Atlantic circulation, permafrost in Siberia, and Australia's Great Barrier Reef.

8. Steffen et al., "Planetary Boundaries"; Colin Waters et al., "The Anthropocene is Function-ally and Stratigraphically Distinct from the Holocene," *Science* 351, no. 6269 (2016).

9. Lenton, "Climate Tipping Points," 595, emphasis added.

10. IPCC 2021, "Summary for Policymakers," in *Climate Change 2021: The Physical Science Basis. Contribution of Working Group I to the Sixth Assessment Report of the Intergovernmental Panel on Climate Change*, edited by V. Masson-Delmotte, et al. (Cambridge: Cambridge Univer-sity Press, 2021): 3–31, 8, 21. Emphasis added.

11. Adeline Johns-Putra, "Climate Change in Literature and Literary Studies: From cli-fi Climate Change Theater and Ecopoetry to Ecocriticism and Climate Change Criticism," *WIREs Climate Change* 7, no. 2 (2016): 226–282; Michael Svoboda, "Cli-fi on the Screen(s): Patterns in the Representation of Climate Change in Fictional Films," *WIREs Climate Change* 7, no. 1 (2016): 43–64; Adam Trexler, *Anthropocene Fictions: The Novel in a Time of Climate Change* (Charlottesville: University of Virginia Press, 2015).

12. John Rawls, *Political Liberalism* (New York: Columbia University Press, 2005), 36–37.

13. This is of course just an analogy. These two facts differ on many counts, starting with the fact that anxiety is not as rational as pluralism (even if this does not necessarily imply that anxiety is irrational; it can be a lucid reaction to an accurate empirical description of the state of the planet).

14. So far, eco-anxiety has been extensively discussed in the media, with a small but growing body of scientific literature on the topic in various disciplines. For a recent review of different forms of eco-anxiety, see Pikhala Panu, "Anxiety and the Ecological Crisis: An Analysis of Eco-Anxiety and Climate Anxiety," *Sustainability* 12, no. 19 (2020).

15. I draw here on the definition of anxiety proposed by André Comte-Sponville in his *Philosophical Dictionary* and adapt it for the topic discussed in this chapter. André Comte-Sponville, *Dictionnaire Philosophique* (Paris: PUF, 2013), 79.

16. For a recent study of ecological threats to human societies, including the risk of collapse events, see C. E. Richards, R. C. Lupton, and J. M. Allwood, "Re-Framing the Threat of Global Warming: An Empirical Causal Loop Diagram of Climate Change, Food Insecurity and Societal Collapse," *Climate Change* 164, no. 3 (2021). There is a growing literature on the topic of societal collapse caused by ecological problems. The emerging transdisciplinary field of collapsology addresses the possible causes of collapse of civilization as we know it, as well as the possible ways to live in a post-collapsed world (Pablo Servigne and Raphaël Stevens, *How Everything Can Collapse: A Manual for Our Times* [Cambridge: Polity, 2020]). Collapsologists are quite influential in the media and contribute to spreading eco-anxiety. Some scholars have criticized this new field because of its survivalist tone and its apolitical discourse. See, for example, Pierre Charbonnier, "Splendeurs et Misères de la Collapsologie. Les Impensés du Survivalisme de Gauche," *Revue du Crieur* 13, no. 2 (2019): 88–95.

17. Henry Shue, "Deadly Delays, Saving Opportunities: Creating a More Dangerous World?" in *Climate Ethics: Essential Readings*, edited by Stephen Gardiner et al. (Oxford: Oxford University Press, 2010), 147–148.

18. Societal collapse and transcendental dangers link eco-anxiety with existential anxiety, a form of anxiety focusing on the threats to the very existence of humans and societies. Global environmental changes can raise deep feelings of ontological insecurity; see Panu, "Anxiety and the Ecological Crisis," 6–7; Dominique Bourg, "Dommages transcendantaux," in *Du risque à la Menace: Penser la Catastrophe*, edited by Dominique Bourg, Pierre-Benoît Joly, and Alain Kaufmann (Paris: PUF, 2013): 109–126.

19. It is, however, important to stress that the most severe cases of mental health effects of climate change are related to the direct experience of severe climate impacts and include post-traumatic stress disorder, depression, anxiety, the exacerbation of psychotic symptoms, and suicidal ideation and suicide completion. Those who are most exposed to such mental health effects rely heavily on the land and land-based activities, such as Indigenous peoples and farmers. See Cunsolo et al. "Ecological Grief and Anxiety: The Start of a Healthy Response to Climate Change?" *The Lancet Planetary Health* 4, no. 7 (2020): e261–e263.

20. Yoann Moreau, *Vivre avec les catastrophes* (Paris: PUF, 2017). To characterize this phenomenon of ubiquitous harmful anthropogenic ecological impacts, Frédéric Neyrat uses the notion of "cosmophagy," a process whereby humans abolish all forms of otherness by "devouring" what remains of the wilderness; we could also refer to this phenomenon as the

"Langoliers scenario," after Stephen King's *The Langoliers*, a novella adapted into a movie in which creatures devour the world in an alternative reality. See Frédéric Neyrat, "Eco-apocalyptic Cinema. Anthropocene, Cosmophagy, Anthropophagy," *Communications* 96, no. 1 (2015): 67–79.

21. Sabine Roeser, "Risk Communication, Public Engagement, and Climate Change: A Role for Emotions," *Risk Analysis* 32, no. 6 (2012): 1033–1040.

22. Johan Rockström and Owen Gaffney, *Breaking Boundaries: The Science of Our Planet* (London: Dorling Kindersley Limited, 2021).

23. Rockström et al., "The World's Biggest Gamble," *Earth's Future* 4, no. 10 (2016): 465–470.

24. In his review of research on eco-anxiety, Pihkala Panu highlights that three major factors discussed in the literature are uncertainty, unpredictability, and uncontrollability (three classic features of anxiety). He also stresses that most forms of eco-anxiety are nonclinical but that some pathological cases that come with anxiety disorders are also discussed. In cases of strong forms of eco-anxiety, mental health care can be required. See Panu, "Anxiety and the Ecological Crisis."

25. Jeff Tollerson, "Top Climate Scientists are Skeptical that Nations Will Rein in Global Warming," *Nature* 599, no. 4 (November 2021): 22–24.

26. Caroline Hickman et al., "Climate Anxiety in Children and Young People and Their Beliefs About Government Responses to Climate Change: A Global Survey," *The Lancet Planetary Health* 5, no. 12 (2021): e863–e873.

27. Hickman, "Climate Anxiety in Children and Young People," 864.

28. As David Miller explains, responsibility can be understood either as "outcome responsibility," that is, "the responsibility we bear for our own actions and decisions," or as "remedial responsibility," that is, "the responsibility we may have to come to the aid of those who need help." He also stresses that although they are conceptually distinct, they are normatively closely connected, since "outcome responsibility provides us with one important way of identifying remedial responsibility." See David Miller, *National Responsibility and Global Justice* (Oxford: Oxford University Press, 2007), 71.

29. Catrioana McKinnon, "Climate Change: Against Despair," *Ethics and the Environment* 19, no. 1 (2014): 31–48; Dominic Roser, "The Case for Climate Hope," in *Politik der Zukunft:: Zukünftige Generationen als Leerstelle der Demokratie*, edited by Nejma Tamoudi, Simon Faets, and Michael Reder (Bielefed: Transcript Verlag, 2020): 65–86; Henry Shue, "Climate Hope: Implementing the Exit Strategy," *Chicago Journal of International Law* 13, no. 2 (2013): 381–402.

30. Roser, "The Case for Climate Hope," 68.

31. McKinnon, "Climate Change: Against Despair," 45.

32. Roser, "The Case for Climate Hope," 77.

33. Roser stresses that both common sense and empirical data tend to support the instrumental value of hope as a motivational factor to achieve uncertain but possible outcomes, but he also acknowledges that "Armchair reasoning can spin both answers as plausible" and that "it is not straightforward to draw clear conclusions from empirical research on hope."

34. As McKinnon explains, the opposite of hope is rather despair, a feeling typically generated by a judgment that the object of hope is impossible or extremely improbable because of the way the world is.

35. Baruch Spinoza, *Ethics: Proved in Geometrical Order*, trans. Michael Silverthorne (Cambridge: Cambridge University Press, 2018), III, Scholium, 132.

36. This may explain why hope was identified by Hickman et al. as an emotion constitutive of climate anxiety, together with worry, fear, anger, grief, despair, guilt, and shame. See Hickman, "Climate Anxiety in Children and Young People," 863.

37. Spinoza, *Ethics*, III, 18, Scholium 2, 109. Emphasis in the original.

38. Comte-Sponville, *Dictionnaire philosophique*, 199.

39. Seth Wynes and Kimberly Nicholas, "The Climate Mitigation Gap: Education and Government Recommendations Miss the Most Effective Individual Actions," *Environmental Research Letters* 12, no. 7 (2017): 1–9.

40. J. Poore and T. Nemecek, "Reducing Food's Environmental Impacts Through Producers and Consumers," *Science* 360, no. 6392 (2021).

41. Augustin Fragnière, "Climate Change and Individual Duties," *WIREs Climate Change* 7, no. 6 (2016): 798–814.

42. Simon Caney, "Two Kinds of Climate Justice: Avoiding Harm and Sharing Burdens," *Journal of Political Philosophy* 22, no. 2 (2014): 125–149.

43. Elisabeth Cripps, *Climate Change and the Moral Agent: Individual Duties in an Interdependent World* (Oxford: Oxford University Press, 2013).

44. Michael Prinzing, "Going Green is Good for You: Why we Need to Change the Way we Think About Pro-environmental Behavior," *Ethics, Policy & Environment* (2020): 1–18.

45. Susanne Moser, "More Bad News: the Risk of Neglecting Emotional Responses to Climate Change Information," in *Creating a Climate for Change: Communicating Climate Change and Facilitating Social Change*, edited by Lisa Dilling and Susanne Moser (Cambridge: Cambridge University Press, 2007): 73.

46. Kai Kuhnhenn et al., "A Societal Transformation: Scenario for Staying Below 1.5°C," Heinrich Böll Foundation and Konzeptwerk Neue Ökonomie (2020).

47. See Michel Bourban, "Ethics, Energy Transition, and Ecological Citizenship," in *Comprehensive Renewable Energy*, 2nd ed., edited by Trever Letcher (Oxford: Elsevier, 2022): 204–220; Michel Bourban, "Climate Justice in the Non-ideal Circumstances of International Negotiations," in *Principles of Justice and Real-World Climate Politics*, edited by Sarah Kenehan and Corey Katz (London: Rowman and Littlefield, 2021); Michel Bourban, "Mitigation Duties," in *Handbook of the Philosophy of Climate Change*, edited by Gianfranco Pellegrino and Marcello Di Paola (Cham: Springer, 2023).

48. This "too little, too late" rationale is clearly illustrated by the results published in a 2021 report from the United Nations Framework Convention on Climate Change (UNFCCC): even if all countries were to respect their current mitigation pledges, total temperature rise by 2100 could reach 2.7°C above preindustrial levels—a substantial overshoot compared to the absolute target of 2°C and the aspirational target of 1.5°C set by the Paris Agreement. UNFCCC, "Nationally Determined Contributions under the Paris Agreement: Synthesis Report by the Secretariat," FCCC/PA/CMA/2021/8 (Glasgow: UNFCCC, September 2021).

CHAPTER FIVE

Death Anxiety and Fossil Fuels

DOMINIC BOYER

Stephanie LeMenager poses an unsettling yet profound question in her marvelous book, *Living Oil*: "Why [does] the world that oil makes remain so beloved?"[1] Peering into the affective depths of American petroculture, she asks what complex of emotions and urges binds us to a mode of life that, with each passing year, reveals itself to be more environmentally catastrophic. LeMenager rightly identifies love for oil and the way of life it has made possible as a fundamental feature of the affective ties that bind. She discusses the "abashed nostalgia" and "petromelancholia" that reference yearnings for the "easy oil" of the mid-20th century. In that era, the American model of modernity globalized, greased by the massive petro/chemical apparatus of the Second World War that sought to rationalize its continued existence through a new postwar dispensation.[2] American modernity advertised unfettered luxury in the form of new time-saving machines, breathtaking speeds and automobility, and magical materials like plastics. If the promise was not seductive enough to encourage willing participation, the American military empire and development apparatus were usually more than willing to step in to help spread American values.

Easy oil promised both prosperity today and an ever-brighter future; in the mid-20th century, experts and the public alike sincerely believed that fossil-fueled economic and technological development could expand infinitely.[3] This was before the consequences of petroculture began to interrupt fantasies of fossil infinitude. Courageous projects like Rachel Carson's *Silent Spring* (1962)

and tragic events like the Santa Barbara oil spill of 1969 drew widespread public attention to mounting evidence of ecosystemic destabilization. At first these
destabilization trends were interpreted as isolated pathologies within an otherwise sound system. But, after the Club of Rome report in 1972, the future outlook of fossil-fueled modernity was clouded by premonitions of widespread
and rapid civilizational collapse were global trends in economic growth and
resource depletion to continue into the 21st century. The "environmentality"[4]
that coalesced in the 1970s ironically saw its greatest victory in the hobbling of
nuclear energy, a cause that the fossil fuel industry vigorously supported. Nevertheless, it became harder to love fossil fuels without qualification after the
1970s and sustainability emerged as a new, if also obscure, object of desire.[5]

Eco-socialist alternatives appeared in the 1970s and 1980s[6] but were actively
repressed both by a pro-fossil mainstream Left politics and by the rightward
swing of the Overton window. The American model doubled down on petromodernity in the form of neoliberal globalization, which, among many other
dispossessive projects, relocated the worst sites of environmental pollution and
waste beyond the view of northern media and northern publics. The shroud-
ing of the world's silent springs allowed the love of oil to endure a few decades
longer, at least in the North, and even to deepen. Over half of cumulative
global greenhouse gas emissions have taken place in the last thirty years, a
time in which the world allegedly "knew better" than to continue burning fossil fuels.

Today it is rare to hear encouraging environmental news. In fact, most days
there is none. The climate emergency is upon us, ceaselessly manifesting in
record-breaking floods, fires, droughts, extinctions, and blooms, a movable
feast of terror that sweeps across the globe with each changing season. Unsurprisingly, "climate anxiety" has become a new affective phenomenon, especially among those unaccustomed to experiencing other kinds of social and
environmental precarity.[7] It is striking how quickly anxiety slides into calamity for some of those with the most resources to endure a chaotic future. Indigenous philosopher Kyle Powys Whyte describes this phenomenon as
settler apocalypticism: the anxious end-of-the-world doomsaying that appears when the North experiences a mere fraction of the existential terror it
visited upon its colonies.[8]

In these times of affective upset, a loving commitment to petroculture can no
longer be understood as rational. Not only stubborn or denialist, the love of
petroculture is often purely hallucinatory in its claims that fossil fuels can still
create a brighter future for all. Perhaps this should be unsurprising. Repressed

love is, to paraphrase Freud, the origin of all neurotic expressions of symptom and anxiety. So, we ought to consider *petroneurosis* as an epistemic and affective companion of our times. Part of this condition is captured well by LeMenager in her diagnostics of nostalgia and melancholia. But in this chapter, I would like to examine the affective states of petroculture further, paying attention more directly to mania and phobia. The 17th century Swiss medical dissertation that gifted us "nostalgia" (grief for the return home) also explored mania as an alternate formulation such that the world only just missed out on "nostomania" as a charismatic concept capturing the emotional landscape of displacement and indenture.[9] I would argue that we should not make the same mistake twice and avoid grappling with "petromania"—an obsessive commitment to petrocultural reproduction—as the irrational core of our present dilemma.

At the same time, I believe that fear of death (thanatophobia) is now a better way of defining the global North's affective relationship to petroculture than love, though, to be sure, affects mingle promiscuously. That fear originates from mania, the urge not to let go despite the inevitability of collapse. The manic disposition in turn spawns more anxious and nervous actions, stoking the broader anxiety culture that this volume analyzes. We see anxiety culture at work, for example, in the nervous investment in new fossil fuel infrastructures to guarantee "economic stability and growth." Even the Biden administration's allegedly "most ambitious climate change plan in U.S. history" continues to actively support oil and gas pipeline projects as part of its business-as-usual.[10] Fossil fuel companies across the world are granted enormous subsidies and tax incentives, and their agents and allies experience a remarkably shallow reservoir of outrage against their actions. In a few places (like Houston), mania revels in its own symptoms and spirals into distinctive and grotesque kinds of perversion.

It is 2024 and the global North has laid its cards on the table. Its political leadership and elite strata have shown that they are willing to sacrifice almost anything to perpetuate petromodernity just a little longer. This manic, hallucinatory state is both what must be understood and what must be undone.

Thanatophobia and the Origins of Petroneurosis

The phenomenon of "death anxiety" has long been a concern of psychoanalysis. Sigmund Freud tarried with anxiety for much of his career. At first, he characterized anxiety as a kind of toxic surplus of libidinal energy. Then it became an affective by-product of repression; for example, "Anxiety is therefore the universally current coinage for which *any* affective impulse is or can be exchanged if the ideational content attached to it is subjected to repression."[11] Finally, late in his career, Freud came to think about anxiety as an affective signaling of emergent dangers, one that indexed traumas past in the effort to spare ego from future trauma. Those traumas came in many forms, but abandonment and castration fears, rather than fear of death per se, motivated them. For Freud, *Furcht* (fear) was object-oriented, whereas *Angst* (anxiety) was an objectless affective state, a readying for danger even when no specific, immediate threat was present.

Melanie Klein, in contrast, argued that all "anxiety has its origin in the fear of death."[12] Like Freud, she wrestled with the apparent paradox between death and experience; in other words, how can the ego truly fear something outside, by definition, of its life experience. Klein's model of object relations overcame this paradox to some degree by positing that the ego could experience (at least partly) death, destruction, dismemberment through objects and thus come to know and to fear those experiences. In this model, anxiety issues from the gap that necessarily remains between the ego's own reservoir of traumas and those that can be only partly known from object relations. In that gap the ego is haunted by an unanswerable question: What *is* the experience of death? The existential unease of death anxiety is something of a permanent companion for the ego; in happy or busy times, or in times of specific *Furcht*, it can drift away into the background. But thanatophobia reemerges all too often in the quiet hours of contemplation.

It is true that the deaths that concern us seem of a different scale than the ego's contemplation of its own demise. The aforementioned anxieties involve both the anticipated intensification of climate catastrophe and the end of the fossil-fueled lifestyle that has destabilized planetary ecosystems. In other words, petroculture and climate change are phenomena whose scales and temporalities radically exceed the epistemic and affective capacities of individuals.[13] They belong to the ranks of what Tim Morton terms "hyperobjects."[14] Still, as Freud did in *Civilization and its Discontents*, I believe there is analytic value in transposing psychoanalytical concepts to transindividual contexts, rendering, in this case, thanatophobia not as an ego-level phenomenon, but rather one that is also collective, discursive, and historical. We need to conceptualize how multiple affective selves inhabiting petroculture anticipate the death of a way of life defined by fossil fuels and what kinds of petroneurosis trail those anticipations.

The multiplicity of petroculture is hard to ignore because there are few lives in the world today wholly untouched by fossil fuels and their petrochemical

by-products. The luxuries and potentialities of modern life are inevitably associated with fossil fuels. In Arjun Appadurai's view, for example, the two great
revolutions defining modernity were transportation and information.[15] Beginning with steam powered ships and locomotives in the 19th century and
evolving toward automobility and routine intercontinental travel in the
20th century, the new speeds and carrying potential of fossil-fueled transport
transformed and intensified travel and exchange from the local scale to the
global. Similarly, the information revolutions beginning with the telegraph
and the telephone and coming to encompass radio, television and the internet have all depended on electricity, two-thirds of which globally is produced
by burning fossil fuels today.

   For death anxiety to really make sense in relation to fossil fuels, we need to
acknowledge to what extent perceptions and experiences not only of a good
life but of life itself are intimately wound up with the use of fossil fuels. A concept like "path dependency" does not adequately capture how much everyday experience—in the global North and everywhere its colonial ventures
touched (e.g., pretty much everywhere)—is saturated with the infrastructures
and effects of carbon modernity. In addition to mobility, trade, and information networks, fossil fuels informed projects of machine manufacture, climate
control, and artificial light, radically shifting experiences of productivity, space,
and time in both domestic and industrial situations across the world.[16] Discussing the experiential effects of artificial light both for good and for ill, Akhil
Gupta explains how it "opened a 'second day' for consumption, recreation,
and schooling (through homework), made it much safer to illuminate tight
urban spaces and the interiors of homes, enabled public spaces to be safer and
more family-friendly," while at the same time it also "enabled longer working
hours on the factory floor. Electricity also enabled shiftwork, such that production units could be open twenty-four hours a day, facilitating the manufacture of goods and the turnover of capital."[17]

   The ubiquity of petroplastics reinforces the logic of fossil fuels. Only 4% of
the world's oil production translates into over 300 million tons of polymers
each year and rising; the average annual per capita consumption of plastic is
35 kg, whereas in the United States, the world's largest plastic consumer, the
figure is closer to 130 kg per person per year. Since the 1950s, plastics have revo-
lutionized the object world of commodities, and their disposability serves as
a model for expansive consumerism and the use of "energy without conscience" more generally.[18] Today, it is difficult to find household objects that
contain no plastic; even foods are not only often wrapped in petroleum by-

products but also frequently contain petrochemical compounds like mineral oil, paraffin wax, tertiary butylhydroquinone (TBHQ), and artificial food colorings. Beyond these kinds of deliberate pervasion, fossil fuels create massive amounts of material waste (e.g., oceanic plastic) and their infrastructures of production and transmission are leaky, constantly distributing errant petrochemicals into the surrounding air, water, and soil.

Karen Pinkus[19] wisely regards fossil fuels as the *vis viva* of modern life, and Cara Daggett[20] shows how their use helped shape modern conceptualizations of work and economy. "Growth," as Tim Mitchell observes, is itself a petroknowledge.[21] Once one aggregates all these forms of presence, the question becomes whether any cultural life exists beyond the concatenated influence of fossil fuels. The fear of the loss of a modern way of life anchors fossil thanatophobia and chains minds and feelings to the current course, even as fossil-fueled civilization advances toward ecological collapse.

The pervasive influence of fossil fuels upon modern life explains their oxygen-like invisibility, a phenomenon that Roman Bartosch characterizes as the "Petroleum Unconscious" given how "The ubiquity of oil and its utter elusiveness as an object of aesthetic contemplation and narrative concern have combined to hinder recognition of petroculture . . ."[22] The unconscious is an apt concept as it marks, for Freud, an unruly yet impactful epistemic domain suppressed from recognition by ego by intrapsychic defense mechanisms. We know that petroleum has increasingly been saddled by negative aesthetics in recent decades, and therefore active repression of the materiality and violence surrounding oil is necessary to permit the ongoing petrocultural love affair with its various kinds of modern enablement and entitlement. European contemporaries, including the great liberal philosophers of freedom, practiced much the same kind of inexcusable silence regarding New World plantation slavery and the transatlantic slave trade in the 17th and 18th centuries.[23] The wealth and luxury slave labor returned to Europe was no secret at the time, so its silencing in elite discourse must be assumed to be an active project of denying the constitutive social and material conditions of elite Europeans' prosperity and privilege. Stated plainly, in the spirit of Frantz Fanon, this was a neurotic situation. Its affective precarity was even recognized at the time, at least by Montesquieu, who penned the following smoking gun in 1748, "It is impossible for us to assume that these people [Negroes] are men, because if we assumed they were men, one would begin to believe that we ourselves were not Christians."[24]

European liberalism and its frantic thirst for freedom originated in a neurotic relationship to Europe's structural violence against Indigenous and

African peoples. Likewise, modern petroculture stands in a neurotic relation-ship to the extractive, dispossessive violence of the wellhead as well as to the environmental and social devastation being wrought by climate change. When neurosis begins to escape its own conditions of suppression, when the rational containment field weakens or perhaps when the experiential contra-dictions (e.g., drought, fire, flood) become too much to bear, neurosis tends to externalize itself in the form of mania (obsessive, hallucinatory reproduction). And just as various feral and manic liberalisms seek to reimpose conditions of white supremacy today, we find petromania surging forth from the anxieties surrounding the necessary demise of the fossil-fueled world order.

Houston (Notes Upon a Case of Obsessional Neurosis)

A full survey of petromania would be an epic task. It is, I believe, a general af-fective condition within the global North (and many elite enclaves in the global South) today for reasons already explained. Its symptom complex is thus at once massive and culturally specific in all locations. So, in lieu of a gen-eral discussion, I offer a specific study of the making of an epicenter of petro-mania: Houston, Texas, home to the largest conglomeration of fossil fuel and petrochemical infrastructure in the Western hemisphere and to some 5,000 energy companies working diligently to make the insanity of fossil fuel use seem not only reasonable and widely beneficial but also inevitable.

The pre-petro history of Houston exemplifies how infrastructures, rela-tions, and attitudes inherited from white settler colonialism assemble the foundations of petroculture. Houston was founded by the real estate–speculating Allen brothers in 1836 on 6,642 acres of woodlands and prairie swamp at the confluence of the Buffalo and White Oak Bayous. The Allens had arrived on the Texan frontier from New York a few years earlier with the in-tention of building a city and a fortune. When the Battle of San Jacinto brought an independent Texas republic into being, they saw the opportunity to create a home for the new government, one astutely marketed by naming it for the war's hero, General Sam Houston. The area around Buffalo Bayou was not their first choice, and it was not unoccupied. Indigenous Akokisa, Atakapa, and Karankawa peoples had already been displaced by violence and mission-ization at the hands of the Spanish, but groups of Cherokee and Creek, them-selves refugees forcibly displaced from their homelands to the east, were encamped near the site of the Allens' purchase. The original attraction of the town to the Anglo settlers was that Buffalo Bayou was navigable (if barely so) by steamboat down to the Gulf of Mexico, making it the deepest inland port in the area. Early settlers lived in tents and huts made of clapboards and pine poles; most walked along mud streets; and most stayed despite endemic disease and flooding, one contemporary opined, "possibly because it was practically impossible to get away."[25] There they deforested the woodlands and anxiously defended their property claims against the spectral forces of "blood thirsty Indians and thieving Mexicans."[26]

Out of the swindles and violence of this resource frontier, the eventual oil capital of the world was born. Yet the first oil obsession to dominate the city was not petroleum, but rather cottonseed oil. The river lands to the southwest of Houston were rife with cotton and sugar plantations, and Houston's combination of railroad and ship access meant that it could be a gathering point for the spoils of local plantation slavery as well as a key transit node within the expanding United States as a whole. By 1882, there were fourteen cottonseed oil companies operating in Texas and producing a total of five million barrels per year, mostly in the Houston area. A decade later, thanks to the local plantation economy, the mills of Houston were producing more cottonseed oil than anywhere else in the world.

The shift to petroleum came in the first decades of the 20th century. Already by 1911, Houston is described by contemporaries as the center of the oil industry, more specifically as "the recognized leader and center of all that involves the handling, financing and exporting of the product of the Texas oil fields."[27] In 1914, a deep water port was completed southeast of Houston's city center, making the 50-mile Houston Ship Channel the capstone, which grew over the course of the next four decades into the largest complex of petroleum refining and petrochemical manufacturing in the Western hemisphere.[28] Already by 1930, 27 tanker lines were operating in Houston, exporting nearly four million tons of petroleum products a year. World War II propelled a surge in the oil-military-industrial complex in Houston; by the mid-1950s, three-quarters of Houston's exports were petroleum derived, feeding the growing global demand for oil. Houston was now a full-formed petropolis with its arteries and muscles lubricated by the cheap fossil fuels that informed every dimension of mid-20th-century urbanism.

Two vectors that crucially expanded and reinforced Houston's fossil heyday were air-conditioning and automobility. The proliferation of relatively cheap window AC units in the early 1950s led the *New York Times* to anoint Houston "The Most Air-Conditioned City" in 1955. Thanks to coal- and gas-powered electricity, the settler logic of domination and displacement could now be extended to tame the weather. The new Houstonian was imagined to be a white-collar worker performing "powerful and intricate brain-work in his air-conditioned office" and "wholly immune to Houston weather except for the mercifully brief moments when he is ducking from house to car, from car to office, and vice versa."[29] That new Houstonian was actually the same old white Houstonian taking advantage of expanding freeway systems to relocate his home outside the dense, gridded metropolitan center. New homesteads in developer-driven cul-de-sacs on the fringes of the expanding megalopolis created quasi-sovereign subdivisions anchored by new large, air-conditioned shopping centers and malls. "Affluent white Houstonians, through their building of suburban climate-controlled houses, businesses, and commercial centers, could avoid both the region's climate and the city core, and the lack of cars and adequate public transportation kept many residences of older neighborhoods from traveling to the outskirts of Houston."[30]

Ninety percent of Houston's growth has occurred since the automobile.[31] Houston sprawled like no city before it, hyperactively lengthening its spines, ignoring infill, eschewing density, swallowing smaller surrounding settlements with relish, eventually reaching 600 square miles, by far the largest area of any US city with a population over one million people. The effect of this growth on urban space was profound, a metastasizing mass of centers and peripheries guided by no design other than the competing opportunisms of various real estate developers and the roads that carried them across the landscape. As architectural theorist Albert Pope has observed, "The center hasn't held in Houston for a long time. With the Medical Center, Post Oak, the Energy Corridor, and The Woodlands we have large multiple centers that all have their own peripheries that bleed into other peripheries and other centers. But more importantly we have smaller multiple centers in terms of subdivisions, office parks, shopping centers, shopping malls—all are part of this polynuclear conurbation. And they are closed. They are not continuous grids. They each have a boundary. In a megalopolis, peripheries are all over the place."[32]

No periphery is ever enough for petroculture. In 1963, NASA's Johnson Space Center (JSC) opened in the Clear Lake area of Houston on land donated by Humble Oil. The JSC has worked avidly to organize still greater concentrations of fossil fuels and technological ingenuities to permit the settler frontier to extend above the Earth, infrastructuring the extraplanetary fantasies of Jeff Bezos and Elon Musk. Houston has been, in all respects, a booster rocket for the Anthropocene trajectory. Today its petroleum complex continues to thrive and the city indulges timeworn settler-liberal dispositions of rampant self-interest, industrial technophilia, racial violence, disregard for environmental consequences, pursuit of productivity and luxury, and desires for mobility and convenience. It may even epitomize modern fantasies of ecological transcendence and domination. But it also symbolizes the hollow ecocidal core of those fantasies. As big as it is, Houston seems somehow less than the sum of its parts. As architect Larry Albert writes, "the more seemingly placeless Houston grows, the more it can seem like Houston. If the generic colonization of sprawling settlements with little regard for local conditions can be said to have a hometown, here it is."[33] Pope likewise describes Houston as the very epitome of "an endless and anonymous sprawl of freeways, office parks, subdivisions, and malls . . . the city that unchecked consumer capital really wants to make."[34]

The anonymity and placelessness of Houston's sprawl is a material expression of petromania. The city grows voraciously, without plan or consideration for who or what it might damage along the way. Meanwhile, it constantly sacrifices its citizens' health and welfare to the interests of the masters of fossil fuels. The Ship Channel remains the spine of Houston's economic prosperity, yet this woefully unregulated space is the site of frequent plant explosions and constant fugitive emissions that cause its frontline communities of color to suffer cancer rates several times the national average.[35]

But to hear the majority of Houston's elite tell it, fossil fuels hover somewhere between a necessary evil and an unmitigated good. A post-fossil fuel future is literally unthinkable to many of them, and when called upon to conceive transition, their minds wander to boondoggles like natural gas as transition fuel or carbon sequestration via enhanced oil recovery or, most recently, to hydrogen, as a way to allow the fossil fuel industry to set its affairs in order. I work at a university defined by its many corporate alliances with the fossil fuel industry and, unsurprisingly, even in the supposed hotbed of environmentality that is American high education, there is much more interest on campus in monetizing new carbon artifacts like nanotubes than there is in decarbonization. The secret of course is that petroculture does not wish to die any more than the ego does. It always wishes to bargain with fate instead of accepting finitude.

But this Houston cannot survive forever. The wrath of climate emergency visited the city in the form of Hurricane Harvey in 2017 with its $125 billion worth of damage and trillions of cubic feet of flood waste. The city government was pressured to finally create a climate action plan. I participated as a consultant in that process, but even those of us that helped author the plan had little faith that the city would actually be able to achieve its goals because of the endless obstacles, slow-walking, and rearguard actions initiated by the city's fossil fuel industry. Four years later, little has changed. In February 2021, when much of the Texas electricity power grid failed largely because of natural gas supply issues, Houston Republican politicians like State Senator Paul Bettencourt took advantage of the crisis to argue for even more fossil-fueled "baseload" energy in place of renewables because of their supposedly greater "reliability."[36]

Although some might describe them as cynics, Houston elites like Bettencourt are sincere maniacs. They derive both purpose and pleasure from their mania. Otherwise, they would be less gleeful in recommending more fossil fuels as the only possible antidote to problems that fossil fuels have created. There is only a thin line between mania and perversion in a place like Houston. The true petropervert revels in the symptoms of self-destruction. As Žižek writes, "The symptom is not only a ciphered message, it is at the same time a way for the subject to organize his enjoyment—that is why, even after the completed interpretation, the subject is not prepared to renounce his symptom; that is why he 'loves his symptom more than himself.'"[37] Perversion may be pleasure, but it is obsessive pleasure that inhibits being present for a world that is dying. To give oneself over to the death of petroculture is the necessary precondition of the post-fossil world that hungers to be born.

Death Acceptance and Post-Fossil Futures

For the later Freud, all anxiety is castration anxiety at its root. Fossil thanatophobia manifests the deep castration anxiety of white colonial patriarchy that its interests and powers will be diminished relative to the interests and powers of the non-white, non-colonial, non-patriarchal, non-human persons who constitute the vast majority of the planetary population. They are not wrong. As Jacques Lacan lectured, anxiety is "what does not deceive, what is beyond doubting."[38] White colonial patriarchy indeed comprehends, in its occasional moments of clarity, that it has entered its senescence. But as we have seen in recent years those moments of clarity are few relative to an abundance of anxious hallucinations: fears of extinction and replacement, wild denials of science and empirical reality, angry demands, intricately insane conspiracy theories, and desperate bargains with phantoms of renaissance like MAGA. Just like Soviet-style socialism in the 1980s, American petroculture is a gerontocracy hallucinating that the mid-20th century can be preserved forever (until it is no more).[39]

How can this epistemic and affective cycle be broken? To return to the silencing of plantation slavery, the situation we find ourselves in today is akin in many ways to the death anxieties that surrounded the end of plantation culture in the Americas.[40] That *Angst* was not dispelled overnight. But eventually affect shifted against the institution that supplied mass wealth and privilege for a certain elite (in no small part because a fossil-fueled apparatus of machines stepped into the gap as a new infrastructure of capital creation). I imagine that the end of fossil fuels will follow a similar route, only hopefully faster as ready-made replacements already exist for our fossil-fueled apparatus and a host of aspirational new elites are poised to try to scale them rapidly. The real fight will be to accomplish decarbonization while also leaving behind the extractivist and dispossessive institutions of European colonization. Petromodernity was the sequel to plantation slavery and its legacies deserve to die with fossil fuels. Instead, let us find our way forward to a better "solarity."[41]

Mania is often the neurotic condition that immediately precedes either implosion and self-destruction or breakthrough and acceptance. In this respect, it is a healthy sign that petromania abounds today. As LeMenager says, the grief of the loss of easy oil is genuine, existential and civilizational and it must be processed as such. Still, we privileged northerners must all do everything within our powers to push through thanatophobia and petromania toward acceptance of the end of fossil fuels. As Roy Scranton puts it, "The biggest problem we face is a philosophical one: understanding that this civilization is *already dead.* The sooner we confront this problem, and the sooner we realize there's nothing we can do to save ourselves, the sooner we can get down to the hard work of adapting, with mortal humility, to our new reality."[42] Beyond acceptance, we need action. "To act," Lacan argues, "is to tear certainty from anxiety." For those fortunate enough to have achieved certainty of the necessary death of petroculture, the time is now.

NOTES

1. Stephanie LeMenager, *Living Oil: Petroleum Culture in the American Century* (New York: Oxford University Press, 2014), 69.

2. Timothy Mitchell, "Carbon Democracy," *Economy and Society* 38, no. 3 (2009): 399–432.

3. Vannevar Bush, *Science: The Endless Frontier* (Washington, DC: United States Government Printing Office, 1945).

4. Timothy Luke, "On Environmentality: Geo-Power and Eco-Knowledge in the Discourses of Contemporary Environmentalism," *Cultural Critique* 31 (1995): 57–81.

5. Allan Stoekl, *The Three Sustainabilities: Energy, Economy, Time* (Minneapolis: University of Minnesota Press, 2021).

6. See, for example, André Gorz, *Energy as Politics*, trans. Patsy Vigderman and Jonathan Cloud (Boston: South End Press, 1980).

7. Sarah Jaquette Ray, *A Field Guide to Climate Anxiety* (Berkeley: University of California Press, 2020).

8. Kyle Powys Whyte, "Indigenous Science (Fiction) for the Anthropocene: Ancestral Dystopias and Fantasies of Climate Change Crises," *Environment and Planning E: Nature and Space* 1, no. 2 (2018): 224–242.

9. Dominic Boyer, "*Ostalgie* and the Politics of the Future in Eastern Germany," *Public Culture* 18, no. 2 (2006): 361–381; Dominic Boyer, "From the Algos to Autonomos: Nostalgic Eastern Europe as Postimperial Mania," in *Postcommunist Nostalgia*, ed. Maria Todorova and Zsuzsa Gille (New York: Berghahn Press, 2010), 17–28.

10. Molly Schwartz, "President Biden has the Most Ambitious Climate Change Plan in US History. Will it be Enough to Save the Planet?" *Mother Jones*, February 3, 2021.

11. Sigmund Freud, *Introductory Lectures on Psychoanalysis*, trans. James Strachey (New York: W.W. Norton, 1966): 501–502.

12. Melanie Klein, "On the Theory of Anxiety and Guilt," in *Envy and Gratitude and Other Works 1946–1963* (London: Hogarth, 1975), 25–42.

13. Imre Szeman, "Conjectures on World Energy Literature: Or, What is Petroculture?" *Journal of Postcolonial Writing* 53, no. 3 (2017): 277–288.

14. Tim Morton, *Hyperobjects: Philosophy and Ecology after the End of the World* (Minneapolis: University of Minnesota Press, 2013).

15. Arjun Appadurai, "Disjuncture and Difference in the Global Cultural Economy," *Public Culture* 2, no. 2 (1990): 1–24.

16. Jonathan Crary, *24/7: Late Capitalism and the End of Sleep* (London: Verso, 2014); David Nye, *Electrifying America: Social Meanings of a New Technology* (Cambridge: MIT Press, 1992); Tanja Winther, *The Impact of Electricity: Development, Desires and Dilemmas* (Oxford: Berg, 2008).

17. Akhil Gupta, "An Anthropology of Electricity from the Global South," *Cultural Anthropology* 30, no. 4 (2015): 557.

18. David Hughes, *Energy Without Conscience: Oil, Climate Change, and Complicity* (Durham: Duke University Press, 2017).

19. Karen Pinkus, *Fuel: A Speculative Dictionary* (Minneapolis: University of Minnesota Press, 2016).

20. Cara Daggett, *The Birth of Energy Fossil Fuels, Thermodynamics, and the Politics of Work* (Durham: Duke University Press, 2019).

21. Mitchell, "Carbon Democracy."

22. Roman Bartosch, "The Energy of Stories: Postcolonialism, the Petroleum Unconscious, and the Crude Side of Cultural Ecology," *Resilience: A Journal of the Environmental Humanities* 6, no. 2–3 (2019): 116–135.

23. Susan Buck-Morss, "Hegel and Haiti," *Critical Inquiry* 26, no. 4 (2000): 821–865.

24. Frantz Fanon, *Black Skin, White Masks*, trans. Charles Lam Markmann (New York: Grove Press, 1967), 250.

25. Benajah Carroll, *Standard History of Houston, Texas from the Study of Original Sources*, Rice University, accessed September 30, 2022, https://archive.org/details/standardhistoryo oocarrrich/page/n1/mode/2up.

26. Carroll, 250.

27. Carroll, 252.

28. Marilyn McAdams Sibley, *The Port of Houston: A History* (Austin: University of Texas Press, 1968).

29. Stanley Walker, "Houston: Coolest Spot in U.S.," *New York Times*, May 15, 1955.

30. Robert Thompson, "'The Air-Conditioning Capital of the World:' Houston and Climate Control," in *Energy Metropolis: An Environmental History of Houston and the Gulf Coast*, ed. Martin Melosi and Joseph Pratt (Pittsburg: University of Pittsburgh Press, 2007), 95.

31. Tom Watson McKinney, "Superhighway Deluxe: Houston's Gulf Freeway," in *Energy Metropolis: An Environmental History of Houston and the Gulf Coast*, ed. Martin Melosi and Joseph Pratt (Pittsburgh: University of Pittsburgh Press, 2007).

32. Raj Mankad, "Is Houston a City? An Interview with Susan Rogers and Albert Pope," *Rice Design Alliance*, July 16, 2014, https://www.ricedesignalliance.org/is-houston-a-city-an-interview-with-albert-pope.

33. Larry Albert, "Houston Wet," (MA thesis: Rice University School of Architecture, 1997), 158.

34. Albert Pope, "Hollow Spaces," *Progressive Architecture*, October 1993, 75.

35. Julianne Crawford, "Environmental Racism in Houston's Harrisburg/Manchester Neighborhood," *Stanford Earth*, March 15, 2018.

36. Jeremy Wallace and Taylor Goldstein, "Responding to Energy Crisis, Texas Lawmakers Call for More Fossil Fuels in Power Grid," *Houston Chronicle*, February 18, 2021.

37. Slavoj Žižek, *The Subline Object of Ideology* (New York: Verso, 1989), 74.

38. Jacques Lacan, *Anxiety: The Seminar of Jacques Lacan, Book X*, ed. Jacques-Alain Miller, tr. A. R. Price (Cambridge: Polity Press, 2014).

39. Alexei Yurchak, *Everything Was Forever Until It Was No More: The Last Soviet Generation* (Princeton: Princeton University Press, 2004).

40. Jean-François Mouhot, "Past Connections and Present Similarities in Slave Ownership and Fossil Fuel Usage," in *The Energy Humanities Reader*, ed. Imre Szeman and Dominic Boyer (Baltimore: Johns Hopkins University Press, 2017), 205–218.

41. Darin Barney and Imre Szeman, "Solarity," *The Southern Atlantic Quarterly* 120, no. 1 (2021): 1–188.

42. Roy Scranton, "Learning How to Die in the Anthropocene," *The New York Times*, November 10, 2013.

CHAPTER SIX

Climate Change Anxiety in Young People

KELSEY HUDSON AND
ERIC LEWANDOWSKI

Young people around the world are increasingly concerned about climate change and demonstrate complex and multifaceted psychological responses. Climate change can evoke a wide range of emotions and reactions, such as fear, grief, guilt, anxiety, anger, hope, optimism, and solastalgia, the emotional distress caused by environmental changes.[1] Negative mental health consequences for young people following climate-related extreme weather events and disasters are well documented, but even those who have not experienced direct impacts of climate change can experience distress simply through their awareness of the climate crisis.

Currently, young people worldwide face direct and immediate threats to their physical and psychological health.[2] Anxiety about climate change can be a natural and adaptive response to the unfolding crisis. Many young people, however, confronting immediate and direct impacts of climate change, such as extreme weather, droughts, land loss, and poor air quality, are at risk of more significant responses like post-traumatic stress, sleep problems, attachment disorders, behavioral and adjustment problems, and substance use problems;[3] grief and identity questioning;[4] disruptions to social support networks;[5] and familial stress.[6] In this chapter, we will describe what is known about climate anxiety, discuss frameworks for understanding young people's anxiety about the climate crisis, and identify ways to empower and support young people as they develop into a climate-changed world.

Defining and Characterizing Climate Anxiety in Young People

To capture the complex feelings that emerge in reaction to environmental and climate-related concerns, terms such as *climate anxiety* and *eco-anxiety* have emerged.[7] These terms describe the process of observing, fearing, and dreading the impacts of climate change, and they are used broadly to describe a number of feelings related to climate change. Climate anxiety relates to the psychological responses specifically associated with climate change, whereas eco-anxiety has been defined as "heightened emotional, mental, or somatic distress in response to dangerous changes in the climate system."[8] Although formal standard definitions do not yet exist for these phenomena and a comprehensive understanding of the phenomenology and prevalence of climate anxiety remains limited, explorations of the various dimensions of climate anxiety suggest that anxiety related to climate change is multifaceted and generally features concerns about the "uncertainty, unpredictability, and uncontrollability" of the course of environmental deterioration.[9] Recently there has been increased attention to young people's emotional distress related to climate change, in part due to the rapid rise of youth climate activism and climate justice movements (e.g., Fridays for Future, Climate Justice Alliance), youth fossil fuel and divestment demonstrations, and lawsuits involving child plaintiffs (e.g., *Juliana v. United States*).

Greater levels of climate anxiety and worry are expressed by young people and young adults compared to older generations. In the United States, 67% of young adults (ages 18–23) reported feeling somewhat or very concerned about the impact of climate change on their mental health compared to 42% of older adults (ages 56–74). Children and teenagers are also expressing concern; a US poll in the summer of 2019 found that 57% of respondents ages 13–17 said that climate change makes them feel afraid.[10] Surveys of children and young people ages 8–16 in the UK have found that 73% are worried about climate change.[11] Approximately 1 billion children—nearly half of the world's child population—live in places that are classified as being at "extremely high risk" to the negative consequences of the climate change, according to UNICEF.[12] Numerous national and international organizations have identified children and young people as a particularly at-risk group in the face of climate change (e.g., American Academy of Pediatrics; World Health Organization). Young people are more vulnerable to the impacts of climate change for many reasons, including the immature state of their physical, psychological, and neurobiological development; their reliance on adults and their physical environments for safety and well-being; and their vulnerability to disease.[13] Children, adolescents, and young adults will also live longer into the climate crisis than older generations and will confront its effects for most of their lives.

Clinical Considerations

Anxiety is a natural psychological and physiological response that signals threat or danger and allows us to prepare, respond, and cope.[14] Given the realities of climate change, there is consensus that emotional responses like anxiety, worry, fear, dread, and other emotions are reasonable and adaptive rather than intrinsically pathological in nature.[15] Similarly, worried thoughts, sleep problems, and difficulty engaging in daily tasks such as working and spending time with family have also been described as within the range of responses.[16] Anxiety about climate change can even be constructive and has been shown to drive people to engage and take action.[17] From a clinical perspective, anxiety about climate change does not immediately reflect a diagnosable mental health problem. Nevertheless, bearing witness to climate-related environmental changes and worrying about the future for oneself, children, species, land, and environmental degradation may cause significant distress that can negatively impact young people's mental health and overwhelm their ability to cope. Overlapping phenomenology has been noted between climate anxiety and clinical anxiety disorders, such as rumination, sleep difficulties, and impaired functioning in daily life;[18] however, because climate anxiety may be seen as a rational response to a real threat, it differs from anxiety disorders, for which anxiety is determined to be disproportionate to the threat. In addition, emotional distress is considered to be clinically significant when it causes impairments in functioning in important domains of life. The distinction between what constitutes normative climate anxiety (and other climate-related emotions like grief or anger) and what should be considered to reflect a psychiatric disorder requires further clarification.

To examine the clinically relevant aspects of climate anxiety, a measure was recently developed by Clayton and Karazsia that identified two subscales: cognitive emotional impairment (e.g., difficulty sleeping, trouble concentrating, crying) and functional impairment (e.g., difficulty completing work tasks, academic responsibilities, impaired relationships) as a result of climate anxiety.[19] In validating this measure, the researchers found that climate anxiety was positively correlated with a combined measure of depression and generalized anxiety symptoms. Using this same measure, Schwartz and colleagues conducted a study examining the relationship between climate anxiety, depressive symptoms, and generalized anxiety symptoms within an emerging adult sample of US students (ages 18–35).[20] Results of this study highlighted that both cognitive emotional and functional impairment were significantly associated with symptoms of generalized anxiety disorder, but only the functional impairment subscale was associated with higher depressive symptoms. A UK-based study of the psychological responses of 16- to 24-year-olds to the COVID-19 pandemic and climate change further illuminated the presence of distress and impairment related to thoughts and feelings about climate change.[21] This study examined the extent to which participants' thoughts or feelings interfered with their well-being or functioning (e.g., trouble falling asleep, feeling distracted by the issue in daily life). Results indicated that the perceived effect of any concern on young people's daily lives was limited, which led the authors to conclude that there was "no compelling evidence" that climate distress has the characteristics of a disorder because it was not seen as interfering significantly with daily activities. In clinical settings, climate change concerns may be intertwined with existing mental health challenges for which people are already seeking treatment. For example, a subset of adults in the United States with obsessive-compulsive disorder reported having obsessions and compulsions that were directly related to climate change and involved concerns about wasting electricity, water, and gas.[22] These findings represent the first initial attempts to establish an empirical basis for understanding the distinctions and interrelationships between climate-related emotions and symptoms of anxiety and depression in young people. This remains a critical area for future research.

Qualitative research involving children and young people highlights that anxiety about climate change may take many forms. For example, a study involving in-depth interviews with 10- to 12-year-old children in the United States found that 82% of the sample expressed sadness, fear, and anger.[23] Similarly, a UK-based qualitative study exploring a small group of 14- to 18-year-olds' thoughts and feelings about the environment identified six themes, including challenging emotions.[24] Expressed emotions within this theme included guilt about having a position of privilege (i.e., not yet being directly affected by the impacts of climate change) and not doing enough, as well as frustration, annoyance, and anger aimed at societal systems and other people. Notably, the participants in this study also expressed "welcomed emotions," such as solidarity, passion, and hope.

Although extensive qualitative and community-based research from low-wealth nations is lacking, interviews with young people and speeches from youth activists from around the world offer a nuanced view of their beliefs and values that cannot be captured in survey data. For example, in a series of interviews on the UNICEF YouTube Channel in which young people described how climate change affects their lives, one young Brazilian activist stated, "Our future, the kids' future, will be affected."[25] As part of her keynote at the Youth-4Climate conference prior to the 26th UN Climate Change Conference of the Parties (COP26), Ugandan youth climate activist Vanessa Nakate implored global leaders to take action and attend to those who will be most affected by climate change: "For many of us, reducing and avoiding is not enough. You cannot adapt to lost cultures, you cannot adapt to lost traditions, you cannot adapt to lost history, you cannot adapt to starvation. You cannot adapt to extinction."

Survey studies involving young people have also illuminated a range of thoughts and feelings about climate change. For example, a survey of young people ages 16–25 from 10 countries in the Global North and Global South found high levels of negative, future-oriented beliefs about climate change, including that "the future is frightening" (75%) and that "humanity is doomed" (56%).[26] This study also found that many young people believe that governments are "failing young people" (65%) and are "betraying future generations" (58%), highlighting the relationship between climate anxiety and perceptions of betrayal by government. Other global studies have found that negative and challenging climate-related emotions are negatively correlated with self-reported mental health in adults (including young adults) in many countries.[27] Thoughts about climate change may also have an existential element, particularly as we are faced with scientific facts about species and biodiversity loss as part of the sixth mass extinction. Anxiety about the future impacts of climate change is affecting young people's family planning. For example, four in ten respondents in the aforementioned global climate anxiety survey reported that they are hesitant to have children.[28] In fact, organizations have formed specifically to support individuals in their reproductive choices (e.g., Conceivable Future).

Climate change influences young people's mental health through multiple pathways and impacts both social and ecological determinants of health.[29] Therefore, social-ecological frameworks incorporating the interplay of individual factors, the physical environment, and the influence of various systems on young people add essential context to understanding youth climate anxiety. Drawing on Urie Bronfenbrenner's social-ecological theory, Crandon and colleagues posit that understanding young people's climate anxiety requires us to "examine the interaction between young people and the systemic contexts in which they live."[30] Climate anxiety, they argue, is caused by complex interactions between multiple systems including individual factors, the micro-system (e.g., family), the meso-system (e.g., community), the exo-system (e.g., media, policy), and macro-system (culture, historical practices). Recent research correlating perceptions of inadequate responses to climate change by governments with greater climate-related distress in young people,[31] as well as young activists stressing the necessity for comprehensive climate action that is both inclusive and equitable, reflect the need to think beyond the individual and seek opportunities to intervene within the broader systems influencing young people's climate anxiety.

Climate Justice

The current and projected impacts of climate change are recognized as social and ecological determinants of young people's health and mental health, which contribute to and interact with other determinants of health, including racism, poverty, housing insecurity, and access to education. The differential impacts of climate change on health and human rights more broadly have been termed *climate justice*, which acknowledges that individuals who are least responsible for contributing to climate change experience some of greatest negative health and mental health consequences, which in turn exacerbates disparities.[32]

Some individuals and communities experience heightened emotional distress beyond anxiety. In particular, those whose livelihood and identities are tied more closely to the land (e.g., farmers and Indigenous Peoples) may experience grief and loss as a result of direct exposure to climate-related changes and stressors.[33] Climate change can also impact young people's individual and group identity. For example, climate change has been described by The National Congress of American Indians as playing a "large role . . . in separating tribal people from their natural resources" and posing "a threat to Indigenous identity."[34] Additionally, although health burdens of environmental degradation and climate change disproportionately affect Black, Indigenous, and People of Color (BIPOC) communities, terms like *climate anxiety* may not adequately capture the feelings or lived experiences of these communities.[35] Discussing the mental health impacts of climate change using terms that mischaracterize and/or minimize young people's experiences may deter them from joining groups or seeking support from providers, who they may perceive as misunderstanding their situation or concern. Future research, intervention, and advocacy work should focus on establishing terminology that is most accurate and meaningful for young people via focus groups, community-based participatory research, and other methods that directly involve individuals themselves in shaping the research questions that affect their communities.

Interventions and Supports

In recognition of the direct and indirect impacts of climate change on young people's mental health, many organizations and professionals in public health, mental health, and medical fields have called for action to support the psychological health of young people. While our understanding of the impact of climate change on young people's mental health is still evolving, resources for individuals struggling with climate anxiety have been developed by researchers, clinicians, and educators, as well as community leaders, advocates, and artists. Although the effectiveness of these approaches for coping with climate anxiety and climate emotions remains to be established empirically, many existing effective treatment approaches for coping with stress, trauma, and/or other mental health challenges can be adapted to support the emotional, cognitive, and behavioral elements inherent to climate anxiety.[36] In fact, several "core components" for helping young people cope with climate change have recently been identified by synthesizing existing literature, obtaining insights from experts, and reviewing existing resources.[37] These components may serve to promote coping and resilience in the face of climate anxiety based on their efficacy for related constructs and include acknowledging and validating feelings, coping strategies and self-care, social connection, connecting with nature, climate justice awareness, and climate action.

Acknowledging Thoughts and Feelings

Evidence indicates that young people who have shared their thoughts and feelings about climate change have felt dismissed and ignored. Acknowledging, normalizing, and validating young people's concerns can make space for them to express their feelings and receive support. Caregivers, educators, and family members can provide opportunities to have these conversations with young people and can listen actively and openly when approached with these concerns. Resources exist to support parents and caregivers in talking with children and young people about climate change; take stock of their own climate emotions, thoughts, and behaviors; model effective coping; and engage in meaningful action.[38]

Coping Strategies and Self-Care

Coping refers to the ways in which young people manage their emotions, think about problems, regulate and direct their behavior, control their physiological arousal, and act on their environments to adjust or decrease stress.[39] In young people, coping styles impact how stress impacts current and future adjustment and psychological well-being and development. In the context of coping with climate change, different coping strategies can affect an individual's sense of agency, self-efficacy, and engagement. Research in Sweden characterized coping strategies of adolescents and preadolescents in the context of climate change.[40] Three coping style were identified: meaning-focused coping, in which behavioral and cognitive responses to distress are guided by engagement in activities that are consistent with and express one's beliefs, values, and existential goals; problem-focused coping, in which efforts are directed at solving the problem that is the source of distress; and emotion-focused coping, in which efforts are aimed at reducing or soothing negative feelings. Compared to problem-focused and emotion-focused coping, meaning-focused coping strategies were associated with better adjustment, higher levels of environmental engagement, positive affect, and self-efficacy. Another study on Swedish adolescents' climate-related coping strategies found that adolescents who were able to establish and maintain positive climate-related communication with parents and friends demonstrated more effective coping than those who had more negative climate-related communication.[41] This work suggests that communication about climate change can impact coping and that different types of coping responses are associated with different emotional outcomes and engagement levels.

Meaning-focused coping strategies can include finding meaning in the climate crisis and cultivating positive or helpful emotions, such as realistic hope and optimism. For example, young people have found meaningful engagement through planting trees (e.g., Plant for the Planet) and providing testimonies to local politicians to shut down coal-fired power plants. Coping also involves taking care of oneself and one's basic needs, such as adequate sleep and nutrition. Leslie Davenport, a climate psychology educator, consultant, and clinician, emphasizes the importance of establishing an ongoing self-care routine to help manage feelings about climate change, engage with the issue, and prevent burnout.[42]

Social Connection and Connecting with Nature

Social support is a protective factor in the face of stress. In the context of climate change, increasing social connection and building connection with community can improve young people's well-being.[43] Social connection can be built by talking with others about climate-related concerns and by becoming involved in groups and organizations, which may increase a sense of meaning and purpose and decrease feelings of isolation. Additionally, a significant body of research suggests that spending time in nature has benefits for young people's psychological well-being.[44] In fact, a recent review of existing groups and interventions for managing eco-anxiety in adults highlighted that connecting with nature was the major focus of a full quarter (26%) of interventions reviewed.[45] Some researchers have described nature as existing on a spectrum, from "nearby nature" to "wilderness";[46] encouraging nature connection on this spectrum is particularly important in areas where access to green space may be limited. Connection with nearby nature can lower levels of distress and contribute to positive moods in young people;[47] in fact, spending as little as 10 to 20 minutes in nature daily may prevent stress and mental health strain.

Climate Justice Awareness and Engagement in Climate Action

Climate justice is a critical consideration in the context of the emotional and psychological impacts of climate change. Such concerns about climate change are interwoven with other issues affecting the everyday lives of BIPOC communities and individuals in low-resource settings in the Global South. Increasingly, climate justice education and exploration are being advocated as part of managing and coping with climate anxiety. For example, exercises and activities exploring privilege, identity, and intersectionality can support young people in identifying and expressing their values on issues of climate justice, which can then be incorporated into actions that support just solutions. It is recommended that interventions and advocacy efforts supporting BIPOC and historically marginalized young people and their communities acknowledge the overlapping and interacting threats that face these communities (e.g., racism, violence, poverty).

Climate action can be an effective way for young people to reduce feelings of helplessness and lack of control by promoting a sense of empowerment and agency. Engaging in collective environmental action has been shown to promote positive feelings and protect against depression symptoms.[48] Recently, youth activism related to climate change and climate justice has become increasingly visible. A leading example is the Fridays for Future climate strikes, in which hundreds of thousands of students in 123 countries left school in an act of peaceful protest about political inaction regarding climate change. Since this time, over 14 million people in 7,500 cities globally have gathered to engage in school strikes and other forms of activism regarding climate change. Young people are also pressing the issue of climate action in court. For example, young people have sued governments to demand increased efforts on climate change in the United States, Portugal, Peru, Colombia, Pakistan, and the Netherlands. In addition, becoming involved in groups focusing on climate change and climate justice can increase social support. Climate action takes many forms, such as individual- and family-level behavioral changes (e.g., clean transportation), supporting officials and policies focusing on climate adaptation and mitigation, or participating in activism (e.g., strikes, protests). Helping young people conceptualize climate action broadly as more than engaging in political protests and strikes can encourage them to affect change in their unique "spheres of influence," including personal life, family, community, academic, or occupational institutions. Notably, youth activism and engagement outside of the climate realm have been associated with both positive and negative mental health effects.[49] Although engaging in activism can help young people manage feelings of helplessness and increase engagement, meaning, and purpose, it can also potentially lead to negative mental and physical health outcomes due to stress, increased exposure to criticism and discrimination, and increased feelings of anger and burnout. Given these potential difficulties, activism or civic engagement should not be *prescribed* as a way to cope with climate anxiety. Instead, young people should be supported in deciding what *types* of engagement are most effective and sustainable for them.

Climate action can provide young people with a source of emotional support and create a network of peer messengers and role models, which can in turn increase the individual and collective agency of others. Researchers, educators, and young people themselves have emphasized the importance of supporting young people in taking political action on climate change, highlighting that activism can help manage anxiety about the future and harness it into determination and optimism. Albert Bandura, a psychologist renowned for his work on knowledge acquisition recently argued that young people's "intuitive principles of change" are closely aligned with his social cognitive theory, which emphasizes the power of social modeling.[50] Seeing other young people participate in individual and collective action helps individuals to build confidence in their own capabilities and sense of agency.

Resources for Coping and Building Resilience

To offer support to the many young people experiencing psychological distress related to climate change, it is critical to think beyond one-on-one encounters and adopt a broader, systems-level approach. Systems thinking will also be necessary to address gaps and inequities in access to mental health services, and it will require communication and collaboration between educators, activists, caregivers, science communicators, and media to deliver information about climate change, while also offering needed support. For mental health services in particular, this may require widespread training of climate-aware providers and the delivery of climate-related psychological health services in school settings. Resources have emerged to support young people to acknowledge their climate emotions, increase coping ability, build efficacy and agency, educate about climate justice, and encourage meaningful action. For example, books on managing distress and anxiety about climate change are available to guide young people in identifying and expressing climate emotions and thoughts, practicing self-compassion and mindfulness, and moving into taking meaningful action.[51] Social media, blogs, and web-based materials serve as important free resources that can help young people understand and process the mental health impacts of climate change (e.g., Gen Dread). Climate psychology–specific organizations have begun to provide free online resources for youth (e.g., Climate Mental Health Network Resources). Social media offers another way for young people to access information about other young people who are managing climate anxiety and are engaged in the environmental crisis (e.g., Eco Tok). On a community scale, the Climate Museum in New York City, which is the first museum in the United States dedicated to climate change, offers exhibitions and events that aim to inspire action on the climate crisis. The Museum's youth programming is dedicated to creating spaces for young people to express their thoughts and feelings about the crisis, as well as to learn about and engage in collective support and action to engender hope, agency, and empowerment. Resources like these promote accurate climate science, offer a space for young people to express their reactions to climate change, and provide ideas for meaningful actions in ways that are accessible to a broad audience of young people and are more economically equitable than many clinical services.

Educational settings represent an important and underutilized opportunity to provide young people with emotional support about climate change. Both educators and students need support systems to help them work through climate anxiety and build coping and resilience. A recent review of research regarding climate anxiety and environmental education highlighted that the first step in acknowledging and managing climate emotions in classroom settings is for educators to acknowledge their own emotional experiences so that they can effectively provide support to students.[52] Educators have called for the development of climate change education that directly involves young people in the "scientific, social, ethical, and political complexities of climate change" and have presented strategies for confronting anxiety and other challenging climate-related emotions in environmental studies and science-based educational settings.[53] Although more accessible and widespread resources are necessary to adequately support educators and students of all educational stages in coping with climate-related content, these resources acknowledge the importance of pairing climate and environmental education with coping and emotional support strategies.

Summary and Future Directions

As young people's climate anxiety is impacted by and developed through multiple pathways, it is critical to use a systems thinking approach to research, advocacy, policy, and intervention development. Our efforts to support young people to cope and build resilience in the climate crisis must be contextualized within the social and ecological determinants of health and mental health, and we must guard against the framing of resilience as a trait residing exclusively within the individual. Existing resources and literature on climate anxiety represent a departure point for efforts to help young people cope with their distress, but significant work remains to adequately characterize the psychological and emotional impacts of climate change. New interventions must account for historical and persisting inequalities and concerns of justice when addressing young people's distress.

Young people have the right to contribute to the decision-making processes that affect them. Thus, it is critical that young people are directly involved in the development of supports and interventions. Such involvement gives power to their voices and supports their sense of agency. In the words of Xiuhtezcatl Martinez, a young Indigenous environmental activist and hip-hop artist, "When it comes to climate change, youth are the future. We are the ones who will be experiencing the consequences from generations who came before us. We have the potential to think outside-the-box when it comes to effective solutions. Hearing youth voices in the conversation on climate change is essential to finding and implementing solutions, demanding actionable solutions from those in office, and leading grassroots efforts from the ground up."[54] Above all, urgent action must be taken to prevent and reduce further climate change impacts to ensure a just and safe future for young people.

NOTES

1. Glenn Albrecht, "Solastalgia: A New Concept in Human Health and Identity," *Philosophy, Activism, Nature*, 3 (2005): 41–55; Panu Pihkala, "Toward a Taxonomy of Climate Emotions," *Frontiers in Climate* 3 (2022), 738154.

2. Adrienne van Nieuwenhuizen et al., "The Effects of Climate Change on Child and Adolescent Mental Health: Clinical Conditions," *Current Psychiatric Reports* 23, no. 12 (2021): 88.

3. Susie Burke et al., "The Psychological Effects of Climate Change on Children," *Current Psychiatry Reports* 20, no. 5 (2018): 35.

4. Ashlee Cunsolo and Neville Ellis, "Ecological Grief as a Mental Health Response to Climate Change-Related Loss," *Nature Climate Change* 8, no. 4 (2018): 275–281.

5. Donice Banks and Carl Weems, "Family and Peer Social Support and Their Links to Psychological Distress Among Hurricane-Exposed Minority Youth," *American Journal of Orthopsychiatry* 84, no. 4 (2014): 341–352.

6. Daniel Garcia and Mary Sheehan, "Extreme Weather-driven Disasters and Children's Health," *International Journal of Health Services* 46, no. 1 (2016): 79–105.

7. Glenn Albrecht, "Chronic Environmental Change: Emerging 'Psychoterratic' Syndromes," in *Climate Change and Human Well-being: Global Challenges and Opportunities*, ed. I Weissbecker (New York: Springer, 2011); Susan Clayton and Bryan Karazsia, "Development and Validation of a Measure of Climate Change Anxiety," *Journal of Environmental Psychology* 69, no. 2 (2020), 101434.

8. Climate Psychology Alliance, *Handbook of Climate Psychology* (2020), https://common slibrary.org/handbook-of-climate-psychology/#:~:text=A%20comprehensive%20guide%20 to%20climate,coping%20strategies%20and%20radical%20hope.

9. Panu Pihkala, "Anxiety and the Ecological Crisis: An Analysis of Eco-Anxiety and Climate Change Anxiety," *Sustainability* 12, no. 19 (2020), 7836.

10. Sarah Kaplan and Emily Guskin, "Most Teens are Frightened by Climate Change, Poll Shows," *The Washington Post*, September 16, 2019.

11. Richard Atherton, "Climate Anxiety: Survey for BBC Newsround Shows Children Losing Sleep Over Climate Change and the Environment," *BBC Newsround*, March 30, 2020.

12. UNICEF, *The Climate Crisis Is a Child's Rights Crisis* (New York: UNICEF, 2021).

13. Francis Vergunst and Helen Berry, "Climate Change and Children's Mental Health: A Developmental Perspective," *Clinical Psychological Science* 10, no. 4 (2021): 767–785.

14. Michelle Craske and David Barlow, *Mastery of Your Anxiety and Panic: Therapist Guide* (Oxford: Oxford University Press, 2006).

15. Ashlee Cunsolo et al., "Ecological Grief and Anxiety: The Start of a Healthy Response to Climate Change?" *Lancet Planet Health* 4, no. 7 (2020): e261–e263.

16. Susan Clayton, "Climate Anxiety: Psychological Responses to Climate Change," *Journal of Anxiety Disorders*, 74 (2020), 102263.

17. Maria Ojala et al., "Annual Review of Environmental and Resources Anxiety, Worry, and Grief in a Time of Environmental and Climate Crisis: A Narrative Review," *Annual Review of Environment and Resources* 46 (2021): 35–58.

18. Clayton, "Climate Anxiety."

19. Clayton and Karazsia, "Development and Validation."

20. Sarah Schwartz et al., "Climate Change Anxiety and Mental Health: Environmental Activism as Buffer," *Current Psychology* 42 (2022): 16708–16721.

21. Emma Lawrence et al., "Young Persons' Psychological Responses, Mental Health, and Sense of Agency of the Dual Challenges of Climate Change and a Global Pandemic," *Lancet Planetary Health* 6, no. 9 (2022): e726–e738.

22. Mairwen Jones et al., "The Impact of Climate Change on Obsessive Compulsive Checking Concerns," *Australian and New Zealand Journal of Psychiatry* 46, no. 3 (2012): 265–270.

23. Susan Strife, "Children's Environmental Concerns: Expressing Ecophobia," *Journal of Environmental Education* 43, no. 1 (2012): 37–54.

24. Rhiannon Thompson et al., "Adolescents' Thoughts and Feelings about the Local and Global Environment: A Qualitative Interview Study," *Child and Adolescent Mental Health* 27, no. 1 (2022): 4–13.

25. "Greta and Eight Young Activists Reveal how the Climate Crisis Is Shaping Their Lives" (video), UNICEF, September 24, 2020, https://www.youtube.com/watch?v=C7dwoqJzETA.

26. Caroline Hickman et al., "Climate Anxiety in Children and Young People and Their Beliefs about Governmental Responses to Climate Change: A Global Survey," *The Lancet Planetary Health* 5, no. 12 (2021): e863–e873.

27. Charles Ogunbode et al., "Negative Emotions About Climate Change are Related to Insomnia Symptoms and Mental Health: Cross-Sectional Evidence from 25 Countries," *Current Psychology* 42 (2021): 845–854.

28. Hickman et al., "Climate Anxiety in Children and Young People."

29. Maya Gislason, Angel Kennedy, and Stephanie Witham, "The Interplay between Social and Ecological Determinants of Mental Health for Children and Youth in the Climate Crisis," *International Journal of Environmental Research and Public Health* 18, no. 9 (2021), 4573.

30. Tara Crandon et al., "A Social-Ecological Perspective on Climate Anxiety in Children and Adolescents," *Nature Climate Change* 12 (2022): 123–131.

31. Hickman et al., "Climate Anxiety in Children and Young People."

32. Patrice Nicholas and Suellen Breakey, "Climate Change, Climate Justice, and Environmental Health: Implications for the Nursing Profession," *Journal of Nursing Scholarship* 49, no. 6 (2017): 606–616.

33. Ashlee Cunsolo et al., "Ecological Grief and Anxiety: The Start of a Healthy Response to Climate Change?" *The Lancet Planetary Health* 4, no. 7 (2020): e261–e263.

34. National Congress of American Indians, "Environmental Sustainability," accessed May 1, 2024, https://www.ncai.org/section/policy/portfolios/environmental-sustainability.

35. Surili Sutaria Patel et al., "Elevating Mental Health Disparities and Building Psychosocial Resilience Among BIPOC Children and Youth to Broaden the Climate and Health Discourse," *Journal of Applied Research on Children: Informing Policy for Children at Risk* 12, no. 1 (2021).

36. Maya K. Gislason, et al. "The Interplay Between Social and Ecological Determinants of Mental Health for Children and Youth in the Climate Crisis," *International Journal of Environmental Research and Public Health* 18, no. 9 (2021): 4573; Lawrence Palinkas et al., "Strategies for Delivering Mental Health Services in Response to Global Climate Change: A Narrative Review," *International Journal of Environmental Research and Public Health* 17, no. 22 (2020): 8562.

37. Larissa Dooley et al., *Climate Change and Youth Mental Health: Psychological Impacts, Resilience Resources, and Future Directions* (Los Angeles: See Change Institute, 2021), https://seechangeinstitute.com/wp-content/uploads/2022/03/Climate-Change-and-Youth-Mental-Health-Report.pdf.

38. See, for example, Elizabeth Bechard, *Parenting in a Changing Climate: Tools for Cultivating Resilience, Taking Action, and Practicing Hope in the Face of Climate Change* (Brasstown, NC: Citrine, 2021); Harriet Shugarman, *How to Talk to Your Kids About Climate Change: Turning Angst into Action* (British Columbia, Canada: New Society, 2020).

39. Bruce Compas et al., "Coping with Stress During Childhood and Adolescence: Problems, Progress, and Potential in Theory and Research," *Psychology Bulletin* 127, no. 1 (2001): 87–127.

40. Maria Ojala, "How do Children Cope with Global Climate Change? Coping Strategies, Engagement, and Well-Being," *Journal of Environmental Psychology* 32, no. 3 (2012): 225–233.

41. Maria Ojala and Hans Bengtsson, "Young People's Coping Strategies Concerning Climate Change: Relations to Perceived Communication with Parents and Friends and Proenvironmental Behavior," *Environment and Behavior*, 51, no. 8 (2019): 907–935.

42. Leslie Davenport, *All the Feelings Under the Sun* (Washington, DC: Magination Press, 2021).

43. Andrea Mah et al., "Coping with Climate Change: Three Insights for Research, Intervention, and Communication to Promote Adaptive Coping to Climate Change," *Journal of Anxiety Disorders* 75 (2020), 102282.

44. Suzanne Tilmann et al., "Mental Health Benefits of Interactions with Nature in Children and Teenagers: A Systematic Review," *Journal of Epidemiology and Community Health* 72, no. 10 (2018): 958–966.

45. Pauline Baudon and Liza Jachens, "A Scoping Review of Interventions for the Treatment of Eco-Anxiety," *International Journal of Environmental Research and Public Health* 18, no. 18 (2021), 9636.

46. Thomas Doherty and Angel Chen, "Improving Human Functioning: Ecotherapy and Environmental Health Approaches," in *Research Methods for Environmental Psychology*, ed. Robert Gifford (Hoboken, NJ: Wiley, 2016).

47. Elizabeth Nisbet, Daniel Shaw, and Danielle Lachance, "Connectedness with Nearby Nature and Well-Being," *Frontiers in Sustainable Cities* 2 (2020).

48. Sarah Schwartz et al., "Climate Change Anxiety and Mental Health: Environmental Activism as Buffer," *Current Psychology* 42 (2022): 16708–16721.

49. Parissa Ballard, Lindsay Hoyt, and Mark Pachucki, "Impacts of Adolescent and Young Adult Civic Engagement on Health and Socioeconomic Status in Adulthood," *Child Development* 90, no. 4 (2019): 1–17.

50. Albert Bandura and Lynne Cherry, "Enlisting the Power of Youth for Climate Change," *American Psychologist* 75, no. 7 (2020): 945–951.

51. For example, Sarah Jaquette Ray, *A Field Guide to Climate Anxiety: How to Keep Your Cool on a Warming Planet* (Berkeley: University of California Press: 2020).

52. Panu Pihkala, "Eco-Anxiety and Environmental Education," *Sustainability* 12, no. 23 (2020): 1–38.

53. David Rousell and Amy Cutter-Mackenzie-Knowles, "A Systematic Review of Climate Change Education: Giving Children and Young People a 'Voice' and a 'Hand' in Redressing Climate Change," *Children's Geographies* 18, no. 2 (2019): 1–18.

54. Julia Woods, "Meet the Youth Climate Activist Suing the U.S. Government," *Environmental Grantmakers Association Blog*, November 17, 2017.

CHAPTER SEVEN

Who Is Afraid of Climate Change?

Exploring Correlates of Climate Change Anxiety Using Machine Learning Models

KRISTINA ALLGOEWER AND

CHRISTIAN MARTIN

Climate change is what the European Commission has called a "megatrend" that is predicted to impact issues as diverse as migration,[1] agriculture,[2] corporate finance,[3] military strategy,[4] urban planning,[5] and many more.

Climate change is also an issue that induces anxiety in parts of the population of countries around the world. According to a recent representative study, respondents in 17 countries viewed global warming as "tremendously dangerous" or a "serious threat."[6] These results are matched by recent survey data collected among people aged 16–25 years in 10 countries. Fifty-nine percent of respondents are "very" or "extremely worried" about climate change, 84% report that they are at least "moderately worried."[7] Eco-anxiety and climate anxiety are the subject of a growing research program within and across various disciplines.[8]

This chapter adds to the growing evidence on climate anxiety by drawing on social science survey data and machine learning methodology. We used data from the 2016 round of the European Social Survey (ESS) as well as from the 2017 and 2021 rounds of the German Longitudinal Election Survey (GLES) to identify correlates of climate change anxiety. Using both theoretically informed regression models and machine learning algorithms, we identified distinct correlates of climate change anxiety.

Climate Anxiety and Voting Preferences:
The Example of Germany

In our theoretically informed models, we predicted voting for different political parties in the German 2017 federal elections by modeling vote choice as a function of basic demographic characteristics along with self-reported degrees of worry about six politically relevant topics, including climate change. We used this model as a baseline to better understand the results of our machine learning classification models. In these, we classified respondents as being worried about climate change to different degrees by allowing the algorithm to find those covariates that minimize the error of this classification, that is, make the best possible predication based on the information available from the data.

Several results stand out. First, in the theoretically informed regression models, clear differences between supporters of different parties emerged. Worry over climate change is a significant positive predictor for vote choice only for the Green Party and, to a lesser extent, the Left Party. Respondents who are less worried about climate change are significantly more likely to vote for the far-right AfD Party. Voters of the two traditionally big parties CDU/ CSU and the SPD have different anxiety profiles, but not markedly so. The only worries that have a significant influence on vote choice for the CDU/CSU are fear of global terrorism and—negatively signed—fear of use of nuclear energy. Put differently, absence of fear of nuclear power is a significant predictor of voting CDU/CSU. Similarly, for the SPD, only two items were significant: fear of the political situation in Turkey and fear of the use of nuclear power. The coefficients are relatively small, as they are for the CDU. Taken together, voters of CDU/CSU and SPD do have distinct anxiety profiles but are mostly marked by the fact that most items that gauge worries are not significant predictors of vote choice for either of the bigger established parties.

In the machine learning models, we used climate change anxiety as the *outcome* to be predicted. The algorithms select variables in the data set that allow for the best predictions of the outcome. We used two different data sources for this step: the 2016 round of the ESS[9] and the 2021 round of the GLES. The variables that the algorithms select as most predictive can be classified into four groups: (a) variables related to climate issues like attitudes on banning fossil fuels or the feeling of personal responsibility to reduce climate change; (b) variables that capture political activism like signing petitions or participating in protests; (c) feelings of anxiety over *other* issues—namely, the COVID-19 pandemic and worries over international terrorism; and (d) postmaterialist values like the importance respondents ascribe to creativity or experiencing new things.

Together, these results paint the picture of climate anxiety as a politically cross-cutting issue that is not easily associated with traditional political party preferences. While climate change anxiety is a good *predictor* of Green Party vote choice in our country example (Germany), climate change anxiety is much less readily *predicted by* standard political variables, including income, age, and preferences over redistribution. Rather, climate change anxiety is best predicted by, among other items, worries over issues that are not predictive of vote choice for the same party (here, the Greens), at least not in our country example, Germany.

Climate change anxiety as a cross-cutting political issue can therefore be expected to exert a nonuniform effect on political parties. For those parties that are clearly associated with policies that combat climate change, increasing anxiety is politically beneficial because it increases their support. On the other hand, parties that are not "owners" of climate change issues will find it hard to increase their support based on other anxiety-inducing issues because some of these issues are predictive of climate anxiety. Climate anxiety as a political issue is also not easily aligned on a traditional left-right scale. Preferences over redistribution or the role of the government in the economy are not predictive of climate anxiety. If climate anxiety is a politically relevant topic—and our models of vote choice suggest that it is—then it is clearly one that plays out on a "new politics" or GAL/TAN-dimension[10] rather than on the established left-right political dimension.

In the remainder of this chapter, we first sketch out theoretical arguments that inform our expectations for the regression models. We then turn to the empirical results, first showing results from regression analysis before turning to the machine learning models and their results.

The Theoretical Arguments

Climate change is a cross-cutting issue because it potentially affects every aspect of human existence. It is much less clear, however, how this pervasiveness translates into individual perceptions. Clearly, not all people are equally worried about climate change, as a cursory glance at any survey on the topic reveals.[11] What is it, then, that makes some people more likely to worry about the effects of climate change than others? Why are some people more afraid of climate change than others? And what are the political consequences of these varying degrees of climate change worry?

Two theoretical strands seem promising in pursuing these questions, that is, postmaterialist value change, and the association of environmental concerns with party politics.

Postmaterialist Value Change and Climate Anxiety

Postmaterialist value change is a theoretical construct associated with the seminal work of Ronald Inglehart.[12] Inglehart hypothesized that a profound value change has taken place among the public in affluent democracies, changing preferences from physical security and material well-being to the pursuit of postmaterialist values like self-expression and autonomy. According to Inglehart, this change is due to the absence of existential threats for the generation that came of age in the 1960s. Being born into the post–World War II environment of seemingly relentless economic growth and increasing material wealth during the *Trente Glorieuses*, supported by growing welfare states and a labor market that increasingly valued and demanded highly educated workers, the postmaterialist generation sought self-actualization and self-determination over material goods.

Among these postmaterialist values was a new appreciation of environmental quality. Economic growth after World War II had been based on industrial mass production and mass consumption,[13] causing a deterioration of air, water, and soil quality. In 1972, the report, "The Limits to Growth," published by the Club of Rome, predicted that nonrenewable resources would be depleted by an increasing world population if consumption patterns did not change.[14] Already 10 years prior to the publication of "Limits to Growth," another famous book, *Silent Spring*, showed how the use of pesticides hurt natural ecosystems.[15] Spring was "silent" because the birds had died and could no longer sing. The way these books were received and their subsequent influence on political and societal debates show that a postmaterialist concern for the environment was established well before the end of the postwar boom.

Concern over environmental deterioration fit perfectly into the values of the newly emerging postmaterialists. Industrial production and the materialist lifestyle could be criticized not only because it pursued the wrong (i.e., materialist) values but also because it proved to be destructive to the very foundation of life. Large-scale industrial production, mass consumerism and a worldview that saw the natural environment as something that could be exploited for the sake of economic growth came to be pitted against the new (and, by extension, more enlightened) values of autonomy, self-expression, and a view of humankind as one element in an interconnected ecosystem with a special responsibility to care for the environment and, if possible, heal what had been destroyed.

The connection between postmaterialist values and care for the environment is robust and still relevant, even after environmentalism has long since entered the societal and political mainstream. Booth, for example, shows that individuals who score higher on postmaterialist values in survey data from the United States show more environmental concern and are more likely to engage in individual actions supporting the environment.[16] In a less optimistic take on the issue, Armingeon and Buergisser show that when citizens are faced with the choice between expenditures for reducing economic inequality and combating climate change, self-interest prevails.[17] To the extent that holding postmaterialist values and material affluence are positively correlated, this translates into a positive association between postmaterialist values and willingness to politically support climate change abatement policies over redistributive policies. This is reflected in Gelissen's finding of a positive correlation between support for environmental protection and individual as well as average country-level postmaterialist value orientation.[18] Focusing on climate change concerns more narrowly, Kvaløy, Finseraas, and Listhaug find a positive correlation with postmaterialist values.[19]

The association between postmaterialist values and care for the environment and, more narrowly, climate change anxiety, also became a politically relevant factor. What then is the association of climate change, climate change anxiety, and political party preferences?

Party Identification and Climate Change Anxiety

Over the last three decades, identification with political parties has diminished in all Western democracies. Party systems that once were analyzed as "frozen" now appear to be "thawing" as new parties emerge and successfully find a foothold in national party systems with the support of voters whose allegiances to traditional parties of the old party families have eroded in the wake of individuation in postindustrial societies.

Two new party families stand out in this process of increased party system volatility and decreasing voter identification. The first party family is the group of green and postmaterialist parties that emerged in the late 1970s and that were particularly successful in Germany, but also in Austria, Finland, Luxembourg, and Belgium, where they form part of the governing coalition. Green parties are also firmly established at the European level where, after the elections to the 2019 European Parliament, "The Greens/

EFA" (European Free Alliance) is today the fourth largest parliamentary group.

The second party family to successfully establish itself across Europe is right-wing populist parties. In an early contribution to a then emerging literature, Piero Ignazi has classified these parties as a new addition to European party systems, distinguished them from other right-wing extremist parties by their more contemporary rhetoric and their avoidance of referencing fascist parties of the time before and during World War II.[20]

Postmaterialist/Green parties on the one hand and right-wing populist parties on the other today hold clearly opposing views on a great many issues, especially those that can be aligned on a GAL/TAN dimension. GAL/TAN stands for a dimension that stretches from "Green, Alternative, Libertarian" to "Traditional, Authoritarian, Nationalist."[21] Among those issues is climate change of which right-wing populist party "platforms are often hostile to policy designed to address climate change, and their leaders and supporters express forms of climate skepticism that place them outside the political mainstream,"[22] whereas Green parties emphasize the fight against the climate change issue and give it more salience in their party manifestos, with neither traditional left or conservative parties being clearly aligned on the issue.[23]

Arguably, Green parties have been more successful in becoming associated with the issue of environmentalism than right-wing populist parties were in owning their preferred issue of immigration. As Abou-Chadi shows, established mainstream parties try to emphasize the issue of immigration when confronted with strong right-wing populist parties in order to take the issue away from them and prove competence on the issue.[24] In contrast, when confronted with strong Green parties, established parties de-emphasize environmental issues, leaving it to the Green parties that are perceived as issue owners with limited possibilities for the established parties to compete on the issue.

This variation between different party families should translate into differences with respect to climate change anxiety. We would expect supporters of Green parties to be more concerned with climate change. At the same time, we might expect to find support for the Greens among the best predictors of climate change anxiety. How do these expectations align with the data?

Empirical Evidence

The Data

We draw on three data sets from two different sources, the GLES and the ESS. We used the 2017 and 2021 postelection surveys from GLES and the 2016 round eight of the ESS. All three data sets are surveys at the individual level. Whereas the GLES data are gathered among eligible and soon-to-be-eligible voters in Germany, interviews for the 2016 ESS round were conducted among residents of 21 European Countries.[25]

Both the GLES and the ESS are high-quality surveys that are representative of the populations from which respondents are drawn. Both the GLES and the ESS contain several hundred variables of substantive interest. Both data sets ask respondents about their worries.[26] This takes place in the form of closed questions, that is, respondents are given a list of different issues and are asked to what degree they are worried about these issues.

The degree of worry over climate change (or, as the 2017 GLES put it, "global warming") has been included in all three surveys used for our analysis. Along with variables about climate change and other worries, the surveys ask a battery of questions regarding individual attitudes and preferences about societally and politically relevant issues. For example, the ESS data contain an item that asks respondents whether they think "Government should reduce differences in income levels." The GLES asks, for example, if a respondent feels that their work is given too little recognition (item q46b), that politicians mainly cater to the rich (q51k), or, simply, if they are using Facebook (q70b).

We will first use a theoretically determined selection of variables from the 2017 GLES to model vote choice for political parties, before we turn to the prediction of climate change anxiety using machine learning models.

Predicting Vote Choice Using Anxiety Data

As a first step, we conducted a series of theoretically informed regression analyses with which we try to identify distinct anxiety profiles across supporters of different political parties in Germany. We used data from the 2017 GLES and modeled whether a respondent voted for a particular party or not as a function of nine variables. With six politically relevant parties in the German party system (CDU/CSU, SPD, AfD, FDP, LEFT, and Greens), this resulted in six regression models.[27]

In the 2017 GLES postelection survey, six items were included to gauge the fears and worries of respondents. In German, the language in which the survey was administered, the question was: "*Wie viel Angst macht Ihnen . . .*" ("How worried are you about . . .") followed by six items:

". . . the refugee crisis?"
". . . global warming?"
". . . international terrorism?"

"... globalization?"

"... political developments in Turkey?"

"... the use of nuclear power?"

Each item can be answered by respondents on a scale that ranges from "1 (Not worried at all)" to "7 (Very worried)." We used only those observations where the answer was not "Don't know" or "No answer," leaving us with between 97.42% and 99.95% valid responses.

We used logit regression analyses to estimate separate models for each of the six parties in the German federal legislature (CDU/CSU, SPD, AfD, FDP, LEFT and GREEN, in the order of their results in the 2017 federal elections). The outcome to be explained in these models was whether a respondent had voted for the party under observation or not. There was over- as well as underreporting of vote choice, as well as of electoral participation. This is a known problem in postelection survey data, and the GLES data are no exception.[28] In the GLES data, respondents underreported voting for the AfD and overreported voting for the Greens.

We ended up with six regression models, one for each of the parties.[29] We wanted to know whether there was any significant difference in the predictive power of different worries for different parties. Using these models, we can gauge if someone who is more afraid of, say, global warming, is more or less likely to vote for, say, the SPD. (As it turns out, being worried about global warming is not a significant predictor for voting for the SPD.)

The theoretical rationale behind this is straightforward. If parties cater to voters with different preferences and these preferences are a function of a set of properties of individual voters, then those same sets of properties can be expected to have an impact not only on vote choice but also on the issues voters are worried about. To give a specific example, Walter, as well as Dancygier and Walter, use individual positions in the labor market to determine preferences over trade, foreign direct investment, and immigration.[30] These preferences are then related to vote choice. For the present context, this work is relevant because labor market position and skill set also determine what voters feel threatened by (or not).

Despite this political economy side of the story, anxiety profiles are obviously more complicated than that. Individual labor market positions do not, for example, easily relate to the degree a respondent is worried by nuclear power, global warming, or international terrorism. Modeling those fears in relation to vote choice allows us to think more broadly about the underlying cultural and economic determinants of different anxiety profiles. Put differ-ently, we can use what we know about political parties and their voters and apply it to our thinking about anxiety.

We added three non-anxiety-related variables to our regression analysis: age, gender, and whether a respondent was surveyed in one of the Eastern German states. Figure 7.1 shows a summary of the results for the worries in the survey, including climate change anxiety. In the figure, the shaded dots show the values of coefficients with standard errors estimated at statistically signifi-cant levels in six logistic regression models. A separate model was fitted for each of the six political parties.

A few results stand out. In contrast to average worries, there is a distinct cluster of worries that are different across voters of different parties. Voters of traditional parties like CDU/CSU and the SPD have different anxiety pro-files, but not markedly so. The only worries that have a significant influence

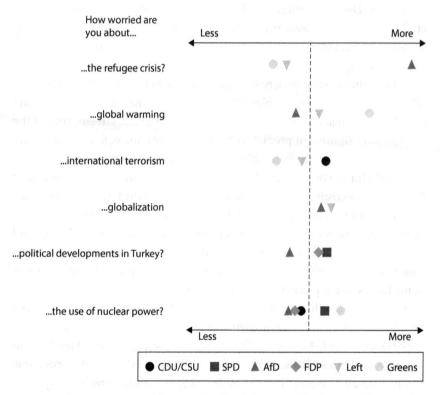

Figure 7.1. Summary of regression results. Shaded data points show coefficients of logit regressions for supporters of different parties.

on the probability of vote choice for the CDU/CSU are fear of global terrorism and—negatively signed—fear of use of nuclear energy. Put differently, absence of fear of nuclear power is a significant predictor of voting CDU/ CSU. Similarly, for the SPD, only two items are significant, fear of the political situation in Turkey and fear of the use of nuclear power. The coefficients are relatively small, as they are for the CDU. Taken together, voters of CDU/CSU and SPD do have distinct anxiety profiles but are mostly marked by the fact that most items that gauge worries are not significant predictors of vote choice for either of the bigger established parties. This reflects their history as big-tent, catch-all parties that gain output legitimacy in the political center.

Something similar is true for another established party in the German system, the FDP. For a majority of postwar West German history, the FDP was the only other party besides SPD and CDU/CSU that was competitive at the federal level. It has played the role of a pragmatic enabler of CDU/ CSU- or SPD-led governments. FDP voters are the ones for whom "anxiety" as a category is least predictive. They only worry about the political situation in Turkey; the other significant result is being not afraid of nuclear power.

In two other parties anxiety is much more predictive, with their voters exhibiting distinct anxiety profiles. These parties are the ones at the opposite end of the postmaterialist–materialist dimension, AfD and Greens. Four of the six issues are significant predictors for Green vote choice, five out of the six items predict AfD vote choice. Not unexpectedly, no single issue is a significant predictor of vote choice where AfD and Greens are on the same side of the anxiety spectrum. On the refugee crisis, voters of the Greens are less worried, voters of the AfD more; for global warming, it is the other way around. International terrorism worries voters of the AfD but is a significant and *negative* predictor for Green voting. Finally, the use of nuclear power is worrisome to voters of the Green Party, whereas exhibiting significantly less fear of nuclear power is predictive of AfD voting.

The results on climate change anxiety and environmental issues more broadly are in line with our theoretical expectations. The results reaffirm the importance of the GAL/TAN or "New Politics" dimension and extend its importance to anxiety issues. Voting for traditional, established parties that compete on an economic dimension is much less readily predicted by anxieties even if those anxieties include foreign policy (developments in Turkey) or macroeconomic issues (globalization).

Predicting Climate Anxiety Using Machine Learning Models

Our next step goes beyond theoretically informed regression analysis. Running regressions is always at risk of missing important determinants of the outcome variable of interest. Machine learning approaches have increasingly been used as a technique that allows researchers to comb through large numbers of variables to identify those that hold the most predictive power when classifying or forecasting outcomes.

Typical applications for machine learning models are situations in which researchers are faced with a large number of variables and limited theoretical expectation as to which variables are particularly predictive. In our case, we are dealing with individual-level data sets that contain several hundred substantive variables. While we have formed some theoretical expectations about correlates of climate change anxiety (as previously discussed), these expectations amount to anything but a full-fledged theoretical model. Arguably, such models are difficult to form in the first place, given the complexity of causal pathways in the social sciences.

Against this backdrop, we used different machine learning models to identify a limited set of variables that are predictive of our outcome quantity of interest, levels of climate change anxiety. These predictors are not theoretically derived and cannot claim to establish causal relationships. Rather, we used the variable identified by the machine learning models as most predictive and brought them back to theoretical considerations about determinants of climate change anxiety.

The conceptual difference between machine learning models and regression analysis is the a-theoretical choice of variables. For example, ordinary least squares (OLS) regressions require researchers to select variables based on theoretical consideration (as we did earlier), but machine learning algorithms choose those variables themselves, applying criteria that maximize the predictive power of their choice.

Classification of ESS Data

We used two different machine learning models to achieve this latter goal in our application of climate change anxiety. With the (cross-national) ESS data, we use a logistic classifier (namely, a 10-fold cross-validation classifier) implemented in the machine learning software WEKA.[31] Two different versions are used: The first one takes the ESS question "How worried are you about climate change?" and tries to predict a respondent's answer in one of the five categories from "not at all worried" to "extremely worried." There is considerable variance on this question. More than a quarter of respondents answer that they are "not at all worried" or "not very worried."

We first arrived at a rate of 59.1% for correctly predicted (classified) respondents. This contrasts with a baseline correct classification rate of 46.3% using the ZeroR classifier.[32] Our classifier selected the following 12 variables as delivering the best prediction based on the information contained in the more than 40,000 observations:

- Born in the country (immigrants are less worried about climate change)
- How worried that the country is too dependent on fossil fuels (more worries connected with more climate change worry)
- How worried about energy supply being interrupted by natural disasters or extreme weather (more worries connected with more climate change worry)
- Thinks the world's climate is changing (those who do are more worried about climate change)
- How much thought given to climate change before today (more thought, more worried)
- Believes climate change is caused by natural processes, human activity, or both (more human activity, more worried)
- To what extent feels personal responsibility is needed to reduce climate change (more responsibility, more worried)
- Climate change causes good or bad impact across the world (those who think it causes bad impact are more worried)
- Against or in favor of banning sales of least-energy-efficient household appliances to reduce climate change (in favor positively correlates with more worries)
- Against or in favor of a European Union–wide social benefit scheme (being in favor positively correlates with more worries)
- Has employment contract unlimited or limited duration (limited duration employees are more worried)
- Important to care for nature and environment (those who think it is important are more worried)

Obviously, many of these items are very closely related to climate change. It would appear unsurprising that respondents who think that climate change is a bad thing are more worried about climate change. This is the reason the algorithm picks these variables—they are predictive of climate change anxiety and can be used to classify respondents' levels of anxiety. But several predictors also are theoretically more interesting—namely, the question about the EU-wide social benefit scheme and the more general question about the importance "to care for nature and the environment." While the first of these is associated with a preference for redistribution at the supranational level, the latter is an item typically associated with postmaterialist values.

In the second version, we reduced the number of categories on the dependent variable to three. These were constructed from the original variable using the responses "not at all worried" and "not very worried" for the first category, the modal category "somewhat worried" for the second category, and the responses "very worried" and "extremely worried" for the third category. We then let our classification algorithm select variables that best predict respondents' membership in one of the three categories. ZeroR classification success is, again, at 46.3%. The machine learning algorithm selected nine variables that predict 65.3% correctly:

1. How worried that the country is too dependent on fossil fuels (more worried connected with more climate change worry)
2. Thinks the world's climate is changing (those who do are more worried)
3. How much thought given to climate change before today (more thought, more worried)
4. Climate change is caused by natural processes, human activity, or both (more human activity, more worried)
5. To what extent feels personal responsibility to reduce climate change (more responsibility, more worried)
6. Climate change causes good or bad impact across world (those who think it causes bad impact are more worried)
7. Favors banning sale of least-energy-efficient household appliances to reduce climate change (in favor of ban correlated with more worries)
8. Gender (more worried if female)
9. Important to care for nature and environment (respondents who think it is important are more worried)

This is a narrower list of variables than for the five-category case. Again, questions related to climate change are highly predictive. Again, the postmaterialist item of care for the environment is predictive, as is gender. Put differently, if we had information on these nine items, we would be able to correctly gauge the climate anxiety of respondents in almost two-thirds of the cases. Theoretically, however, the results seem limited. It is not at all surprising, let alone informative for other politically relevant questions, that preferences for more efficient household appliances are predictive of climate change anxiety.

We therefore let the algorithm select predictors among variables that are *not* related to climate change. To do so, we restricted the number of variables from which the algorithm can select its predictors to those that do not have an obvious connection to climate change. The rationale for this restriction is that we hope to find predictors that carry some theoretical importance and on which we might miss out by focusing on the cluster of climate change variables. Using this approach, the algorithm selected two groups of variables to predict climate anxiety.

First, we found a cluster of items along the materialist/postmaterialist dimension, with all variables supporting the notion that holding stronger postmaterialist values is associated with climate change anxiety. Specifically, the algorithm picked 21 items, for example, "It is important to think new ideas and be creative" (positive), "It is important to be rich and to have money and expensive things" (negative), "It is important to try new and different things in life" (positive), "It is important to behave properly" (negative).

The second cluster revolves around political activism items. Predictive items are: "I have worn or displayed campaign badge/sticker in the last 12 months," "Signed a petition in the last 12 months," "Taken part in lawful public demonstration in the last 12 months," "Boycotted certain products in the last 12 months," and "Posted or shared anything about politics online in the last 12 months."

On the one hand, individuals who score highly on the postmaterialist scale are more concerned over climate change. On the other hand, variables that capture political activism are among the best predictors for climate change worries. Variables that capture more traditional means of political participation, especially variables that capture the closeness to political parties, are much less predictive. This can be interpreted in a way that casts climate change worry as a left political topic, but one that is owned more by the Green, postmaterialist left than by traditional socialist or social democratic parties. This is corroborated by the findings on political activism.

Prediction with GLES Data

The next data source was from the most recent wave of the 2021 GLES. The dependent variable is the degree to which a respondent is worried about climate change, measured on a 1 to 7 scale where 1 stands for "not at all worried" and 7 for "very much worried."[33] Independent variables are all non-identification variables in the GLES with a sufficient number of observations. Here, "Sufficient" means not containing so many missing values as to render calculations impossible. For example, the variable d19, "Are you worried about losing your business" (authors' translation), has only 211 non-missing observations because most respondents are not self-employed. The variable was therefore omitted from the analysis as were others that had too many missing observations. Although it is possible that they contain valuable information, their sparsity simply did not allow for inclusion in the analysis. Following this approach, we are left with 168 covariates.

We treated the dependent variable as continuous and fit a linear lasso[34] using the plug-in selection method. We opted for this method because it tends to parsimoniously select those variables that best approximate the data generating process.

Using this method, we are left with eight variables:

1. Feeling sympathy toward supporters of the Green Party
2. Supporting groups that fight climate change
3. Supporting further European integration
4. Supporting stricter measures against climate change
5. Supporting higher levies on fossil fuels
6. Anxiety about international terrorism
7. Anxiety about the COVID pandemic
8. Not being a self-declared member of the "Querdenker" movement, an antivaccine and antimask group that has been spreading disinformation as well as staging protests against vaccine mandates and COVID-related restrictions.[35]

The lasso produced an R-squared of 0.671 in the training data and 0.669 in the validation data, with a mean square error of 0.934 and 0.950, respectively. This error can be interpreted as the accuracy of the prediction based on the selected variables. The accuracy is considerably higher than those produced by other lasso selection methods. We are therefore confident that the plug-in method is not only the most parsimonious one in terms of variable selection but also the one with the highest predictive power.

Conclusion

We have used data from the GLES, rounds 2017 and 2021, and data from the ESS round 2016, to identify correlates of climate change anxiety. To do that, we first formulated theoretical expectations revolving around (a) the connection between postmaterialism and concern for the environment and, more specifically, climate change; and (b) the emergence of a new dimension in politics along which the conflict over climate change concern and, more generally, postmaterialist issues is politically organized and relevant. We then turned to theoretically informed regression models with which we predicted vote choice in Germany based on anxiety. In a second step, we allowed machine learning algorithms to pick variables among a large number of possible covariates that best predict climate change worries.

Several results stand out. First, in the theoretically informed regression models, clear differences between supporters of different parties emerge. Worry over climate change is a significant positive predictor for vote choice only for the Green Party and, to a lesser extent, the Left party. In the machine learning models, the variables that the algorithms pick as most predictive of climate change anxiety can be classified into four groups: (a) variables related to climate issues like attitudes on banning fossil fuels or the feeling of personal responsibility to reduce climate change; (b) variables that capture political activism like signing petitions or participating in protests; (c) feelings of anxiety over other issues, namely the COVID-19 pandemic and worries over international terrorism; and (d) postmaterialist values like the importance respondents ascribe to creativity or experiencing new things but also political attitudes related to positions on a GAL/TAN-dimension, like support for EU integration.

Together, these results paint the picture of climate anxiety as a politically cross-cutting issue that is not easily associated with traditional political preferences. While climate change anxiety is a good predictor of Green Party vote choice in our country example (Germany), climate change anxiety is much less readily *predicted by* standard political variables, including income, age, and preferences over redistribution.

Climate anxiety will, therefore, not be easily absorbed into the standard structure of party competition and political competition more generally. While green parties have successfully positioned themselves to become issue owners of environmental concerns, the clustered nature of anxieties points to a more complex relationship between anxieties and political preferences. This is also reflected in the importance of items that capture political activism beyond party politics and elections.

NOTES

1. Richard Black et al., "Migration, Immobility and Displacement Outcomes Following Extreme Events," *Environmental Science & Policy* 27, no. 1 (2013): S32–S43; Lori Hunter, Jesse Luna, and Rachel Norton, "Environmental Dimensions of Migration," *Annual Review of Sociology* 41 (2015): 377–397.

2. Ariel Ortiz-Bobea et al., "Anthropogenic Climate Change Has Slowed Global Agricultural Productivity Growth," *Nature Climate Change* 11, no. 4 (2021): 306–312; Tim Wheeler and Joachim von Braun, "Climate Change Impacts on Global Food Security," *Science* 341, no. 6145 (2013): 508–513.

3. Yannis Dafermon, Maria Nikolaidi, and Giorgos Galanis, "Climage Change, Financial Stability and Monetary Policy," *Ecological Economics* 152 (2018): 219–234; Stefano Battison et al., "A Climate Stress-Test of the Financial System," *Nature Climate Change* 7, no. 4 (2017): 283–288.

4. Solomon M. Hsiang, Marshall Burke, and Edward Miguel, "Quantifying the Influence of Climate on Human Conflict," *Science* 341, no. 6151 (2013): 1235367.

5. Johannes Langemeyer et al., "Urban Agriculture? A Necessary Pathway Towards Urban Resilience and Global Sustainability?" *Landscape Urban Planning* 210 (2021); Briony Norton et al., "Planning for Cooler Cities: A Framework to Prioritise Green Infrastructure to Mitigate High Temperatures in Urban Landscapes," *Landscape and Planning* 134 (2015): 127–138.

6. Vodafone Institute for Society and Communications, *The Global Future Pulse. Sustainability* (Berlin, 2021), accessed May 2, 2024, https://www.vodafone-institut.de/en/publication/majority-thinks-tackling-climate-change-is-responsibility-of-governments/.

7. Tosin Thompson, "Young People's Climate Anxiety Revealed in Landmark Survey," *Nature* 597, no. 7878 (2021): 605.

8. Pikhala Panu, "Anxiety and the Ecological Crisis: An Analysis of Eco-Anxiety and Climate Anxiety," *Sustainability* 12, no. 19 (2020).

9. Unfortunately, the most recent (2018) round of the ESS did not include a module to gauge items related to climate change.

10. GAL/TAN stands for a dimension that stretches from "Green, Alternative, Libertarian" to "Traditional, Authoritarian, Nationalist."

11. For example, in the 2021 German Longitudinal Election Survey used in this paper, almost 4% of respondents say that they are "not worried at all" about climate change. A cumulative 19% of survey participants responded that they are worried at values of 3 or less on a 1 to 7 scale, where 1 is "not worried at all" about climate change and 7 is "very worried."

12. Robert Inglehart, *The Silent Revolution: Changing Values and Political Styles Among Western Publics* (Princeton: Princeton University Press, 1977); Robert Inglehart, *Culture Shift in Advanced Industrial Society* (Princeton: Princeton University Press, 1989).

13. Kiminori Matsuyama, "The Rise of Mass Consumption Societies," *Journal of Political Economy* 110, no. 5 (2002): 1035–1070.

14. Donella Meadows et al., *The Limits to Growth: A Report for the Club of Rome's Project on the Predicament of Mankind* (New York: Universe Books, 1972).

15. Rachel Carson, *Silent Spring* (New York: Houghton Mifflin, 1962).

16. Douglas Booth, "Postmaterialism and Support for the Environment in the United States," *Society & Natural Resources*, 30, no. 11 (2017): 1404–1420.

17. Klaus Armingeon and Reto Buergisser, "Trade-Offs Between Redistribution and Environmental Protection: The Role of Information, Ideology, and Self-Interest," *Journal of European Public Policy* 28, no. 4 (2021): 489–509.

18. John Gelissen, "Explaining Popular Support for Environmental Protection: A Multilevel Analysis of 50 Nations," *Environment and Behavior* 39, no. 3 (2007): 392–415.

19. Berit Kvaløy, Henning Finseraas, and Ola Listhaug, "The Publics' Concern for Global Warming: A Cross-National Study of 47 Countries," *Journal of Peace Research* 49, no. 1 (2012): 11–22.

20. Piero Ignazi, "The Silent Counter-Revolution," *European Journal of Political Research* 22, no. 1 (1992): 3–34.

21. Ryan Bakker et al., "Measuring Party Positions in Europe: The Chapel Hill Expert Survey Trend File, 1999–2010," *Party Politics* 21, no. 1 (2015): 143–152.

22. Matthew Lockwood, "Right-Wing Populism and the Climate Change Agenda: Exploring the Linkages," *Environmental Politics* 27, no. 4 (2018): 712–732. For the US context, see Daniel Fiorino, "Climate Change and Right-Wing Populism in the United States," *Environmental Politics* 31, no. 5 (2022): 801–819. For a more nuanced view of populist parties and climate change, see Vieth Selk and Jörg Kemmerzell, "Retrogradism in Context. Varieties of Right-Wing Populist Climate Politics," *Environmental Politics* 31, no. 5 (2022): 755–776.

23. Fay Farstad, "What Explains Variation in Parties' Climate Change Salience?" *Party Politics* 24, no. 6 (2018): 698–707.

24. Tarik Abou-Chadi, "Niche Party Success and Mainstream Party Policy Shifts—How Green and Radical Right Parties Differ in Their Impact," *British Journal of Political Science* 46, no. 2 (2016): 417–436.

25. Namely, Austria, Belgium, Switzerland, Czechia, Germany, Estonia, Spain, Finland, France, United Kingdom, Hungary, Ireland, Israel, Iceland, Italy, Lithuania, Netherlands, Norway, Poland, Portugal, Russia, and Sweden.

26. Unfortunately, there were no questions relating to worries over climate change in the most recent round (2018) of the ESS.

27. Given that our dependent variable is binary (voted for party 1 through 6, yes or no), we used survey logistic regression analysis, i.e., a survey design-weighted maximum likelihood estimator that estimates coefficients and standard errors of our covariates to achieve the highest probability to correctly predict the outcome variable.

28. Christian Martin, "Electoral Participation and Right-Wing Authoritarian Success: Evidence from the 2017 Federal Elections in Germany," *Politische Vierteljahresschrift* 60, no. 2 (2019): 245–271.

29. We also used a multinomial logit model with vote choices for the six different parties as the categorical outcome variable; the results are virtually identical with the ones reported. In the interest of clarity, we omit the multinomial logit results.

30. Stefanie Walter, "Globalization and the Demand-Side of Politics: How Globalization Shapes Labor Market Risk Perceptions and Policy Preferences," *Political Science Research and Methods* 5, no. 1 (2017): 55–80; Rafaela Dancygier and Stefanie Walter, "Globalization, Labor Market Risks, and Class Cleavages," in *The Politics of Advanced Capitalism*, ed. Pablo Baramendi et al. (Cambridge: Cambridge University Press, 2015), 133–156.

31. Frank Eibe, Mark Hall, and Ian Witten, *Data Mining: Practical Machine Learning Tools and Techniques* (Burlington, MA: Morgan Kaufman, 2016).

32. ZeroR uses no information from the data except for the distribution of the dependent variable. It then classifies every respondent as being within the modal category.

33. In the original German questionnaire, the item is worded as "*überhaupt keine Angst*" to "*sehr große Angst.*"

34. Lasso stands for Least Absolute Shrinkage and Selection Operator. It is a regression technique that seeks to select a limited number of variables out of many variables to arrive at an estimate of a quantity of interest, i.e., the dependent variable. It does so by "shrinking" coefficients (hence the name) until some of them become zero. A random split of the sample into training and validation data is used to check the performance of different selection algorithms.

35. This variable is the only one out of the eight that loses significance once it is used in a full-sample regression. The variable is heavily skewed with more than 99% of respondents answering that they do not belong to the "Querdenker" movement.

PART THREE

POPULATION HEALTH
AND SOCIAL WELL-BEING

Introduction

JOHN P. ALLEGRANTE

Anxiety is typically recognized as a clinical medical or psychiatric disorder that affects the individual. According to the US National Institute of Mental Health, anxiety disorders at the individual clinical level frequently share features of excessive fear and anxiety and related behavioral disturbances.[1] With an estimated 31% of adults who will experience an anxiety disorder in their lifetime, the prevalence of anxiety as a diagnosis has been rising over recent decades. In 2019, the US National Center for Health Statistics reported that the percentage of adults 18 years and older who experienced symptoms of anxiety in the past two weeks ranged from 16.6% for those aged 30–44, to 15.2% for those 45–64, to 11.6% for those 65 years and older, and was as high as 19.5% for those age 18–29, with women more likely than men to experience mild, moderate, or severe symptoms of anxiety.[2] Moreover, *The Lancet* reported that the global prevalence and burden of depressive and anxiety disorders has risen sharply in response to the COVID-19 pandemic.[3]

It is against this backdrop that the four chapters contained in Part III explore anxiety and its relationship to population health and social well-being from a variety of perspectives that go beyond anxiety as a medical idiom. In the first chapter, Nicholas Freudenberg presents an overarching public health perspective on the problem of anxiety. Using several public health concepts, he examines the causes of anxiety and its health and social consequences at the population level. He notes that "in the last 20 years the world has experienced a cascade of anxiogenic crises—the COVID pandemic, escalating climate change, rising economic inequality, [and] growing political conflict and polarization." But as Freudenberg concludes, "No credible evidence suggests that the observed and perceived increases in several types of anxiety in the last few decades are due to changes in human biology or neurochemistry. Instead, it is the result of human decisions, by individuals, institutions, businesses, and policymakers, decisions that pushed more people into anxiety and diminished their capacity to avoid or end it."

Next, gun violence in America is the topic of Sonali Rajan's essay in Chapter 9. Rajan, a behavioral health researcher in education, begins her essay by providing a personal account of her first experience with gun violence as a teenage high school student and then goes on to explore the landscape of the human carnage from Columbine to Uvaldi that the quintessentially American epidemic of gun violence has produced in US schools and beyond. She analyzes the complex causes of gun violence and discusses the myriad cultural, social, and political challenges to bringing about the kinds of meaningful legislative and other gun safety reforms that could mitigate the anxiety many parents now feel about sending their children to school.

The third chapter in this section, "Adolescent Anxiety: Iceland as Canary in the Coal Mine," addresses the issue of the growing prevalence of anxiety among adolescents and its impact on substance use. In their review of what can be learned from this small Nordic nation, Meyers, Thorisdottir, Sigfusdottir, Asgeirsdottir, and Allegrante point out that first we must ascertain the existence of an anxiety culture—especially among youth—and then seek to make sense of it. To do so, they argue, it is "paramount to understand the relationship between adolescents and their environment." They conclude by noting that adolescents perceive the world to be changing, and that perhaps young people—like the proverbial canary in the coal mine—are telling us through their own increasing reports of anxiety that they are noticing.

Finally, Part III concludes with a chapter by sinologists Angelika Messner, Roman Marek, and Zhao Xudong, who write about anxiety and global health through the lens of the Chinese cultural context and lived experience. They point out, for example, that patients in China who suffer from generalized anxiety disorder are more likely to complain of somatic symptoms than their Western counterparts. Notwithstanding such comparative differences in medical concepts about anxiety, its treatment, and its outcomes, they suggest that rapid cultural, social, economic, and technological transformation may not be the driving forces behind cultural anxiety. But rather "the loss of traditional social communities [that] has caused a deterioration of care systems, thereby affecting the young and the old, the rich and the poor alike."

NOTES

1. See the National Institute of Mental Health, "Any Anxiety Disorder," accessed May 17, 20204, https://www.nimh.nih.gov/health/statistics/any-anxiety-disorder.

2. Centers for Disease Control and Prevention, "Symptoms of Generalized Anxiety Disorder Among Adults: United States, 2019," September 2020, https://www.cdc.gov/nchs/products/databriefs/db378.htm.

3. COVID-19 Mental Disorders Collaborators, "Global Prevalence and Burden of Depressive and Anxiety Disorders in 204 Countries and Territories in 2020 Due to the COVID-19 Pandemic," *Lancet* 398, no. 10312 (2021): 1700–1712.

CHAPTER EIGHT

A Public Health Perspective on Anxiety

NICHOLAS FREUDENBERG

Anxiety describes an individual state of mind, a clinical disorder that warrants medical diagnosis, and a collective modifiable psychological characteristic of populations such as families, communities, and nations. Some tasks, such as developing optimal treatment for individuals with anxiety disorders or organizing health care institutions to provide such care (topics considered elsewhere in this volume) require clear distinctions among these various meanings for anxiety. However, developing effective public health policies and programs to prevent and reduce the overall social burden of anxiety, the topic of this chapter, may profit from considering the range of states of anxiety, their common drivers, and the benefits and costs of cross-cutting policies and programs.

The goal of public health is to improve the health of populations and reduce inequities or disparities in health across communities, populations, and nations. Public health professionals develop and implement policies, programs, and services that contribute to these goals, and public health researchers provide evidence that can inform effective and equitable interventions.

Like other disciplines and professions such as education, social work, and law that have academic and theoretical roots as well as a practical mission to improve the world, public health operates at multiple levels from the individual, family, and peer network to the community, region, nation, and world. Developing effective public health policies and programs requires synthesizing evidence, academic insights, and methodologies across these levels, disciplines, and theories.

In this chapter, I use several public health concepts to examine the causes and consequences of anxiety—considered as both a state of mind of individuals and populations and a medical diagnosis—as an influence on the health of populations. The goals are to examine the causes and health and social consequences of anxiety at the population level to suggest strategies for preventing anxiety using types of prevention from primordial prevention (averting a problem before it develops) to tertiary prevention, which treats manifestations of illness to prevent further deterioration and disability.

More broadly, I hope to spark an interdisciplinary, intersectoral conversation that can inform the creation of a research and action framework for population-level strategies for the prevention and treatment of anxiety. Jabareen defines conceptual frameworks as "interlinked concepts that together provide a comprehensive understanding of a phenomenon" and argues that by grounding and linking concepts to their intellectual and social origins, scholars can deepen our understanding of the "real world."[1]

Table 8.1 defines some of the key public health concepts used in this chapter to examine the causes and consequences of anxiety in the 21st century.

Ecological Models

In public health, ecological models recognize multiple levels of influence on health, including biological, psychological, and sociodemographic characteristics, as well as family, cultural, community, and environmental influences. Public health ecological models enable researchers to map the intersecting influences of factors that operate within and across distinct levels of social organization and design interventions that acknowledge and leverage these multiple influences. This approach can inform analyses of the determinants of anxiety at various levels (Figure 8.1). A key concept is that social conditions and societal allocations of wealth and power can operate as anxiogenic influences, defined as life experiences and living conditions that can cause, trigger, or exacerbate anxiety as a state of mind, a medical diagnosis, or a characteristic of a population.[2]

The Social Determinants of Health

Building on the historical roots of public health from the 19th century, beginning in the early 21st century, a body of scholarship on social determinants of health (SDOH) has emerged. SDOH theory posits that the "circumstances in

TABLE 8.1.

Public Health Concepts Relevant to Study of Anxiety

Anxiogenic influences	Exposures, environments, or policies that increase anxiety.
Anxiolytic influences	Exposures, environments, or polices that decrease anxiety.
Collective action	Action taken together by a group of people whose goal is to enhance their condition and achieve a common objective. Many public health advances such as clean drinking water, safe food, and improved and safer working conditions have come about as a result of the collective action of social movements, reformers, and concerned citizens.[a]
Commercial determinants of health	Commercial determinants of health are the social, political, and economic structures, norms, rules, and practices by which business activities designed to generate profits and increase market share influence patterns of health, disease, injury, disability, and death within and across populations.[b] Social media companies; gig employers; food, alcohol, and tobacco companies; and health care institutions pursue business or political strategies that heighten anxiety.
Ecological health model	Provides a comprehensive framework for understanding the multiple and interacting determinants of health and health behavior as they operate at varying levels of social organization and are used to inform the design of multilevel interventions.[c]
Fundamental causes	Rose[d] described fundamental causes as "the cause of the causes" of other health problems.
Precautionary principle	The public health principle that the burden of proof for potentially harmful actions by industry or government rests on the assurance of safety, and where credible threats of serious damage exist, scientific uncertainty must be resolved in favor of prevention.[e]
Primordial prevention	In 1978, Strasser[f] proposed the term *primordial prevention* for actions that could avert global health problems from unfolding. Primordial prevention seeks to modify fundamental causes in ways that prevent the range of adverse consequences from developing. Other levels of prevention include primary, which uses clinical and public health approaches to prevent disease or injury before it occurs; secondary, which aims to reduce the impact of a disease or injury that has already occurred by early intervention at the individual or community level; and tertiary, which softens the impact of an ongoing illness or injury with lasting effects by rehabilitation, emotional support, or disease management.[g]
Social determinants of health	Social determinants of health (SDOH), according to the US Department of Health and Human Services, *Healthy People 2030*, are "the conditions in the environments where people are born, live, learn, work, play, worship, and age that affect a wide range of health, functioning, and quality-of-life outcomes and risks."[h] Many such social determinants, including housing quality, access to health care, food access, and social isolation, have been linked to anxiety and other psychological states.[i]

(continued)

TABLE 8.1. (*continued*)

Public Health Concepts Relevant to Study of Anxiety

Syndemic theory	A syndemic is defined as two or more health conditions that interact synergistically and impose a high burden of disease. Syndemic theory posits that individual epidemics are "sustained in a community/population because of harmful social conditions and injurious social connections."[j]
Systems thinking/systems science	Systems thinking analyzes the ways that a system's constituent parts or the parts of many systems interrelate and how systems work over time and within the context of larger systems to ameliorate or exacerbate social problems. In public health, systems thinking (and its more formal scientific foundation, systems science) are used to, for example, understand how systems of work, health care, and school interact to influence conditions like anxiety.[k] Systems thinking looks for both positive and negative unintended consequences of working across systems and seeks to identify cross-cutting interventions, policies, and programs that can more effectively reduce a problem such as anxiety.

a. Dorothy Cilenti, et al., "System Dynamics Approaches and Collective Action for Community Health: An Integrative Review," *American Journal of Community Psychology* 63, no. 3–4 (2019): 527–545.

b. Nicholas Freudenberg, et al., "Defining Priorities for Action and Research on the Commercial Determinants of Health: A Conceptual Review," *American Journal of Public Health* 111, no. 12 (2021): 2202–2211.

c. Lucie Richard, Lise Gauvin, and Kim Raine, "Ecological Models Revisited: Their Uses and Evolution in Health Promotion Over Two Decades," *Annual Review of Public Health* 32 (2011): 307–326.

d. Geoffrey Rose, *Rose's Strategy of Preventive Medicine* (Oxford: Oxford University Press, 1992).

e. Bernard D. Goldstein, "The Precautionary Principle Also Applies to Public Health Actions," *American Journal of Public Health* 91, no. 9 (2001): 1358–1361.

f. Toma Strasser, "Reflections on Cardiovascular Diseases," *Interdisciplinary Science Reviews* 3, no. 3 (1978): 225–230.

g. Lisa A. Kisling and Joe M. Das, "Prevention Strategies," in *StatPearls* (Treasure Island, FL: StatPearls Publishing, 2022).

h. "Social Determinants of Health," US Department of Health and Human Services, Office of Disease Prevention and Health Promotion, Healthy People 2030, https://health.gov/healthypeople/priority-areas/social-determinants-health.

i. Manuela Silva, Adriana Loureiro, and Graca Cardoso, "Social Determinants of Mental Health: A Review of the Evidence," *European Journal of Psychiatry* 30, no. 4 (2016): 259–292.

j. Merrill Singer and Scott Clair, "Syndemics and Public Health: Reconceptualizing Disease in Bio-Social Context," *Medical Anthropology Quarterly* 17, no. 4 (2003): 423–441.

k. Gemma Carey, et al., "Systems Science, and Systems Thinking for Public Health: A Systematic Review of the Field," *BMJ Open* 5, no. 12 (2015):e009002.

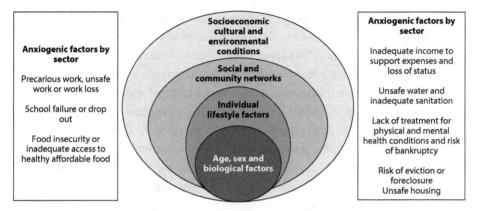

Figure 8.1. Social determinants of health and anxiety. Based on the Social Determinants of Health. See "Social Determinants of Health," US Department of Health and Human Services, Office of Disease Prevention and Health Promotion, Healthy People 2030, https://health.gov /healthypeople/priority-areas/social-determinants-health.

which people grow, live, work, and age, and the systems put in place to deal with illness" are shaped by political, social, and economic forces.[3] Improving the health of populations and closing the gaps in health among various groups that characterize most societies requires changes in the political, economic, and social factors that harm health and a more equitable distribution of the benefits and costs of the allocations of wealth and power.

One theme of the SDOH literature is that proximate causes of ill health have deeper causes, what social epidemiologists label the "cause of the causes." Rose identified poverty, social exclusion, poor housing, and poor health systems as the causes of ill health in the current era.[4] The most basic determinants of patterns of ill health and disease have been labeled fundamental causes, defined by Link and Phelan in 1995 as the social, economic, and political structures that explain why class inequities in health persist even as social conditions change.[5] More recently, Clouston and Link have written that the goal of this approach was to "understand the persistence of associations between socio-economic status (SES) and morbidity and mortality despite the fact that the diseases afflicting humans, and the risk and protective factors influencing those diseases, changed substantially across time and place."[6] In this view, as conditions change, people of higher SES have the resources and capacities to adapt to these changes while those with lower SES do not. Applied to anxiety, this suggests that reducing the differing manifestations of anxiety across time and place requires addressing the economic and political structures that trigger these varying responses in different populations and settings.

An important aim of this approach is to determine whether multiple preventable diseases are influenced through multiple mechanisms. In this chapter, I make the case that recent changes in the political and economic system known as modern capitalism have served as a fundamental cause of increases in anxiety—as well as many other health conditions. In this view, reducing anxiety will require changes in this political and economic system. Syndemic theory posits that when two or more health outcomes (e.g., diabetes, depression) have intersecting causes and consequences, interventions that address the multiple and upstream determinants may be more effective than categorical, downstream ones.[7] Conditions that have been associated with anxiety include depression, diabetes, COVID-19 infection, HIV, malaria, and tuberculosis and may warrant application of syndemic theory.[8]

A more recent focus within the SDOH approach is to analyze commercial influences on health, which are defined as the actions, norms, and ideas of market and business actors such as corporations, trade associations, lobbying firms, and advertising and public relations firms that influence patterns of health and disease.[9] Figure 8.2 summarizes this approach.

Banks, for example, contribute to financial anxiety by foreclosing on houses, refusing to renegotiate debt, and promoting speculative financial instruments. Social media companies promote "fear of missing out" to generate additional clicks and advertising revenue,[10] and drug companies market anti-anxiety drugs. In 1999, for example, GlaxoSmithKline launched an almost $100 million ad campaign to promote Paxil, a prescription drug for anxiety disorders and depression, as a remedy for the disease of "being allergic to people." "Every marketing director's dream," claimed Paxil's marketing director, "is to find an unidentified or unknown market and develop it." In the year after this ad campaign was introduced, Paxil's sales rose by nearly 20%.[11]

Given the pervasiveness of anxiety, it is not surprising that corporations look to market products and services purported to reduce anxiety. However, when marketers of tobacco, alcohol, cannabis, tranquilizers, firearms, or large and powerful SUVs and pickup trucks claim that their products reduce anxiety and cover up or fail to disclose their risks, government has an opportunity and an obligation to set rules that limit these harms.

Another relevant public health lens for the study of anxiety is systems thinking, or systems science. Arnold and Wade have defined systems thinking as "a set of synergistic analytic skills used to improve the capability of

Structural influences on commercial determinants of health

Structural influences describe recurrent and patterned arrangements of power and influence which shape opportunities in a society; distinctive and stable arrangements of institutions whereby humans interact in a society.

Component	Definition	Relationship to anxiety
Political and economic system	Patterned network of relationships constituting a coherent whole that exists between institutions, groups, and individuals	Type of economic and political system (system of production, resource allocation and distribution of good and services within a society or geographic area), labor market
Stratification	Society's categorization of its people into groups based on socioeconomic and other factors	Social class and mobility, distribution of economic resources and political power by class, race/ethnicity, or caste, patterns of business ownership, patterns of inequity
Organization	Stable structure of relations inside a group, which provides a basis for order and patterns relationships for members	Forms of business organization and institutional arrangements for regulation of commercial activities
Governance	Rules and processes by which a society steers itself towards goals	Trade and investment treaties, intellectual property rights and protections, tax codes and legal codes, business law
Norms	Standards or patterns of behavior, based on prevailing beliefs and values, considered normal or expected in a particular society	Self-regulation of business sector, free and competitive markets, role of state in privatization and deregulation

Actor influences on commercial determinants of health

Actor influences describe capacity of individuals and organizations to act independently and make their own choices.

Components	Definition	Examples
Market-oriented practices	Actions businesses take to maximize returns on investment, revenues, profits, shareholder value and market share.	Product design, manufacturing processes, pricing, supply chain management, marketing, advertising and promotion, retail distribution, pricing, investment/divestment, tax management
Policy and political-oriented practices	Actions and strategies businesses use to increase their power and influence and decrease uncertainty	Campaign contributions, lobbying, sponsored research, philanthropy, corporate responsibility activities, public and government relations

Living conditions, lifestyles, environments, services, and norms that shape patterns and distribution of Individual and population levels of anxiety and anxiety disorders

Figure 8.2. Applying the commercial determinants of health framework to the study of anxiety.

identifying and understanding systems, predicting their behaviors, and devising modifications to them in order to produce desired effects."[12] Rejecting reductionist models, systems thinking acknowledges that the causes of health problems cut across systems and sectors, that cause and effect often have complex reciprocal relationships, and that unidimensional or single-level interventions often have unintended adverse consequences. Figure 8.3 illustrates this framework.

Several dimensions of changes in the incidence, prevalence, and distribution of anxiety, both as a state of mind and a medical diagnosis, suggest the value of systems thinking as an analytic framework.

First, over the last few decades, several varieties of anxiety, some associated with clinical diagnoses and others with population-level effects but each with different proximate causes and symptoms, have been documented. On the clinical side these include generalized anxiety disorders, obsessive compulsive disorders, panic disorders, post-traumatic stress disorders, and social anxiety disorders.[13] Varieties of anxiety with more social causes include, among others, health anxiety,[14] COVID anxiety,[15] race and racism-related anxiety,[16] climate anxiety,[17] financial anxiety,[18] social media–generated anxiety,[19] housing anxi-

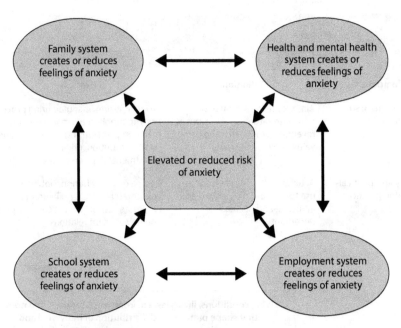

Figure 8.3. Systems thinking approach to anxiety.

ety,[20] and food anxiety.[21] Any outcome associated with such a diverse array of exposures and triggers is unlikely to have a single cause or to be amenable to a single intervention. Thus, a systems perspective offers opportunities for more cross-cutting investigations and prevention and treatment strategies.

Second, given the multiple exposures linked to anxiety, prevention and control strategies that use the insights of systems science—the value of locating interventions at the nodes that connect systems to increase their impact, the importance of anticipating unintended positive and negative consequences for interventions across systems, and the potential for modeling how changes in one system can influence changes in health across populations and systems—can magnify impact and address drivers of both prevalence and inequities.

Finally, a *collective action* lens informs an examination of how different actors from social movements and civil society groups to governments can act to modify the structures and systems that contribute to anxiety, that is, how they can begin to modify the fundamental causes of anxiety. The goals of such changes are to prevent or reduce exposure to anxiogenic influences, defined as environments or substances that cause anxiety, and to increase exposures to anxiolytic environments or substances, which inhibit anxiety. In addition, public health interventions can mitigate the adverse health impact of such exposures and modify systems or practices that distribute the harmful consequences of anxiety inequitably by race/ethnicity, class, gender, immigration status, or other stratifications.

The creation of a public health framework for the prevention of anxiety builds on centuries of debates within psychology, psychiatry, philosophy, neuroscience, and other fields on the origins of anxiety. In the current era, the dominant scientific view is that anxiety is the result of a chemical imbalance in the brain that can be corrected with biochemical interventions. But in the 17th century, the English physician Richard Napier identified the principal sources of anxiety among his patients as worries over love, marriage, death, and especially debt.[22] In the 1890s, the sociologist Emile Durkheim argued that anomie, a social condition defined by an uprooting or breakdown of social values and standards, separated individuals from their communities and led to an increase in suicide and other psychological problems.[23] The mid-20th-century psychologist Erich Fromm attributed anxiety in the modern world to unchecked capitalism, unemployment, and the potential for a nuclear holocaust.[24] According to Fromm, separation from a familiar and comfortable world elicits feelings of anxiety and powerlessness, which can then turn into fear and destructiveness,[25] an analysis that resonates in the current period. By locating new approaches to addressing anxiety in the historical and intellectual context of these prior debates, public health professionals can contribute new insights and new approaches to research, theory, and practice.

Current Approaches to Prevent Anxiety

Each of the public health concepts introduced in this chapter provides insights into the development of strategies, policies, and programs to prevent anxiety or reduce its adverse impact. None, however, is sufficient on its own to develop comprehensive, sustainable, and effective interventions. Like other complex public health problems with multiple causes and consequences, preventing anxiety requires the use of blended frameworks and approaches that are grounded in a particular place and time and subject to change as conditions change. By synthesizing existing evidence into a unifying framework, identifying gaps in the knowledge that can be filled with new research, evaluating existing policies and programs that prevent or mitigate anxiety in order to develop a body of practice-based evidence, and developing and testing new intervention strategies, public health researchers, policy makers, practitioners, and advocates can contribute to reducing the high burden of anxiety-related morbidity, mortality, and health inequities.

What might be the core components of such a comprehensive policy strategy in the coming decades of the 21st century in the United States and other high-income but highly inequitable societies?

First, educators and public health professionals in particular can contribute to reframing the public understanding of anxiety as a mostly individual problem to one that is rooted in social, political, and economic structures. As long as the current biomedical model that attributes the causes of anxiety to biochemical and neurological imbalances and the solutions to correcting such imbalances through pharmacological, behavioral, or other biological interventions persists, our society's capacity to prevent anxiety will be limited.

A clear example of this individualistic approach is the recent formulation of the idea of "good anxiety."[26] In this view, anxiety is "actually essential to our survival, " as one neuroscientist writing about "good anxiety" put it.[27] Her anxiety, she explained, "had driven me to make the changes to my lifestyle that were now great sources of joy."[28] By taking up "exercise, clean diet and meditation," she has "learned how to use anxiety to improve my life."[29] She concludes, "Anxiety can be good . . . or bad. It turns out that it's really up to you."[30]

One strategy for challenging this reductionist approach is to present evidence on the broader causes of anxiety and propose alternative analyses that spotlight opportunities for preventing the social structures, policies, life circumstances, and conditions that trigger and perpetuate anxiety. In doing this, public health policies can begin to construct and reflect an alternative public understanding of anxiety.

Second, health professionals can ground their approaches to prevention in the daily lives and day-to-day experiences of people experiencing or at risk of anxiety. Whatever the role of endogenous genetic, neurochemical, or biological vulnerabilities, at both the individual and populations levels, anxiety is triggered by actual and perceived experiences: loss of employment, housing, health insurance, or food security; fear of threats to one's health or environment; social exclusion; political, interpersonal, or sexual violence; or other sources. Only by understanding the objective and perceived anxiogenic exposures for various populations can public health and other professionals engage multiple constituencies in reducing such exposures or modifying their individual or collective perception.

Third, effective approaches must take on the multiple sources of anxiety in people's lives. Reducing one of a dozen causes might be a good starting point, but to improve people's lives will require diminishing anxiogenic forces at multiple levels and across multiple sectors. For many populations, for example, employment, housing, and food insecurity come in a package and so anxiety-reducing strategies must address each of these triggers. In this case, systems thinking can help inform a broader policy perspective and more effective intervention strategies. Growing income inequality triggers employment, housing, and food outcomes so strategies that reduce this gap—minimum wage, universal free child care, or fair and equitable taxation—could reduce all three sources of anxiety as well as many other health problems.

Systems science also suggests that interventions that take place at the nodes of two or more systems can have a greater, more synergistic impact than those in a single system. For example, a school-based mental health program within a school health center can reach children, teachers, and families to modify interpersonal dynamics (e.g., shaming and punishing children), institutional practices (e.g., requiring high-stakes testing), and access to services (developing effective links and referrals to community mental health providers) in ways that reduce exposure to anxiogenic forces in family, school, community, and health care systems.[31]

Fourth, effective approaches must identify and tackle the fundamental drivers of anxiety. Fundamental drivers in the current era are essential dynamics of 21st century capitalism such as globalization, financialization, deregulation, rising income inequality, and a view of markets rather than government as the force most responsible and qualified to solving social and health problems.[32] Changing these dynamics will require building links to the social movements that have the vision, mission, and capacity to bring about transformative as well as incremental changes. Black Lives Matter; the #MeToo movement against sexual abuse, sexual harassment, and rape culture; the Sunrise Movement and other climate change groups; Moms Demand Action, the anti-gun violence group; and Fight for $15, a grassroots alliance of low-wage workers, are just a few of the movement organizations tackling the drivers of anxiety. Defining a shared agenda to take on the social, economic, and political cause of anxiety and then taking a collective action to advance this agenda is a daunting challenge, but in fact public health advances have always required such alliances and past public health successes can be a rich source of guidance.[33]

Finally, public health professionals, researchers, and advocates must join other reformers and activists to insist another world is possible. At the individual and societal levels, anxiety can lead to paralysis or action. Those who benefit from the status quo, those who have worked to shape public norms and values to endorse business-as-usual, insist that the world we have is both the best world possible and inevitable. Their success in enlisting support for this faith-based belief that contradicts world history is a major obstacle to enlisting people in transformative action to tackle fundamental drivers of ill health, including anxiety. Hope for the future, the belief that another world is possible, is the surest antidote to despair and paralysis. By acting in small and not-so-small ways, by nurturing and celebrating successes, and by disseminating these success stories widely, public health professionals can begin to show that other less anxious worlds are possible.

Conclusion

While it might be reassuring to some to think that we could eliminate anxiety by putting an anxiolytic drug in the drinking water, in reality this approach is unlikely to be feasible, effective, or ethical. Moreover, it risks unintended side effects. Biomedical and individual-level responses to anxiety are necessary but not sufficient. On their own, they have failed to reverse increasing incidence of anxiety or to prevent the growing inequities in the health and social burdens it imposes, especially on low income communities and nations. By monopolizing the public resources and private capital available for reducing anxiety, drug companies, hospitals, mental health professionals, and others have diverted attention from taking on the social, economic, and political causes.

Absent the (so far) imaginary magic bullet, comprehensive public health approaches to reducing and better managing anxiety will require changing policies, programs, and practices of individuals, communities, and institutions at multiple levels, in multiple systems, and informed by multiple disciplines and theories. Eventually, this approach has the potential to bring about meaningful reductions in the incidence, prevalence, and severity of both individual and population-level anxiety.

Humans have always suffered from anxiety. In just the last century, the Great Depression, World War II, the Cold War, colonial wars, globalization, and changes in the world's political and economic systems have regularly triggered anxiety. No reliable evidence allows researchers to compare the population impact of these events over time and place.

But in the last 20 years the world has experienced a cascade of anxiogenic crises—the COVID pandemic, escalating climate change, rising economic inequality, growing political conflict and polarization, often accompanied by targeted hate campaigns against groups such as immigrants, Muslims, Asian Americans, women, LGBTQ people, Blacks and Latinx, Indigenous people, and others. Might there be a tipping point for anxiety, where the capacity of communities and nations to recover and of individuals to treat or manage their anxiety is so diminished that recovery is no longer possible?

Years of research on the consequences of rising carbon levels in the atmosphere show that for climate change, such a tipping point has already been identified and now serves as a catalyst for global, national, community, and individual-level action to reduce carbon emissions. Could such an approach inform a public health approach to anxiety? In public health, the precautionary principle is a fundamental value that asserts, even in the absence of definitive evidence on the benefits of proposed remedies, if the consequences of inaction are known and substantial, action is required.[34]

No credible evidence suggests that the observed and perceived increases in several types of anxiety in the last few decades are due to changes in human biology or neurochemistry. Instead, it is the result of human decisions, by individuals, institutions, businesses, and policymakers—decisions that pushed more people into anxiety and diminished their capacity to avoid or end it. Along with several prior generations of public health researchers, Frieden has observed that public health interventions that change systems and structures are more likely to be effective and to yield measurable improvements in health and health equity than those that change only individuals or health care delivery.[35]

Thus, to reduce anxiety, we will need to take on the most fundamental social, economic, and political systems and policies that have led to increases in anxiety. To use another metaphor, rather than hiring more lifeguards and ambulance drivers to rescue anxious people who have jumped or fallen into the swirling currents of the river, we need instead to build the policies, programs, and practice fences that will keep them from falling into the river in the first place.[36] By building these structures with other partners, together we can replace the age of anxiety with the age of hope for a healthier, more just world.

NOTES

1. Yosef Jabareen, "Building a Conceptual Framework: Philosophy, Definitions, and Procedure," *International Journal of Qualitative Methods* 8, no. 4 (2009): 49–62.

2. Lucie Richard, Lise Gauvin, and Kim Raine, "Ecological Models Revisited: Their Uses and Evolution in Health Promotion Over Two Decades," *Annual Review of Public Health* 32 (2011): 307–326.

3. Michael Marmot et al., "Closing the Gap in a Generation: Health Equity Through Action on the Social Determinants of Health," *The Lancet* 372, no. 9650 (2008): 1661–1669.

4. Geoffrey Rose, *Strategy of Preventive Medicine* (Oxford: Oxford University Press, 1992).

5. Bruce G. Link and Jo Phelan, "Social Conditions as Fundamental Causes of Disease," *Journal of Health and Social Behavior*, Spec. no. (1995): 80–94.

6. Sean A. P. Clouston and Bruce G. Link, "A Retrospective on Fundamental Cause Theory: State of the Literature and Goals for the Future," *Annual Review of Sociology* 47, no. 1 (2021): 131–156.

7. Finn Diderichsen, Ingelise Andersen, and Jimmi Mathisen, "Depression and Diabetes: The Role of Syndemics in the Social Inequality of Disability," *Journal of Affective Disorders Reports* 6 (2021): 100211.

8. William V. Bobo et al., "Association of Depression and Anxiety with the Accumulation of Chronic Conditions," *JAMA Network Open* 5.5 (2022): e229817–e229817; Kai Yuan et al., "A Systematic Review and Meta-Analysis on Prevalence of and Risk Factors Associated with Depression, Anxiety and Insomnia in Infectious Diseases, including COVID-19: A Call to Action," *Molecular Psychiatry* 27, no. 8 (2022): 3214–3222.

9. Nicholas Freudenberg, *At What Cost Modern Capitalism and the Future of Health* (Oxford: Oxford University Press, 2021).

10. James A. Roberts and Meredith E. David, "The Social Media Party: Fear of Missing Out (FoMO), Social Media Intensity, Connection, and Well-Being," *International Journal of Human–Computer Interaction* 36, no. 4 (2020): 386–392.

11. Allan V. Horowitz, *Anxiety: A Short History* (Baltimore: Johns Hopkins University Press, 2013), 140–141.

12. Ros D. Arnold and Jon P. Wade, "A Definition of Systems Thinking: A Systems Approach," *Procedia Computer Science* 44 (2015): 669–678.

13. Seon-Cheol Park and Yong-Ku Kim, "Anxiety Disorders in the DSM-5: Changes, Controversies, and Future Directions," *Advances in Experimental Medicine and Biology* 1191 (2020): 187–196.

14. Gordon J. G. Asmundson et al., "Health Anxiety: Current Perspectives and Future Directions," *Current Psychiatry Reports* 12, no. 4 (2010): 306–312.

15. Nader Salari et al., "Prevalence of Stress, Anxiety, Depression Among the General Population During the COVID-19 Pandemic: A Systematic Review and Meta-Analysis," *Globalization and Health* 16, no. 1 (2020): 57.

16. Daniel B. Lee, Enrique W. Neblett, Jr., and Veronica Jackson, "The Role of Optimism and Religious Involvement in the Association Between Race-Related Stress and Anxiety Symptomatology," *Journal of Black Psychology* 41, no. 3: 221–246.

17. Shuquan Chen et al., "Anxiety and Resilience in the Face of Natural Disasters Associated with Climate Change: A Review and Methodological Critique," *Journal of Anxiety Disorders* 76 (2020): 102297.

18. Gilla K. Shapiro and Brendan J. Burchell, "Measuring Financial Anxiety," *Journal of Neuroscience, Psychology, and Economics* 5, no. 2 (2012): 102–193.

19. Betul Keles, Niall McCrae, and Annmarie Grealish, "A Systematic Review: The Influence of Social Media on Depression, Anxiety, and Psychological Distress in Adolescents," *International Journal of Adolescence and Youth* 25, no. 1 (2019): 79–93.

20. Ankur Singh et al., "Housing Disadvantage and Poor Mental Health: A Systematic Review," *American Journal of Preventive Medicine* 57, no. 2 (2019): 262–272.

21. Andrew M. Taylor and Hannah D. Holscher, "A Review of Dietary and Microbial Connections to Depression, Anxiety, and Stress," *Nutritional Neuroscience* 23, no. 3 (2020): 237–250.

22. Michael MacDonald, *Mystical Bedlam: Magic, Anxiety, and Healing in Seventeenth-Century England* (Cambridge: Cambridge University Press, London, 1983), 67.

23. Emile Durkheim, *Suicide: A Study in Sociology* (New York: The Free Press, 1897 [1951]).

24. Horowitz, *Anxiety: A Short History*, 94.

25. Erich H. Fromm, *Escape from Freedom* (New York: Holt, Reinhart and Winston, 1941).

26. Wendy Suzuki, *Good Anxiety: Harnessing the Power of the Most Misunderstood Emotion* (New York: Atria Books, 2021).

27. Suzuki, *Good Anxiety*, 4.

28. Suzuki, *Good Anxiety*, 5.

29. Suzuki, *Good Anxiety*, 6.

30. Suzuki, *Good Anxiety*, 9.

31. Catherine Diamond and Nicholas Freudenberg, "Community Schools: A Public Health Opportunity to Reverse Urban Cycles of Disadvantage," *Journal of Urban Health* 93, no. 6 (2016): 923–939.

32. Nicholas Freudenberg et al., "Defining Priorities for Action and Research on the Commercial Determinants of Health: A Conceptual Review," *American Journal of Public Health* 111, no. 12 (2021): 2202–2221.

33. Theodore M. Brown and Elizabeth Fee, "Social Movements in Health," *Annual Review of Public Health* 35 (2014): 385–398.

34. Kumanan Wilson and Katherine Atkinson, "Toward Neo-Precaution: A New Approach to Applying the Precautionary Principle to Public Health," *American Journal of Bioethics* 17, no. 3 (2017): 44–46.

35. Thomas R. Frieden, "A Framework for Public Health Action: The Health Impact Pyramid," *American Journal of Public Health* 100, no. 4 (2010): 590–595.

36. John McKinley, "The Case for Refocusing Upstream: The Political Economy of Illness," in *The Sociology of Illness: Critical Perspectives*, ed. Peter Conrad (New York: St. Martin's Press, 1997).

CHAPTER NINE

Anxiety and School Gun Violence in America

SONALI RAJAN

Twenty-five years ago, one teacher and 12 high school students were killed by two of their classmates at Columbine High School in Littleton, Colorado. The perpetrators were armed with multiple firearms, including a semiautomatic handgun. They injured another 21 individuals before killing themselves. The Columbine shooting left an indelible impression on the nation's psyche; such violence in a school was unimaginable to many at the time.

My own memory of that day is vivid. Just four weeks earlier, a drunk driver killed my high school music teacher as he drove home from our late-night orchestra rehearsal. The days that followed felt dark and heavy, like I was enveloped in a fog of deep sadness. It was all any of us could think about: his young family, the violent and sudden manner in which he was taken from this world, the loss of a mentor who had encouraged and championed his students and who reminded us to not give up on our biggest dreams. It had been a difficult month. On the morning of the Columbine shooting, my brilliant and intuitive mother, who always seemed to know what my sisters and I needed well before we did, encouraged us to stay home from school. She called it a "reset day"—a chance to catch up on sleep and homework and eat a warming lunch. It was self-care before self-care was popularized, if you will.

My sisters and I were crowded around our kitchen table. I was trying to work through a chemistry problem set, balancing redox reactions. It was unusually cool for April in upstate New York; spring buds on the massive maple tree in our front yard were starting to emerge, yet it was chilly enough to warrant wearing a thick sweatshirt. I remember trying to focus on my homework, my feet tucked neatly under me while I sifted through paragraph after paragraph about oxidation numbers and limiting reagents. But my mind kept drifting. My parents would often tune in to National Public Radio in our home while we studied; like white noise, it was easy to tune it out. On that day the news was playing on the radio in the background. But suddenly, my sisters and I started piecing together unfamiliar phrases ("black trench coats" . . . "shooting" . . . "multiple causalities"). Like hail colliding with a windshield—sudden, forceful, jarring—the words kept tumbling out of the radio. *Guns. Students. Hiding. Teachers. Dead.*

It was unthinkable to me—to all of us, really—that something like this could happen. Schools universally, after all, are spaces to learn and grow and challenge oneself and places to spend time with friends and navigate the emotional complexities of adolescent life. At least I had, until that moment, the enormous privilege of believing that was the case. As I would come to learn, that was not so—and still is not—for many children across the United States. And as I would also come to learn, Columbine was not the first school shooting of its kind, and nor would it be the last. On that gray April afternoon, the news of the school shooting at Columbine High School felt inconceivable. Surely, we—the authorities—would do everything we could to prevent that kind of violence from ever happening again.

The Endemic of School Gun Violence in the United States

Over the last twenty-five years since Columbine, school gun violence persists. This time, as I write this, I am sitting at a different kitchen table. Now with my bright-eyed son next to me (his feet tucked under him, just like mine) as he draws a picture—"a spaceship, Mama." I give him a tight squeeze while scrolling through a spreadsheet that captures data on every intentional school shooting over the past several years, catching my breath every now and then as I remember that each cell represents students and school staff who have died or been injured in such acts of unthinkable, senseless violence.

Just a few years ago, 17 students and school personnel were killed and 17 more injured in another school shooting—this time in Parkland, Florida—where the perpetrator was armed with an AR-15 semiautomatic rifle. And less than three months after that, one of the deadliest school shootings took place at Santa Fe High School in Texas, where eight students and two teachers were killed and 13 more were wounded. This time the perpetrator used a

12-gauge pump-action shotgun and a .38-caliber revolver, both legally owned by his father.

I choose to highlight these more recent shootings because they are fairly familiar to the American public and—because of social media and global news coverage—many elsewhere. Perhaps the details of the weapons used or the manner in which these shootings ultimately ended are less known, but my hunch is that any person who keeps even a casual eye on the news is likely to know of these tragedies to some degree.

But I could just as easily highlight the school shooting at Freeman High School in Rockford, Washington, in the months before Parkland, where the perpetrator used an AR-15 style semiautomatic rifle to kill one student and injure three more. Or, just three weeks prior to the Parkland shooting, when a high school student in Marshall County, Kentucky, shot 16 people at Marshall County High School, killing two, with a pistol he obtained from his stepfather's unlocked cabinet. Or the Rancho Tehama Elementary School shooting in Corning, California, which took place just before the American Thanksgiving holiday in November 2017. This time the perpetrator used a homemade AR-15-style rifle to injure three people. Or the shooting at Highland High School in Palmdale, California, that occurred just one week before the Santa Fe High School shooting in May 2018 and resulted in one injured student. These shootings, too, matter and are as deeply tragic and equally traumatic to the communities in which they occur as the shootings that receive the relentless media attention.

The challenging question is: How should these incidents be defined? The definition of *school shooting* varies markedly by researcher and organization. For example, some experts have focused on operationalizing "mass shootings,"[1] whereas others include any type of gunfire on school grounds.[2] Some are interested in school shootings on any type of school campus (including preschools and institutions of higher education), and still others are focused specifically on acts of gun violence where a shooter's intent can be determined.[3] The nuance and variation in definition matters. Regardless of definition, gunfire of any kind in any school is not normal. Nor should it be expected, or—worse—justified.

Over the past two decades, there were approximately 60 "active school shootings" in K-12 schools in the 20 years since the Columbine massacre (incidents where the shooter's intent to harm at least four people has been established).[4] During this same period there have also been hundreds of instances of gunfire on school grounds.[5] This could mean an accidental discharge of a gun that unwittingly injured a student in the process or a gun massacre perpetrated by an individual with deliberate harmful intent, resulting in multiple fatalities. Indeed, *The Washington Post* has estimated that since 1999, more than 370,000 children "have experienced gun violence at school since Columbine."[6] Their work has drawn important attention to the ramifications that different types of gun violence at school (e.g., witnessing gunfire and hearing gunshots, or both) has on youth well-being.

My colleagues and I recently made a case for a range of possible exposures to violence involving a gun to also be considered in the dialogue about gun violence prevention.[7] Specifically, we argue that the following experiences should be included when operationalizing "gun violence exposure": injury from a gun, being threatened by a gun, witnessing gunfire, and hearing gunshots. Because we also know youth gun violence exposure can and does occur outside of school spaces (in homes and within neighborhoods),[8] equipping schools to be prepared to support students who have had a friend or family member who has been shot and who have had a close friend or a sibling, or both, carry a gun is equally important.

Unfortunately, very little is empirically known about the long-term impact of any type of school shooting on school communities, particularly among students in K-12 schools who are in varying critical stages of physical and socioemotional development; that is, we have limited research that has explicitly studied this phenomenon. We know lingering trauma exists. In early 2019, two student survivors of the Parkland massacre and one of the parents of the Sandy Hook Elementary School mass shooting victims all died by suicide.[9] We know how post-traumatic stress, anxiety, and other indicators of trauma impact the lives of survivors.[10] An article in *Essence* magazine poignantly captured the brutality of what we now expect of children: "when students who have witnessed gun violence enter school, they are expected to perform as though traumatic and life-altering events have never occurred."[11]

One can extrapolate from the research on the impact of violence on child development to recognize that firearm violence in schools—however it is defined—fundamentally disrupts critical learning and childhood or adolescent development.[12] Yet, most current discussions among policymakers about gun violence prevention continue to occur independently from conversations about educational best practice and without consideration of the full impact of gun violence exposure on child health and well-being. More disconcerting, many of the proffered solutions to the problem of gun violence in school spaces have been proposed without the input of educators or the insight of a solid research base informing these proposals.[13]

The result? Gun violence in schools persists. And because many evidence-informed actions proposed to stem gun violence are thwarted by political arguments grounded—sometimes erroneously—in a limited interpretation of the American Second Amendment, gun violence is likely to persist.

Anxiety Culture and Our Collective Response to School Gun Violence

The natural human response to any tragedy is to do everything possible to reduce the likelihood that it could ever happen again. We ask: What could we have done to prevent this? For example, in the early 1980s, we sought to address the high rates of injury and death due to drunk driving.[14] As a society, we came to political consensus to set legal limits for blood alcohol concentration levels for drivers, made sure that cars were designed with state-of-the-art safety features, invested in public education efforts, and worked closely with law enforcement to ensure that roads were kept safe. As a result, car crashes resulting from drunk driving declined significantly.[15] The efforts are not perfect—as the loss of my beloved music teacher two decades ago painfully illustrates—but such societal changes together resulted in immeasurably safer communities across the United States.

Conversely, in our efforts to keep schools safe from gun violence, we have responded in ways that have little or no existing evidence base and are likely having a negative impact on child health outcomes, on student learning, on teacher burnout, and on the well-being of school personnel. Indeed, we have turned to a response grounded in anxiety instead of science or, one might argue, compassion. This has shaped our K-12 schools in such a way that schools now serve as spaces that are structured and "prepared" to anticipate this kind of violence—a culture of anxiety, if you will.

We have taught children how to turn off the lights and shelter and hide quietly in their school bathrooms while they practice active shooter drills.[16] We have armed teachers.[17] (At present, 28 states allow school personnel to be armed with guns.[18]) We have invested tens of millions of dollars into the hardening of schools, equipping classrooms with bulletproof white boards and students with bulletproof backpacks.[19] We have installed metal detectors, security cameras, and implemented locker and person searches; in essence, we have criminalized our school spaces.[20] We have taught students and school staff how to administer first aid in the case of traumatic blood loss from a bullet wound.[21]

But meaningful prevention ought to occur across a spectrum, where the prevention of school gun violence should effectively consider its root causes. In this way, we can think about preventing school gun violence—not just in the moment of a violent act—but by discovering what might lead a child to choose to carry a gun or to fundamentally feel unsafe or disenfranchised from their school community. K-12 schools must recognize the anxiety caused by the anticipation of school gun violence as they consider more generative and effective ways to prevent this kind of violence.

Framing the Problem Through the Lens of Anxiety Culture

In early 2019, I had the opportunity to sit on a panel at Columbia University's School of Journalism to discuss the issue of gun violence. As faculty members, my colleagues and I often sit on panels such as this, which is typically an opportunity for Columbia students and faculty across disciplines to learn more about preventing gun violence. But in this instance, the organizers had specifically brought together panelists with a range of perspectives on the topic of gun safety.

One of the panelists, Cabot Phillips, was a known conservative commentator. As I entered the room, he immediately came over to greet me. Cabot had a firm handshake and was impeccably dressed. Having done a little online sleuthing prior to the panel, I knew he would come prepared to make his case, not just for less gun regulation but also to speak to the importance of the Second Amendment, the Constitutionally guaranteed right to bear arms and what that means for many Americans. I thought it took some confidence to agree to sit on a panel where the other speakers and most, if not all, of the audience held strongly left-leaning opinions on this issue. In other words, I and others were there to advocate for legislative reforms and other measures that would limit access to guns.

Toward the end of the nearly hour-long discussion, the conversation became more animated as each of us found our stride. In the heat of one particular exchange, Cabot quoted a statement to me that the National Rifle Association (NRA) also often makes: "Over the past 20 years, gun ownership has increased and gun violence has decreased." I sharply responded, "that's not true," and proceeded to quote the most recent statistics from the Centers for Disease Control and Prevention that illustrate the growing epidemic of gun violence.[22] To which Cabot replied, "you can't count gun suicides . . . if you just look at gun homicides, gun violence has decreased."

I did not have a good response. How could he simply discount one of the most devastating forms of gun violence? But because our panel was nearly out of time, we had no further opportunity to pursue the conversation.

Hours after the panel concluded, I kept coming back to that moment. Was Cabot correct in seeking to differentiate between types of gun violence?

The Types of Gun Violence

To some extent, Cabot had a point. The effective prevention of homicides looks different from the effective prevention of suicides, although there is some critical overlap, particularly with regard to gun access. Perhaps unsurprisingly, research has clearly illustrated that gun possession puts an individual at risk for homicide and also increases the likelihood that someone who is suicidal will commit suicide with a gun. Thus, reducing access to firearms is likely to decrease risk in both cases.[23]

In truth, no clear consensus exists about how to operationalize gun violence. The available information is limited. Depending on the side one takes on this issue, it is far too easy for any of us to cherry-pick information for the sake of making a point. So, how do we go about generating a workable definition, and why does this matter? As my panel experience illustrated, defining gun violence by type and considering the location and the number of casualties play a role in our understanding of this issue.

Broadly speaking, several types of incidents qualify as gun violence: homicide, suicide, attempted suicide, and accidental shootings. Mass shootings often include homicide, homicide attempts, suicide, and/or attempted suicide. How are these defined? *Firearm homicide* is when a person intentionally kills someone with a gun. *Firearm suicide* is the intentional act of causing one's own death. A *suicide attempt* is when someone tries to kill themselves, but they do not die. And *accidental shootings* are instances where a person accidentally injures or kills themselves or others with a firearm. Mass shootings can include multiple forms of gun violence, therefore there is some variation in how mass shootings are defined. For example, the FBI has typically operationalized *mass murders* (a subset of mass shootings) as incidents where four or more people have been killed in one particular act of violence (excluding the shooter).[24] A more commonly used definition of *mass shooting* is any incident where four or more people have been shot but not necessarily killed (and not including the shooter).[25] There has also been some disagreement over whether mass shootings that are connected to another shooting incident should include the ancillary incident in its count. (Perhaps one of the most well-known examples of this is the Sandy Hook shooting. Prior to shooting multiple children and school personnel at the elementary school in Newtown, CT, the perpetrator killed his mother in her home.)

Nevertheless, if we lump all these gun violence incidents together (considering injury or death from a firearm to be our two outcomes of interest), the numbers are staggering. The average of data from the last 5-year period means 113,150 individuals are shot with a gun in the United States every year. Of these, an estimated 36,500 are killed, and more than 76,000 individuals every year are gunshot survivors.[26]

The majority of people who die by gun violence die by suicide.[27] This translates to an estimated 22,265 people each year.[28] "Completion rates" for suicide with a gun are very high given the lethality of a firearm.[29] As such, a relatively small number of people (3,650) survive a firearm suicide attempt. Conversely, while accidental shootings result in a high number of injuries each year (32,850 on average), fewer than 400 people die from accidental shootings. Within these data and specific to children, nearly 1,500 children are killed with a gun each year and another 6,294 are injured. More than a third of the children who die from gun violence die from suicide with a gun, and of those children who are injured with a gun, nearly half (46%) are shot during accidental shootings.[30]

The term *school shooting* is also operationalized in various ways. For example, Everytown for Gun Safety, a nonprofit organization dedicated to "ending gun violence and building safer communities," has been tracking all school shooting incidents since 2013. They broadly define school shootings as "any time a gun discharges a live round inside (or into) a school building, or on (or onto) a school campus or grounds, where 'school' refers to elementary, middle, and high schools (K-12) as well as colleges and universities."[31]

Various news media outlets (most notably, *The Washington Post* and *CNN*) have also defined and subsequently tracked school shootings. *The Washington Post* data in particular consist of all school shootings since Columbine, and they have been continually adding to this data set since its initial publication in April 2018. Specifically, *The Washington Post* includes nearly every form of gun violence but excludes suicides that occurred privately (in other words, those that did not cause a threat to another child), as well as accidental discharges that did not cause an injury to anyone other than the person handling the gun.[32] Their data differ from most data sources because they not only document how many are injured or killed by gunfire on school property and during school hours, but by using these data they have been able to estimate how many children have been affected by these shootings (specifically, how many children have witnessed gun violence or actively hid from such violence in an effort to stay safe). As of May 2022, *The Washington Post* had documented over 311,000 children who have been exposed to gun violence in K-12 schools in the United States since the shooting at Columbine.[33] For some time, the US Department of Education had been documenting the number of students expelled specifically because they were caught bringing a firearm to school, but they stopped reporting those data in 2010. Data on school discipline are all still documented and made publicly available for nearly every school in the United States. Unfortunately, the reasons for these punishments (e.g., if the reasons are firearm-related) are not known, so the data are limited from the perspective of understanding firearm violence in schools.

What We Can Conclude

Summarizing the problem is complicated. Some overarching conclusions about school shootings can be drawn if we look across these data sets. First, all types of gun violence do occur on school grounds, but the prevalence of mass shootings in particular at schools is actually very small. Less than 1% of all school gun violence is due to mass shootings. Although mass shootings comprise a small percentage of the actual number of gun violence incidents, they also comprise the majority of injuries and deaths from school gun violence. Thus, of all the children who are injured or die during a school shooting scenario, the majority take place during mass shootings. So, state and federal policies that actively reduce access to the most lethal types of firearms might go the farthest toward preventing this particular type of school shooting.[34]

Second, the various data sources about school shootings also show that more than 60% of school shooting incidents take place in majority-minority schools, that is, schools that predominantly serve students of color. Thus, even though the news media narrative about mass shootings in schools focuses on schools that are predominately white, the gun violence burden is largely borne by Black children. A staggering statistic from *Everytown* is that Black students make up 15% of the K-12 US school population, but 24% of those students who are killed or injured on school grounds are Black.[35] Consider that Black students are also disproportionately impacted by other forms of trauma in comparison to their white peers,[36] and so the racial disparities in gun violence

among children must be considered as we invest in the prevention of gun violence across communities.

Third, as we are already seeing, conceptualizing school shootings by the
number of injuries and deaths is somewhat crude. It ignores a large body of
literature on adverse childhood experiences (ACEs), childhood development,
and exposure to violence more broadly. Indeed, my colleagues and I argue that
exposure to gun violence occurs in other forms that must also be accounted
for: being threatened by a gun, hearing gunshots, witnessing gunfire, knowing a friend or family member who has been shot, and having a close friend
or a sibling who carries a gun.[37] Most available research has focused on how
children experience these various interactions, but teachers and other school
staff may have had these experiences as well. Undoubtedly, these experiences
have an impact and likely affect a child's ability to learn and an educator's ability to engage fully with their students and colleagues.

When I have had the chance to share this in different settings, inevitably
someone comments, "but it's the injuries and death that really *matter.*" And to
a degree, I understand that sentiment. In fact, much of my work has focused
solely on injuries and deaths. But exposure to these other forms of gun violence can actually be predictive of future gun violence. According to a recent
paper: "It is important that we include this in our understanding of gun violence exposure since research has shown that certain forms of gun violence
can be thought of as a social contagion, spreading via peer-to-peer networks.[38]
*Thus, individuals are often more likely to be injured or killed with a firearm if
someone they know has also been injured or killed with a firearm.*"[39]

To prevent future gun violence, we need to be responding to and supporting children and their school communities who may have had experiences
with other, less talked about—and less frequently measured—forms of gun
violence. And this is, in fact, a more generative way of utilizing the construct
of anxiety culture in the context of gun violence prevention to further effective solutions.

What does this mean? The original question was how best to define school
gun violence. Perhaps the most useful effort would involve supporting data collection efforts, similar to what *The Washington Post* has done, where we recon-
ceptualize our notion of "gun violence" to include a range of experiences with
firearms. Indeed, I would argue that we need a systematic data collection effort
for all schools within the K-12 system that documents all forms of gun violence
exposure among students and staff. Schools need to be able to understand what
is happening to their students and staff so that they can best support them. We

know if a child has been shot or killed, but what about the children who witness gunfire in school or on their way to and from school? What about children who witness gunfire in their communities? What about school staff who have also been exposed to gunfire in some form? And how does all of this contribute to the larger community anxiety about gun violence?

Supporting schools to document this information and subsequently making these data available to other school districts would do two things: (1) it would allow schools to better understand the forms of violence that their communities are being exposed to and reconsider ways our government (at the federal, state, and municipal levels) could best support them in the aftermath of violence; and (2) it would highlight the prevention of gun violence as a serious public health *and* educational priority. Instead of responding to the anticipation of possible school gun violence with metal detectors, what if we equipped schools with critical knowledge and information about the type and range of experiences their students and staff have endured? Instead of adding to these potentially traumatic experiences through reactive strategies such as active shooter drills, what if we provided support for the school community, for example, by a larger physical mental health staff so that they could better support students and staff who have experienced trauma?

In 2016, Data Quality Campaign published a report titled "*Time To Act: Making Data Work for All Students.*" The authors of the report highlighted four key best practices for schools to collect and then utilize data: (1) measure what matters; (2) make data use possible; (3) be transparent and earn trust; and (4) guarantee access and protect privacy.[40]

Based on these principles, we need to ensure we have an accessible and protected data system in place so that school nurses, psychologists, social workers, teachers, and school administrators can readily access and document the various forms of gun violence their students have experienced. We document whether a student needs glasses for reading or is eligible for other support services. In the same way we can integrate data on child exposure to gun violence into existing data systems for schools. By "measuring what matters" (in this case, understanding the various types of gun violence students have been exposed to), we can better support students and schools alike. Likewise, we can provide school staff with an opportunity to disclose information about their experiences with gun violence and provide them with additional support as needed to ensure they are best able to do their job.

This information can be used to speak accurately to the prevalence of gun violence in our schools and the range of gun violence experiences our children, teachers, and school staff may be experiencing. Schools can subsequently consider embracing what is known as a "trauma-informed" lens[41] by placing an emphasis on enabling students and staff to build supportive nurturing relationships, remove punitive discipline strategies, and invest in curricular efforts that foster social-emotional learning among students, among other such efforts.[42] School administrators can guide the content of professional development efforts for school staff to include educating staff about ACEs more generally, providing crisis management guidance, and educating staff on specific ways to engage with parents and caregivers.

Schools could also choose to integrate information about youth gun violence exposure into an Individualized Education Program (IEP), so that students who might be experiencing poor health outcomes in the aftermath of having been exposed to gun violence in any form, might receive specialized instruction and related services. These data can also help schools set budget priorities.

Ultimately, exposure to gun violence in various forms is linked to a range of poor health and learning outcomes. For schools and school districts looking to improve testing scores, attendance levels, and graduation rates, it is in their best interest—and of course the interest of each child—to reduce the impact of trauma exposure.

Reimagining Solutions: Where Do We Go from Here?

Our society has talked at length about poor mental health as a precursor to gun violence, but we have not equipped schools with the resources to sufficiently address and respond to indicators of poor mental health. The National Association of School Psychologists recommends, at a minimum, no more than 500 students per psychologist. Recent estimates indicate that most school districts in the United States do not meet even this most basic standard.[43] We have hypothesized what the possible behavioral predictors of school gun violence are (e.g., a history of being bullied, exposure to video games, among many others), but we have invested limited federal dollars into research that would allow us to rigorously test these hypotheses.[44]

The leadership of the NRA was famously quoted just one week after the gun massacre at Parkland High School in 2018 as saying "[we need to] figure out a way to harden our schools," a sentiment grounded in the NRA's commitment to American freedom.[45] What if, instead, we did not treat schools as fortresses sheltering scared children and anxious teachers who are clouded by anxiety and an anticipation of fear? What if we reimagined our schools as open, inviting, inclusive, joyful spaces? Schools where children and staff were not simply existing in classrooms absent from violence but who were also thriving, learning, and truly free?

What if we were all collectively equipped with a level of knowledge about gun violence in schools so we could understand this issue with clarity? What if we supported our school—and by extension its staff and students—by providing them with sufficient resources and tools? What if we invested in and implemented comprehensive preventive efforts at the school and community levels that could more likely get to the heart of what precipitates gun violence in the first place? What if it became the norm for schools to embrace a trauma-sensitive lens to better meet the needs of students who have been exposed to gun violence within and outside of their classrooms? What if our government implemented policies at the state and federal levels that were informed by actual data, made it harder for youth to have access to guns, and ensured that the deadliest forms of firearms stayed out of the hands of those with a history of violence? What if we engaged parents, pediatricians, school staff, and others in these conversations? What if we framed the prevention of gun violence, not just as a public health emergency but as a national educational priority? What if we called on our elected officials and leaders of professional organizations to champion the safeguarding of America's schools in a visionary way? What if we took bold, collective action on this issue? What if we recognized that movement forward would result from action on all these fronts?

What if our collective response did not prepare our schools for the inevitability of the next school shooting but rather drew on the notion of anxiety culture that this book attempts to conceptualize as a way in which the eradication of gun violence in schools becomes a genuine possibility? These are the guiding questions we should and can use to reimagine how our schools can be kept safe from school gun violence while ensuring that our children thrive.

NOTES

1. Jaclyn Schildkraut and H. Jaymi Elsass, *Mass Shootings: Media, Myths, and Realities* (Santa Barbara, CA: Praeger Publications, 2016).

2. Everytown for Gun Safety, "Gunfire on School Grounds in the United States," 2022, https://everytownresearch.org/maps/gunfire-on-school-grounds/.

3. Paul M. Reeping et al., "State Firearm Laws, Gun Ownership, and K-12 School Shootings: Implications for School Safety," *Journal of School Violence* 21, no. 2 (2022): 132–146.

4. Reeping et al., "State Firearm Laws," 132–146.

5. Everytown for Gun Safety, "Gunfire on School Grounds in the United States."

6. John Woodrow Cox et al., "School Shootings Database," *The Washington Post*, May 27, 2022, https://www.washingtonpost.com/graphics/2018/local/school-shootings-database/.

7. Sonali Rajan et al., "Youth Exposure to Violence Involving a Gun: Evidence for Adverse Childhood Experience Classification," *Journal of Behavioral Medicine* 42, no. 4 (2019): 646–657.

8. See Pilar Bancalari, Marni Sommer, and Sonali Rajan, "Exposure to Endemic Community Gun Violence: A Systematic Review," *Adolescent Research Review* 7 (September 2022): 383–417; Sam Bieler and Nancy La Vigne, "Close-Range Gunfire Around DC Schools," *Urban Institute*, 2014, https://www.urban.org/sites/default/files/publication/22906/413216-close-range -gunfire-around-dc-schools.pdf; Melissa Tracy, Anthony A. Braga, Andrew V. Papachristos, "The Transmission of Gun and Other Weapon-Involved Violence Within Social Networks," *Epidemiologic Reviews* 38, no. 1 (2016): 70–86; and Amma W. Wright et al., "Systematic Review: Exposure to Community Violence and Physical Health Outcomes in Youth," *Journal of Pediatric Psychology* 42, no. 4 (2017): 364–378.

9. H. Yan and M. Park, "1 week. 3 suicides. 1 Tragic Connection to School Massacres," *CNN*, March 26, 2019, https://www.cnn.com/2019/03/26/us/school-shootings-suicides/index.html.

10. Valentina Cimolai, Jacob Schmitz, and Aradhana Bela Sood, "Effects of Mass Shootings on the Mental Health of Children and Adolescents," *Current Psychiatry Reports* 23, no. 3 (2021): 12.

11. Erica Ford, "Reducing Gun Violence by Healing Trauma," *Essence*, October 23, 2020, https://www.essence.com/op-ed/life-camp-inc-mobile-trauma-unit/.

12. Rajan et al. "Youth Exposure to Violence Involving a Gun."

13. Sonali Rajan and Charles C. Branas, "As We Reimagine Schooling, Let's Reimagine Gun Violence Prevention, Too," *Hechinger Report*, December 10, 2020, https://hechingerreport.org/as -we-reimagine-schooling-lets-reimagine-gun-violence-prevention-too/.

14. "Public Health Approach to Gun Violence Prevention," *Educational Fund to Stop Gun Violence*, 2021, https://efsgv.org/learn/learn-more-about-gun-violence/public-health-approach -to-gun-violence-prevention/.

15. "On 50th Anniversary of Ralph Nader's 'Unsafe at Any Speed,' Safety Group Reports Auto Safety Regulation Has Saved 3.5 Million Lives," *The Nation*, December 1, 2015, https://www .thenation.com/article/archive/on-50th-anniversary-of-ralph-naders-unsafe-at-any-speed -safety-group-reports-auto-safety-regulation-has-saved-3-5-million-lives/.

16. Mai ElSherief et al., "Impacts of School Shooter Drills on the Psychological Well-Being of American K-12 School Communities: A Social Media Study," *Humanities & Social Science Communications* 8, no. 315 (2021).

17. Sonali Rajan and Charles C. Branas, "Arming Schoolteachers: What Do We Know? Where Do We Go From Here?" *American Journal of Public Health* 108, no. 7 (2018): 860–862.

18. RAND Corporation, "The Effects of Laws Allowing Armed Staff in K-12 Schools," 2020, https://www.rand.org/research/gun-policy/analysis/laws-allowing-armed-staff-in-K12 -schools.html#:~:text=State%20implementation%20data%20valid%20as,part%20of%20a%20 specific%20program.

19. Seth J. Prins and Kajeepeta Sandhya, "Visible Security Measures in Schools: Research Summary," 2019, https://criticalsocialepi.org/pdf/Prins%20Visible%20Security%20Measures%20 in%20Schools.pdf; Abigail Hankin, Marci Hertz, and Thomas Simon, "Impacts of Metal Detector Use in Schools: Insights From 15 Years of Research," *Journal of School Health* 81, no. 2 (2011): 100–106; and Bryan R. Warnick and Ryan Kapa, "Protecting Students from Gun Violence. Does 'Target Hardening' Do More Harm Than Good?" *Education Next* 19, no. 2 (2019): 22–28.

20. Prins and Kajeepeta, "Visible Security Measures in Schools: Research Summary."

21. Joseph Tobias et al., "Protect our Kids: A Novel Program Bringing Hemorrhage Control to Schools," *Injury Epidemiology* 8, no. S1 (2021): 31.

22. Centers for Disease Control and Prevention, CDC WONDER, accessed July 4, 2024, https://wonder.cdc.gov/.

23. See Charles C. Branas et al., "Investigating the Link Between Gun Possession and Gun Assault," *American Journal of Public Health* 99, no. 11 (2009): 2034–2040; Elinore J. Kaufman

et al., "State Firearm Laws and Interstate Firearm Deaths From Homicide and Suicide in the United States: A Cross-Sectional Analysis of Data by County," *JAMA Internal Medicine* 178, no. 5 (2018): 692–700; James H. Price, Amy J. Thompson, and Joseph A. Dake, "Factors Associated With State Variations in Homicide, Suicide, and Unintentional Firearm Deaths," *Journal of Community Health* 29, no. 4 (2004): 271–283; and Paul M. Reeping et al., "State Gun Laws, Gun Ownership, and Mass Shootings in the US: Cross Sectional Time Series," *BMJ* 364 (2019): l542.

24. William J. Krouse and Daniel J. Richardson, "Mass Murder with Firearms: Incidents and Victims, 1999–2013," Congressional Research Service, June 30, 2015, https://sgp.fas.org/crs/misc /R44126.pdf.

25. Federal Bureau of Investigation, "Active Shooter Safety Resources," https://www.fbi.gov /about/partnerships/office-of-partner-engagement/active-shooter-resources.

26. AHRQ, "Healthcare Cost and Utilization Project."

27. AHRQ, "Healthcare Cost and Utilization Project."

28. AHRQ, "Healthcare Cost and Utilization Project."

29. David M. Studdert et al., "Handgun Ownership and Suicide in California," *New England Journal of Medicine* 382, no. 23 (2020): 2220–2229.

30. AHRQ, "Healthcare Cost and Utilization Project."

31. Everytown for Gun Safety, "Gunfire on School Grounds in the United States."

32. Cox et al., "School Shooting Database."

33. Cox et al., "School Shooting Database."

34. Louis Klarevas, Andrew Conner, and David Hemenway, "The Effect of Large-Capacity Magazine Bans on High-Fatality Mass Shootings, 1990–2017," *American Journal of Public Health* 109, no. 12 (2019): 1754–1761.

35. Everytown for Gun Safety, "Gunfire on School Grounds in the United States."

36. Joya N. Hampton-Anderson et al., "Adverse Childhood Experiences in African Americans: Framework, Practice, and Policy," *American Psychologist* 76, no. 2 (2021): 314–325.

37. Rajan et al., "Youth Exposure to Violence Involving a Gun."

38. Charles C. Branas, Sara Jacoby, and Elena Andreyeva, "Firearm Violence as a Disease—'Hot People' or 'Hot Spots'?" *JAMA Internal Medicine* 177, no. 3 (2017): 333–334.

39. Ben Green, Thibaut Horel, and Andrew V. Papachristos, "Modeling Contagion Through Social Networks to Explain and Predict Gunshot Violence in Chicago, 2006–2014," *JAMA Internal Medicine* 177, no. 3 (2017): 326–333. Emphasis added.

40. Data Quality Campaign, *Time to Act: Making Data Work for Students*. April 2016, https:// dataqualitycampaign.org/wp-content/uploads/2016/04/Time-to-Act.pdf.

41. Shandra M. Chafouleas et al., "Toward a Blueprint for Trauma-Informed Service Delivery in Schools," *School Mental Health* 8, no. 1 (2016): 144–162.

42. See Rajan and Branas, "As We Reimagine Schooling;" and Nichola Shackleton et al., "School-Based Interventions Going Beyond Health Education to Promote Adolescent Health: Systematic Review of Reviews," *Journal of Adolescent Health* 58, no. 4 (2016): 382–396.

43. National Association of School Psychologists, "Shortage of School Psychologists," 2021, https://www.nasponline.org/research-and-policy/policy-priorities/critical-policy-issues /shortage-of-school-psychologists.

44. Sonali Rajan et al., "Funding for Gun Violence Research is Key to the Health and Safety of the Nation," *American Journal of Public Health* 108, no. 2 (2018): 194–195.

45. Remarks by Wayne LaPierre, executive vice president and CEO of the National Rifle Association, at the Conservative Political Action Conference, February 22, 2018, https://www .democracyinaction.us/photos18/cpac18/nra022218spt.html.

CHAPTER TEN

Adolescent Anxiety

Iceland as Canary in the Coal Mine

CAINE C. A. MEYERS,

INGIBJORG EVA THORISDOTTIR,

BRYNDIS BJORK ASGEIRSDOTTIR,

INGA DORA SIGFUSDOTTIR,

AND JOHN P. ALLEGRANTE

The well-being of young people is of primary concern to practitioners, policymakers, and researchers alike. As we progress further into an era enshrined in ubiquitous technological, political, and societal change, many wonder what effects this will have—and perhaps has already had—on the well-being of young people. Moreover, there is a growing sense of urgency about what consequences might be beyond the horizon if anxiety among young people is neither understood nor addressed as it fits into the greater context of adolescent well-being.

In many places around the world, evidence has accumulated to suggest that the well-being of young people is declining. This decline is primarily characterized as reports of increases in symptoms of anxiety and depression.[1] Anxiety disorders are already among the leading conditions diagnosed in children, with a telling 31.9% of children having received a diagnosis of at least one anxiety disorder in their lifetime.[2] This number is often higher for girls.[3] While anxiety is just one element of the adolescent experience, it has garnered and continues to deserve special attention given its reach among young people. It shares similar social predictors to that of other elements (both emotional and behavioral) of well-being in young people, such as anger, depression, suicide, and substance use, and if left unaddressed, or perhaps worse, *misunderstood*, there is a risk for downstream consequences that extend well into adulthood.[4] This could be especially detrimental at a societal level with a third of young people at risk for developing at least one anxiety disorder in their lifetime. Mental health problems that occur earlier in life are known to increase the risk of poorer mental health throughout the remainder of the life.[5]

Addressing the issue of increased anxiety among young people necessitates a deconstruction of the factors that give rise to both negative and positive emotional and behavioral outcomes, especially as they fit into the context of well-being. Until recently, understanding the scope of these factors has been a challenge, largely due to the lack of a comprehensive framework that incorporates researchers, policymakers, and professionals who are concerned with the growth, development, and well-being of young people.[6] Nonetheless, it has been thoroughly studied within a social context of mental health, generating sufficient knowledge to understand how most adolescents relate to their environment and are reciprocally influenced by it. From the lens of an anxiety culture, which assumes that something about society is related to or perhaps is directly causing an elevation in symptoms of anxiety in adolescents, it is paramount to explore what factors might be at play. Furthermore, it is incumbent upon us to understand what can be done at both the individual and population levels to address these trends by drawing insight from a theoretical framework that seeks to answer these questions at all levels of the individual and their respective society(ies). The country of Iceland may provide critical knowledge into this phenomenon, having been the birthplace of such a framework more than two decades ago and now a world-class leader in population-based prevention work in adolescent substance use.

This chapter will traverse the unique situation that occurred among Icelandic youth and expand upon why this country's perspective is worth hearing about when we speak of anxiety culture. Further, this chapter will seek to convince readers that to first ascertain the existence of an anxiety culture, especially among youth, and to subsequently make sense of it, it is paramount to understand the relationship between adolescents and their environment. Thus, the goal of this chapter is to elucidate some of the mystery around why youth appear to be experiencing more anxiety today by drawing from the work in Iceland since the late 1990s. We believe we can offer several insights as well as caveats.

Iceland as Canary in a Coal Mine

The story begins over two decades ago when a public health crisis occurred among Icelandic adolescents. As regular as clockwork, the streets of the nation's capital, Reykjavik, filled with groups of intoxicated teens—some as young as 13 years old—every weekend. At the same time, reports from the European

Union placed Icelandic youth among those with the highest rate of substance users in Europe. In response to the growing concern, a group of social scientists, policymakers, and practitioners, among others, who worked with children and adolescents, corroborated their concerns around the crisis and sought to adopt a new approach supported by research and community collaboration. This endeavor required a fundamental shift in thinking about teenage behavior and the role of their environment, as well as a collective political will to do things differently. Focused on bringing about a systems change and drawing from sociological theories, the group created a population-level survey to be administered at the school level to monitor the trends of adolescent substance use and to understand the factors associated with this behavior. This endeavor, named *Youth in Iceland*, brought the team a unique insight into the lives of teenagers. The study included factors beyond the young person as an individual, such as their families, schools, peer groups, leisure habits, and the social structures around them. These are otherwise known as the risk and protective factors of substance use among this age group.

An initial sobering analysis of the data indicated that more than 80% of 15- and 16-year-olds had tried alcohol at least once in their lives and 42% had been drunk in the last 30 days in Iceland. Seventeen percent had tried cannabis. It also revealed that specific attributes in the environmental and social structures of adolescents were potential candidate risk and protective factors for substance use. With this knowledge, a shift occurred in prevention efforts, focusing on upstream prevention under the name of the Icelandic Prevention Model. Grounded in evidence, the aim was to prevent problems of adolescent substance use before they arose. The model encouraged more time spent with family, more investment in structured leisure time for activities like sports, arts, and music, and greater monitoring of children's whereabouts and their activities, among other efforts. Above all, the prevention model shifted the burden of responsibility from the young individual to the community and maximized opportunities within the environment of children to engage more in healthy activities. Two decades later, teen substance use in Iceland is among the lowest in Europe. (Figure 10.1).

After having reduced teenage substance use in Iceland, the team shifted their focus to the broader well-being of children and adolescents, which now includes self-reported metrics of anxiety. The infrastructure used for the Icelandic Prevention Model serves today as a means of population-wide surveillance of the health, behavior, and overall well-being of all the youth in Iceland, in addition to now being one of many data registries linked to the

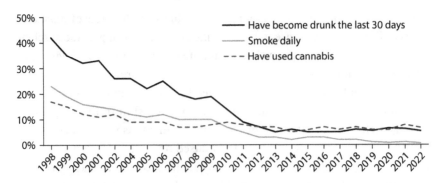

Figure 10.1. Trends of teenage substance use between 1998 and 2022 in Iceland. Source: Adapted from Kristjansson et al., "Development and Guiding Principles of the Icelandic Model for Preventing Adolescent Substance Use," *Health Promotion Practice* 21, no.1 (2020): 65–69.

genetic, developmental, and behavioral profiles of Icelandic youth, allowing for longitudinal research into the biopsychosocial interplay of factors of more than 4,000 adolescents.[7] This has made Iceland somewhat of a "canary in a coal mine" that is situated in the middle of the North American and Eurasian continents. Because the contemporary adolescent culture in Iceland draws much influence from both continents by reason of the rise of globalization, any clues from what is happening in Iceland may transcend to other advanced economies of the world. Researchers and policymakers in Iceland who are constantly monitoring the population trends will have a first glimpse into any changes that may affect the lives and well-being of young people. Thus, if there is a global cultural shift trending toward a culture of anxiety, Iceland is most likely to be among the first to see it and to understand what underlying factors are at play and their implications. Furthermore, Iceland can act quickly with the data-driven approach inherent to the Icelandic Prevention Model. Not only does this make Iceland a bellwether in adolescent research and policymaking, it also demonstrates how Iceland is a canary in a coal mine. If Iceland sounds the alarm, then it may be an indicator that something similar is happening among young people globally and others may wish to take notice.

The Social Conditions of Adolescent Well-Being and Behavior

While much of the following has been previously alluded to, this section will provide further nuance into the nature of adolescent well-being from a social context. Adolescence is a monumental period of development in which the interplay between a young person's biological predispositions and environment emerge and take form.[8] It is a time in which adolescent social development, including behavior, is highly sensitive to their surroundings, thus setting precedence for their emotional and mental well-being later in life.[9] As children transition into adolescence, a greater desire for independence emerges and they begin to spend significantly more time navigating their social lives with their peers.[10] The emotional landscape and behavior of adolescents become heavily influenced by their peer group, while at the same time, family dynamics, school, and community influences continue to contribute to varying degrees. This relationship was evidenced in Iceland during the implementation of the prevention model and continues to be evidenced as concepts and processes of this work are now being scaled globally.[11]

Predictive social factors for teenage behavior emerged across four domains: family, peer group, school, and leisure time (Figure 10.2). The people living in Iceland learned that by changing the environment young people inhabit through these four domains, the likelihood of the protective factors within the four domains changed as well, resulting in a measurable decrease in substance use. Interestingly, despite substance use being the primary outcome of interest, theft and vandalism also decreased, perhaps indicating there are horizontal effects to these efforts.

Of course, the social conditions of adolescent well-being and behavior cannot be written about without consideration for the modern-day context, especially as we anticipate and observe changes to the landscapes and subsequent dynamics of adolescent social exchange with increased social media use. In under 20 years, social media has become an integral part of the lives of young people, with almost all adolescents using some form of social media. In Iceland, approximately 48% to 58% of girls and 24% to 29% of boys in grades eight to ten use social media three hours or more daily.[12] Despite now being more than a decade after the debut of social media and its integration into most lives, there remains much speculation about whether, and to what extent, it transforms the dynamics of traditional youth relationships. As such, its role is largely uncertain. It is also uncertain whether an actual transformation of relationships would even carry any sort of negative consequences.

Only recently has a framework been developed to study and think about the nature of these relationships, particularly peer relationships, within the context of social media.[13] In this framework, Nesi and colleagues point out that social media has potentially created an environment where peer-relationship dynamics have become amplified, in that adolescents have become more

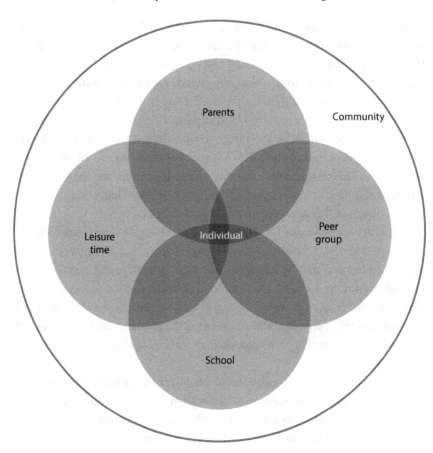

Figure 10.2. The young individual in relation to aspects of their social environment.
Source: Adapted from Kristjansson et al., "Development and Guiding Principles of the
Icelandic Model for Preventing Adolescent Substance Use," *Health Promotion Practice* 21, no.1
(2020): 65–69.

frequently subject to peer contact, to public displays of the self, and to feedback from others. In turn, this may be increasing distress among teens around
peer acceptance and identity formation, thereby also increasing negative
self-evaluation, social comparison, as well as negative perceptions of support
from friends. Because adolescents are already highly sensitive to these peer-
related stressors, it may be plausible that the amplification of these peer attributes is related to the observed decreases in mental well-being.

Latest Trends in Iceland

In 2013, parents, school psychologists, and researchers working with the Icelandic Prevention Model, among others, sounded the alarm that something else was changing with regard to the well-being of adolescence in Iceland. Both observations and anecdotal reports suggested a potential increase in anxiety among young people. Since the Icelandic Prevention Model is based on a constant dialogue between policymakers, researchers, and practitioners, it was possible to apply the data-driven approach to examine if that really was the case. A rise at one time point is enough to raise awareness among those working with and for youth.

To be able to gauge the change in symptoms of anxiety and to understand if teens with high symptom levels follow a similar pattern over time, a cut-off score was created based on the top 5% in the year 2006. The scale is from zero to nine and those that score between seven and nine are considered as having high symptoms. This does not translate to clinical symptoms, however, but is meant to be a measure of change over time.

Some unsettling trends were uncovered in self-reported symptoms of anxiety in teens between the ages of 15 and 16 years old, particularly among girls, among whom symptoms appear to have been on a fairly steady incline since 2006.[14] This upward trend continued in the past decade while more or less stabilizing in boys.

Based on this criterion, 8.2% of girls were estimated as having high symptoms of anxiety in 2006 compared to 2.2% of boys. In 2022, the proportion of girls reporting high symptoms has increased to 20.3% with the proportion of boys having increased to 3.5% (Figure 10.3). When we use mean scores (Figure 10.4) as an indicator for increased symptoms of anxiety, the change is not as visible. This suggests that, overall, the groups comprise students with both high and low symptoms, and we may be witnessing a polarization where more students report little to no anxiety and more students report feeling very anxious.

Considering these numbers, there are several potential explanations for this general upward trend. For example, climate anxiety is speculated to be an emerging phenomenon where adolescents' perceptions of the future are becoming increasingly despondent—so much so that these perceptions may be producing a negative impact on their well-being.[15] This has not been directly measured in Iceland. Others suggest that it is the ongoing exposure to negative

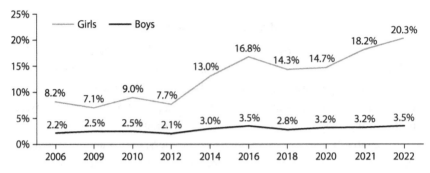

Figure 10.3. Proportion of Icelandic 15- to 16-year-olds reporting high symptoms of anxiety (cut-off score >7) between 2006 and 2022.

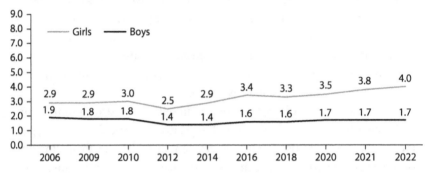

Figure 10.4. Mean symptoms of anxiety as reported by 15- to 16-year-olds in Iceland between 2006 and 2022.

world events, political polarization, and global inequities through social media and other forms of media, such as the news.[16] Again, some make the case that social media may have created an environment that amplifies the stressors associated with adolescent peer dynamics (recall Nesi and colleagues).[17] Indeed, all of this, including the fact that it has become more normalized to talk about feelings, could reasonably contribute to more self-reported symptoms of anxiety among adolescents. And, of course, there are other plausible reasons out there that have not been mentioned. The challenge remains in disentangling the relationships that underly these observations, as well as their magnitudes and direction. If there is a case to be made for an anxiety culture, perhaps it can then be best characterized by the uncertainty of it all coupled with the awareness that something is happening. Young people, especially girls, are reporting that they feel more anxious (both physically and socially), but the underlying reasons remain a mystery.

To stick with the metaphor, this is much like the canaries in the coal mines, who were used by coal miners to detect primarily carbon monoxide even though other gases very well could have been present. The miners never really knew which gas it was that the canaries were being distressed by. Regardless, any distress indicated that swift action was necessary to save the canaries and the human coal miners. In the case of the miners, this meant exiting the mine before the gas levels killed them. In the case of Iceland, this has meant further exploration deeper into the mines, so to speak, of the adolescent experience in relation to the broader cultural and social environment.

Are the Social Conditions of Contemporary Adolescence an Explanation?

Understanding predictors within the social conditions of young people is integral to ensuring their well-being. Furthermore, regardless of the inherent causal relationships that determine adolescent behavior and well-being (that have yet to be fully deconstructed), certain elements within the social environment of young people lie somewhere along the causal chain and have predictive value. The four key domains of the Icelandic Prevention Model can be revisited to look for clues to explain the decrease in adolescent well-being today. Iceland has already begun doing this work.

Since the implementation of the model, the time young people spend with their parents has increased, and stable parental support and parental monitoring has been rising in Iceland. Therefore, changes in family dynamics can be ruled out as a potential explanation with a high degree of certainty. Likewise, young people continue to engage in high-quality leisure activities such as sports, music, and art. Thus, this too can be ruled out with a degree of certainty. Peer relationships, however, have undergone a noticeable change, which might be worth exploring. In 2006, 66% of girls ages 15 to 16 reported that it was very easy to discuss personal issues with their friends compared to 33% of boys. Today, the number for girls has decreased to 42% and for boys to 30% (Figure 10.5). Likewise, in 2006, 23% of boys reported that it was very easy to receive caring and warmth from friends compared to 61% of girls. Figure 10.6 shows that trends of receiving caring and warmth from friends has fluctuated for girls, peaking in 2012, before declining again until 2022, below baseline, whereas for boys, trends have initially increased, before approximately returning to baseline.

These trends raise some crucial questions and in fact provide some tantalizing clues as to why we are observing a significant rise in self-reported

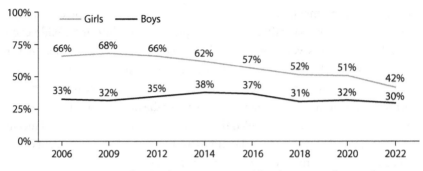

Figure 10.5. Percentage of Iceland 15- to 16-years-olds who reported it was "very easy" to discuss personal matters with friends between 2006 and 2022.

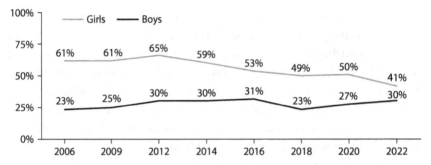

Figure 10.6. Percentage of 15- to 16-years-olds who reported it was "very easy" to receive caring and warmth from friends between 2006 and 2022.

symptoms of anxiety—especially among girls. Since adolescence is heavily characterized by peer relationships, and these dynamics demonstrably play a significant role in shaping the emotional well-being of young people, a decrease in perceptions of peer support may result in increased anxiety among adolescents. The question is: Why have perceptions changed over the past decade, more so for girls than boys?

Connected More Than Ever—But, Not Really

Being "connected more than ever," is somewhat of a cliché, but it is appropriate in light of the recent findings around changes in perceived peer support among teens. Although the term *connected* typically refers to social media use (i.e., being connected online), it does not necessarily imply that social media is the underlying or sole perpetrator responsible for the observed increases in adolescent anxiety. Nonetheless, it intuitively feels like a good place to start, especially bearing in mind the framework of Nesi and colleagues, which as you may recall, hypothesized that social media may be transforming the nature of peer relationships by reason of amplifying peer-related stressors.[18] This starting place is also supported by recent findings in Iceland that provide some insight around social media use, particularly the type of social media use associated with these stressors, and its effects on adolescent well-being. Adolescents who spent more time passively engaged in social media (e.g., scrolling with no purpose) were at a greater risk for decreased well-being compared to those who spent more time actively engaged in social media (e.g., using social media with a purpose to connect).[19] In fact, peer support emerged as a protective factor for those actively engaged in social media use against decreased well-being. This provides considerable evidence that something about changes in peer dynamics could be affecting the well-being of young people, and it may be related to social media use. None of this constitutes definitive evidence that social media is first on the causal chain to decreased adolescent well-being. It could be (and is likely to be) just one piece of a much bigger puzzle on the long chain with reciprocal relationships and feedback loops.

The amount of time young people spend using social media that could otherwise be spent in more intimate spaces with peers and in pursuit of other, perhaps more rewarding, activities is interesting to consider. We hypothesize that communication and the nature of social interactions among adolescents have been changing over the past decade, characterized primarily as a loss of intimacy between peers in exchange for the traditional peer-related stressors being amplified through social media use. In other words, peer support remains an important protective factor in the lives of young people, not only against substance use and other negative behaviors but also against poor well-being, which may include symptoms of anxiety. This can, in part, explain why girls appear to be affected more since not only are they more sensitive to the traditional peer-related stressors than boys[20] but girls reported a decrease in perceived peer support over the past decade whereas boys reported relatively no changes. The caveat is that this has been written today by drawing from the best available evidence, which unfortunately remains subject to many limitations. It also does not address the possible effects among gender diverse adolescents. More research needs to be done on those who do not identify within the gender binary of boy or girl. Albeit there is no reason to believe that peer support would not be an important protective factor in the lives of gender nonbinary adolescents as well because adolescence is a critical developmental period for the shaping of one's identity.

Speculations abound on how different factors in the social environment of children and adolescents can be linked to anxiety. *Anxiety culture* might not be the correct term to describe changes to the society, unless it is written about carefully. Facing obstacles, coping with changes, and solving dilemmas are all part of the human experience and, as previous generations have demonstrated, we are resilient. Even if young people report more symptoms of anxiety compared to that of the cohorts before them, it does not necessarily mean that they perceive these symptoms as negative. Anxiety serves an adaptive purpose. Therefore, the narrative that is provided to them ought to be carefully considered. Research has shown that culture and society can have an impact on one's willingness and ability to express emotions honestly; therefore, it does not necessarily mean that there has been an inherent increase in symptoms of anxiety.[21] Perhaps it has simply become normalized to talk about feelings and to recognize feelings. Overall, these observations might simply be indicative of a bigger, global cultural change, which encompasses a fundamental change in means of communication, thereby altering certain protective dynamics of peer relationships.

Insight from the COVID-19 Pandemic

The day-to-day routines that had defined adolescence for most children were significantly disrupted by the COVID-19 pandemic in Iceland, despite being a country with relatively flexible restrictions for children and youth compared to other non-Nordic countries. Although the public health responses by Icelandic officials typically favored preserving the lives of youth and adolescents to the greatest extent possible, temporary lockdowns were enforced, and children were required to attend school virtually from home, refrain from hanging out with friends, and cease engaging in other group activities (e.g., sports, music, art) during this time. The strain on children created under these circumstances were of grave concern for Icelandic officials as the pandemic intersected with the increased prevalence for mental health problems among adolescents within the country.

Two studies found evidence for decreased adolescent well-being during the pandemic.[22] In addition, the Icelandic Ombudsman for Children collected and published stories from children recounting what it was like to be a child in the pandemic.[23] This provided children the opportunity to emphasize how their lives had become different. On average, they expressed feeling content during this time; they observed less tension in their homes during the mornings, spent more time with their families at home, and caught up on sleep. Among the greatest reported burden of the pandemic, however, was restrictions against seeing peers.

Anecdotally, family dynamics improved during the pandemic, but friend dynamics were negatively affected. Empirically, we see that adolescent well-being decreased overall during the pandemic. Taken together, this further provokes the thought that peer relationships play a large role in adolescent mental and emotional well-being, even during collective societal strain, such as a pandemic.

For the sake of transparency, much of the foregoing discussion remains speculation, and the toll on adolescent mental health after the pandemic remains unknown. It is difficult to surmise whether it will have an overall positive or negative effect on the well-being of children, and despite much speculation favoring the latter, it is uncertain whether it will accelerate the already increasing prevalence of mental health problems among this age group or taper off. The early evidence suggests that even after restrictions have been eased, mental health has not improved. Not all children, however, come from the same homes. Those living in unfavorable home conditions have been disproportionately negatively affected by the pandemic. Nevertheless, it remains an important topic to touch upon given its global reach. With time we may see what societal or cultural elements are the strongest predictors of adolescent well-being, which includes symptoms of anxiety, with some data already alluding to these answers. As a collective, we need to be prepared, especially in light of the knowledge that, prior to the pandemic, rates of these self-reported symptoms were already rising.

What We Can Expect and What Needs to be Done

What does the future hold? If it is true that young people are losing important intimate connection in exchange for amplified peer-related stressors, then this upward trend will likely continue in the absence of something being done— especially among girls. Furthermore, we can expect an additional rise in self-reported symptoms of anxiety that may not necessarily be representative of anything clinical or negative, given the ongoing normalization of talking about feelings across many cultures. Whether they become clinical (negative), however, may be contingent on the narrative that is superimposed onto them.

At the beginning of this chapter, the modern era was characterized as being a time enshrined in ubiquitous change. Inevitably, this comes with uncertainty, and uncertainty can, among other things, manifest as anxiety on an individual level. And it can do so on collective cultural and social levels as well.

The world *is* changing, and perhaps young people are simply telling us, whether knowingly or not, that they are noticing. Because they may not necessarily know how to respond to these feelings, it is important to provide them with the right messages and tools.

Those who work with children and youth and those who are raising children in these ever-challenging circumstances can help by discerning between what is adaptive and what is cause for further concern. Anxiety as a result of perceiving less support from friends is probably adaptive rather than clinically significant. It is a *signal* that a critical necessity of well-being is missing, and so a behavioral change—such as less time spent passively scrolling on social media and more time intimately and actively engaged with peers— may need to happen. As such, young people will likely benefit from parents and caregivers encouraging more time spent intimately with friends and using social media actively to engage with friends rather than using it passively. They may also benefit from parents and caregivers actively creating more circumstances in their lives that increase the likelihood of this happening, without necessarily removing social media from their lives.

Policymakers and practitioners can improve the lives of young people by increasing and advocating for increases in mental health care resources. Primarily, they can help teach young people that emotions are adaptive. Young people should not be taught to fear anxiety. Instead, they should be taught that although it is increasingly more acceptable to acknowledge and talk about feeling anxious about themselves and about the world, it is important to learn how to cope and how to accept and respond to these emotions in a healthy manner. In fact, perhaps this message would even resonate with those trying to make sense of this phenomenon. Rather than something to be feared, a societal manifestation of anxiety or a society that supposedly creates anxiety may in fact be a collective signal that something ought to change.

In conclusion, four elements make up a young person's social environment. Peers, family, leisure habits, and school all have strong predictive value for the well-being and behavior of adolescents. Iceland is unique in that the work done to understand how their young people relate to and are affected by these domains began over 20 years ago, and the results of this work have already translated well beyond just a successful reduction in teenage substance use. The impact on Iceland, which consistently ranks as one of the happiest places or best places to live on earth, at the collective society level has been considerable, even in the face of the same global changes other countries are facing. Iceland has experienced one of the quickest industrial revolutions and cultural changes ever, has lost cultural environmental beacons such as glaciers to climate change, is situated on a volcanic island that creates a lot of uncertainty and vulnerability, and is repeatedly subjected to six months of dark, dreary winter weather every year. Yet Icelanders gracefully hold on to this top spot. Anyone serious about improving the lives of young people, which must include addressing their mental well-being, needs to understand how their own children relate to these four domains. While the recommendations provided here are certainly worth pursuing, more needs to be done. When it comes to the future of our young people, it is incumbent upon us to make a global effort to ensure that each child lives in a society or has access to a society that strives to take care of them. This necessitates building the infrastructure to monitor the well-being of young people everywhere and to build an evidence-based foundation for intervention work. The absence of these critical social supports for well-being in adolescents—that indeed extend into adulthood—may in fact be the driver of the culture of anxiety we are observing. The absence of protective factors among peers, leisure habits, school, and family, which are embedded in the broader community, creates insecurity and uncertainty in everyone's lives. The canary is sounding the alarm; it is time to fix the coal mine.

NOTES

1. See Stephan Collishaw, "Annual Research Review: Secular Trends in Child and Adolescent Mental Health," *Journal of Child Psychology and Psychiatry* 56, no. 3 (2015): 370–393; Natalie Durbeej et al., "Trends in Childhood and Adolescent Internalizing Symptoms: Results from Swedish Population Based Twin Cohorts," *BMC Psychology* 7, no. 1 (2019): 50; Inga D. Sigfusdottir et al., "Trends in Depressive Symptoms, Anxiety Symptoms and Visits to Healthcare Specialists: A National Study among Icelandic Adolescents," *Scandinavian Journal of Public Health* 36, no. 4 (2008): 361–368; and Ingibjorg E. Thorisdottir et al., "The Increase in Symptoms of Anxiety and Depressed Mood among Icelandic Adolescents: Time Trend between 2006 and 2016," *European Journal of Public Health* 27, no. 5 (2017): 856–861.

2. Kathleen Ries Merikangas, Erin F. Nakamura, and Ronald C. Kessler, "Epidemiology of Mental Disorders in Children and Adolescents," *Dialogues in Clinical Neuroscience* 11, no. 1 (2009): 7–20.

3. Kathleen Ries Merikangas et al., "Lifetime Prevalence of Mental Disorders in US Adolescents: Results from the National Comorbidity Study-Adolescent Supplement (NCS-A)," *Journal of the American Academy of Child and Adolescent Psychiatry* 49, no. 10 (2010): 980–989.

4. See Bryndis Bjork Asgeirsdottir et al., "Protective Processes for Depressed Mood and Anger among Sexually Abused Adolescents: The Importance of Self-Esteem," *Personality and Individual Differences* 49, no. 5 (2010): 402–407; Inga-Dora Sigfusdottir, George Farkas, and Eric Silver, "The Role of Depressed Mood and Anger in the Relationship Between Family Conflict and Delinquent Behavior," *Journal of Youth and Adolescence* 33, no. 6 (2004): 509–522; and Inga Dora Sigfusdottir et al., "Suicidal Ideations and Attempts among Adolescents Subjected to

Childhood Sexual Abuse and Family Conflict/Violence: The Mediating Role of Anger and Depressed Mood," *Journal of Adolescence* 36, no. 6 (2013): 1227–1236.

5. Ronald C. Kessler et al., "Age of Onset of Mental Disorders: A Review of Recent Literature," *Current Opinion in Psychiatry* 20, no. 4 (2007): 359–364.

6. Thorhildur Halldorsdottir et al., "A Multi-Level Developmental Approach towards Understanding Adolescent Mental Health and Behaviour: Rationale, Design and Methods of the LIFECOURSE Study in Iceland," *Social Psychiatry and Psychiatric Epidemiology* 56, no. 3 (2021): 519–529; and Inga Dora Sigfusdottir et al., "Stress and Adolescent Well-Being: The Need for an Interdisciplinary Framework," *Health Promotion International* 32, no. 6 (2017): 1081–1090.

7. Drs. Thorhildur Halldorsdottir and Inga Dora Sigfusdottir have written extensively on this framework. See Sigfusdottir et al. "Stress and Adolescent Well-being," 1081–1089; and Halldorsdottir et al. "A Multi-Level Developmental Approach," 519–529.

8. Tomás Paus, Matcheri Keshavan, and Jay N. Giedd, "Why Do Many Psychiatric Disorders Emerge during Adolescence?" *Nature Reviews. Neuroscience* 9, no. 12 (2008): 947–957.

9. Natasha H. Bailen, Lauren M. Green, and Renee J. Thompson, "Understanding Emotion in Adolescents: A Review of Emotional Frequency, Intensity, Instability, and Clarity," *Emotion Review* 11, no. 1 (2019): 63–73.

10. Wendy E. Ellis and Lynne Zarbatany, "Understanding Processes of Peer Clique Influence in Late Childhood and Early Adolescence," *Child Development Perspectives* 11, no. 4 (2017): 227–232.

11. The Icelandic Prevention Model is currently being implemented in hundreds of communities worldwide with support and guidance from the Icelandic research consultancy, Planet Youth. See https://planetyouth.org.

12. See page 25 of Rannsóknir og greining (Icelandic Centre for Social Research and Analysis), "Ungt fólk 2022: Landið" ("Youth in Iceland 2022: The Country"), https://rannsoknir.is/wp-content/uploads/2022/04/Ungt-Folk-8.-til-10.-bekkur-2022-Landid.pdf (Icelandic text). A previous study by Ingibjorg E. Thorisdottir et al., "Longitudinal Association between Social Media Use and Psychological Distress among Adolescents," *Preventive Medicine* 141 (December 2020): 106270, https://doi.org/10.1016/j.ypmed.2020.106270, found that the impact of time spent on social media and all outcomes of psychological distress was stronger for Icelandic girls than boys and that increased social media use was positively related to symptoms of depressed mood over time.

13. Jacqueline Nesi, Sophia Choukas-Bradley, and Mitchell J. Prinstein, "Transformation of Adolescent Peer Relations in the Social Media Context: Part 1—A Theoretical Framework and Application to Dyadic Peer Relationships," *Clinical Child and Family Psychology Review* 21, no. 3 (2018): 267–294.

14. See Thorisdottir et al., "Increase in Symptoms of Anxiety," 856–861.

15. Elizabeth Marks et al., "Young People's Voices on Climate Anxiety, Government Betrayal and Moral Injury: A Global Phenomenon," *SSRN Scholarly Paper* (ID 3918955) (Rochester, NY: Social Science Research Network, 2021), https://doi.org/10.2139/ssrn.3918955.

16. Amandeep Dhir et al., "Online Social Media Fatigue and Psychological Wellbeing—A Study of Compulsive Use, Fear of Missing out, Fatigue, Anxiety and Depression," *International Journal of Information Management* 40 (June 2018): 141–152.

17. Nesi, Choukas-Bradley, and Prinstein, "Transformation of Adolescent Peer Relations in the Social Media Context."

18. Nesi, Choukas-Bradley, and Prinstein, "Transformation of Adolescent Peer Relations in the Social Media Context."

19. Ingibjorg Eva Thorisdottir et al., "Active and Passive Social Media Use and Symptoms of Anxiety and Depressed Mood Among Icelandic Adolescents," *Cyberpsychology, Behavior and Social Networking* 22, no. 8 (2019): 535–542.

20. Inga Dora Sigfusdottir and Eric Silver, "Emotional Reactions to Stress Among Adolescent Boys and Girls: An Examination of the Mediating Mechanisms Proposed by General Strain Theory," *Youth & Society* 40, no. 4 (2008): 571–590.

21. Bernardo Paoli, Rachele Giubilei, and Eugenio De Gregorio, "Tears of Joy as an Emotional Expression of the Meaning of Life," *Frontiers in Psychology* 13 (2022): 792580.

22. See Thorhildur Halldorsdottir et al., "Adolescent Well-Being amid the COVID-19 Pandemic: Are Girls Struggling More than Boys?" *JCPP Advances* 1, no. 2 (2021): e12027; and Ingibjorg Eva Thorisdottir et al., "Depressive Symptoms, Mental Wellbeing, and Substance Use among Adolescents before and during the COVID-19 Pandemic in Iceland: A Longitudinal, Population-Based Study," *The Lancet Psychiatry* 8, no. 8 (2021): 663–672.

23. See Umboðsmaður Barna (Icelandic Ombdusman for Children), "Frásagnir barna af heimsfaraldri" ("Children's Stories of the Pandemic"), https://www.barn.is/frasagnir-barna-af-covid-2/ (Icelandic text).

CHAPTER ELEVEN

Anxiety and Global Health

Chinese Perspectives

ANGELIKA MESSNER,

ROMAN MAREK, AND

ZHAO XUDONG

*Everyday life in current China . . . entails extensive concerns for
well-being and deep-seated fears of vulnerability*[1]

The temporal or geographical comparison regarding the prevalence of mental
disorders is challenging. One inevitably runs into difficulties concerning the
comparability of diagnostic tools, cultural specificities, and ethical factors.[2]
Therefore, the consideration of cultural issues has been addressed for diagnosis criterions of anxiety disorders and trauma- and stressor-related disorders
in both DSM-5 and ICD-11. For instance, patients suffering from generalized
anxiety disorder (GAD) in non-Western societies are more likely to complain
of somatic symptoms than their Western counterparts.[3] However, some of the
somatic symptoms reported by GAD patients in Hong Kong are not even included in the DSM, such as palpitations, difficulty breathing, and sweating.[4]
Here, a concrete case might illustrate the importance of integrating cultural
context to understand a patient's perspectives on stress, coping styles, and
family dynamics. This case highlights some unique features of rapidly changing traditions and living conditions in China, for example, the so-called 4-2-1
family structure (4 grandparents, 2 parents, 1 child) due to the one-child policy (一孩政策) during the past decades, as well as the Confucian family concept with its moral emphasis on filial piety. In the following case, all these
factors intertwine and contribute to the psychopathology of an anxiety
disorder.

A Clinical Vignette

A 32-year-old man was initially referred by the emergency department for recurrent, excessive anxiety over a three-month period, physically associated with intermittent chest pain, shortness of breath, sweat, and oral dryness. The symptoms lasted several hours each day, worsening in the afternoons, just before returning home from his office. Prior to seeking help in the emergency department, the patient had experienced several stressful life events. Three years ago, he got married and cofounded a security company. His business thrived and he had already begun setting up a new company. However, he suffered a series of misfortunes: his father-in-law was diagnosed with terminal liver cancer, which led to depression in his wife (i.e., the patient's mother-in-law) and eventually to her unexpected death by suicide. Yet, the father-in-law's diagnosis turned out to be wrong, and he was discharged from hospital with a favorable prognosis. Thereupon, he quickly started a new romantic relationship with another woman who subsequently moved into the family home. This behavior was considered "immoral, shameless, and ungrateful" by many of the family's acquaintances and friends. The situation deeply hurt his daughter (the patient's wife), causing the latter to "lose face" (*diūliǎn* 丢脸), and leading to conflicts among family members. One year prior to the onset of the patient's symptoms, his wife gave birth to a son. Several months later, the 2007 financial crisis began to affect the patient's business. The family stressors were exacerbated by China's 4-2-1 family structure since the patient and his wife both represented the only offspring in their generation. Emotions were additionally intensified by the Confucian emphasis on the family as a focus of moral behavior, expressed by filial piety and continuation of the family line. The patient was diagnosed with a generalized anxiety disorder and treated with medications and family therapy. After two months of treatment, he recovered.

The case highlights the influence of general sociological trends and cultural specificities on an individual's psychological condition. Since China's rapid modernization processes weakened collective structures and fueled inequalities, the subject of anxiety in China began to draw the attention of both Chinese and Western sociologists.[5] Chinese sociologists, who were studying the concept of increasing consumerism in the late 20th century and the rise of individualism in both rural and urban settings,[6] addressed the issue of anxiety in the context of China becoming a "fractured society" (*duànliè shèhuì* 断裂 社会).[7] For example, anxiety disorders are more common in "left-behind children" (i.e., children who live separately from their parents as their parents work in more developed areas) in China.[8] Recently, the topic of anxiety in China also entered the realm of mass media. Based on epidemiological studies,[9] media reports quickly jumped to the conclusion that "Anxiety is on the Rise in China."[10] This first wave of attention to anxiety in China mostly explained the phenomenon by the "breathless pace of economic reform."[11] Then, in the course of the global COVID-19 pandemic, a second wave of global public attention hit China. This time, not only was yet another rise of anxiety observed[12] but also the emergence of an open expression of feelings, resulting in a public discourse on psychological problems.[13] Thus, within a relatively short time, anxiety in China became the subject of two distinct global waves of attention. The distinction lies not only in the alleged causes of (presumably) rising levels of anxiety in China but also in the discourses, *topoi*, or metanarratives the two waves touched. While the first wave discussed anxiety in the context of age, gender, and in the rhetoric of (social, economic, cultural, political, etc.) transition (*zhuanxingqi* 转型期),[14] the second wave quickly identified the pandemic as the culprit. It remains to be seen whether this media coverage also perpetuated the *topos* of China as "the other," as something alien to "us," where people feel and express their emotions differently (i.e., less than "us"). Thus, while the development of anxiety levels in China is interesting as such, the discussion of these levels might prove to be just as—or even more— interesting. Do Chinese people have their own unique perception of anxiety? Is anxiety in China different from anxiety in Western culture? How do Chinese people understand (their) anxiety?

Anxiety in the Chinese Language

As discussed elsewhere in this book, the term *anxiety* (just like *anger*, *angst*, *anguish*) derived from the Proto-Indo-European root *h_2engh-, meaning narrow, tight, to constrict, to compress, be distressed, or be anxious. The Chinese character for narrowness or tightness is 悶 (*mēn*). Initially, many Chinese characters were intended to visually represent their meaning. In the course of time, these early pictograms were continuously systematized and evolved in the so-called character radicals that are used in contemporary written Chinese. Today, the majority of Chinese characters comprise a combination of two (or more) of these components. Usually, one of the radicals indicates the meaning or the category of a character, while the other specifies its pronunciation. But there is more to this combination of components and radicals creating a single sign, because often the radicals involved convey a little story within themselves. For example, the Chinese character 悶 for tightness is composed of two radicals: 門 (*mén*) for "gate," "door," "entrance," "opening;" and 心 (*xīn*), representing the heart. Thus, this character depicts the heart constrained between two doorposts. In Japanese, the (identical) Kanji character 悶 means "to be in agony," "to worry."[15] It is interesting to note that the radical used to constrain the heart is the door (門), and not, for example, the more common radical 囗 (*wéi*), a character already combining two radicals to convey the meaning "enclosure." Could it be that the character should indicate a more floating, transient character of "narrowness" since it takes only one step forward or backward to escape the tightness of a doorframe? Or does the character indicate that the feeling of tightness forms part of a *rite de passage*, that it is a feeling connected to the transition from one sphere to the other, when you still cling to the old and are hesitant to enter the new? Of course, these thoughts remain highly speculative, but it is of note that the Chinese character for "threshold" also combines our two doorposts (門) with the character meaning "or," "perhaps," "possibly," "else," or "maybe": 閾.

Concerning expressions and descriptions of anxiety, Chinese language has a rich vocabulary. Just to mention a few: 焦慮 (*jiāo lǜ*): anxiety, fear; 惶 (*huáng*): frightened; 慮 (*lǜ*): worry and concern; 憂 (*yōu*): worry, fear, concern, sorrow, care; 憂慮 (*yōu lǜ*): to worry/anxiety (about); 愁苦 (*chóu kǔ*): distress. The Chinese language character commonly used to convey the meaning of "anxiety" (恐, *kǒng*) brings us back our heart (心) in action, this time combined with the character 鞏 (*gǒng*) meaning "to bind" or "to guard."

In a historical perspective, the character 恐 appears quite often in literary and medical texts, for example conveying the meaning of "sincere worriedness" (*chéng kǒng* 誠恐) in the sense of a doctor worrying about the well-being of his or her patients. This worriedness is not to be confused with general fear of bandits or demons, or the anxiety (*kǒngjù* 恐懼) of a woman in the throes of childbirth whose newborn might die. The difference between anxiety (恐, *kǒng*) and fear (懼, *jù*) is not fundamental, even though this distinction is rudimentarily discussed in ancient medical texts. However, anxiety (恐, *kǒng*) is consistently associated with the physical realm.

Concepts of Anxiety from Chinese Perspectives: Localizing of Emotions

In Chinese culture, a "body-cartography" associates internal organs with characteristic traits and emotional dispositions. The canonical medical textbook of classic Chinese literature, the *Huángdì Nèijīng* 黃帝內經 (*The Inner*

Canon of the Yellow Emperor, 206 BCE–220 CE), identifies the five viscera as orbs where essences accumulate (*wǔ jīng suǒ bìng* 五精所並). The five viscera are: the heart, the liver, the lungs, the kidney, and the spleen. The liver is identified as the source of worry, while the kidneys are identified as the source of fear:

> When the essences (*jing* 精) and *Qi* 氣 [of all five yin-organs] conglomerate in the heart, it will give rise to joy (*xi* 喜); when it concentrates in the lungs, it will give rise to sorrow (*bei* 悲), when it concentrates in the liver, it will give rise to worry (*you* 憂); when it concentrates in the spleen, it will give rise to dread (*wei* 偎); when it concentrates in the kidneys, it will give rise to fear (*Kong* 恐) 五精所並：精氣並於心則善，並於肺則悲，並於肝則憂，並於脾則畏，並於腎則恐，是謂五並，虛而相並者也[16]

Thus, the *Huángdì Nèijīng* 黃帝內經 localizes anxiety in various parts of the body, most importantly in the heart, the gall bladder, and the kidneys.[17] A "sinking gallbladder" (*danluo* 胆落) manifests itself in anxiety and panic (*zhānghuáng* 張皇), while fright and panic (*jīngjù* 驚懼) as much as hopelessness (*shīwàng* 失望) will increase.[18] Moreover, for example, a "small" (shrunken, tightened, contracted) gall bladder (*dǎn xiao* 膽小) is associated with timidity, anxiety, even cowardice (*qiè* 怯). In contrast, courage (*yǒng* 勇) derives from a "big" (swollen) gall bladder. This association is established as early as in the aforementioned *Huángdì Nèijīng*. Since anxiety is often accompanied by palpitations, a frightened heart and a trembling gall bladder are seen as indications for a weakened gall bladder (*dǎn qiè* 胆怯). In addition, tuberculosis—the so-called consumptiveness (*láo qiè zhī zhèng* 痨怯之症)—is also accompanied by anxiety and is thus associated with injured (*shāng* 傷) heart- and lung-*Qi*, and with an overall damaged *Qi*, for example, after childbirth. We will therefore examine the concept of *Qi* in the following paragraph.

The localization of emotions is a difficult task. Yet, it is even harder to measure, quantify, and visualize bodily perceptions of emotions. Jari K. Hietanen and colleagues from the University of Tampere in Finland started an interesting project involving special algorithms that could analyze visual representations in body silhouettes (Figure 11.1).[19] They asked 701 persons to indicate bodily sensations associated with different emotions using a "unique topographical self-report method." The bodily sensations associated with anxiety were an increased activation in the upper chest, especially around the heart, and in the middle of the body, combined with a decreased activation in the legs, indicating a more depressing, constraining emotion. When comparing

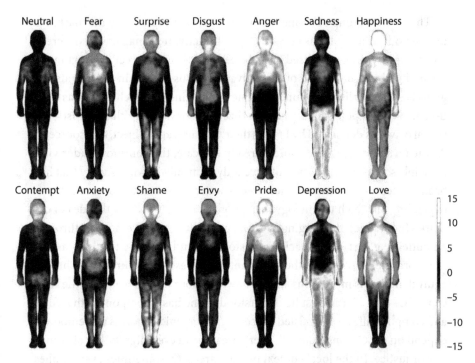

Figure 11.1. Bodily topography of basic and nonbasic emotions associated with words. Lighter shades indicate increased emotions and darker shades indicate decreased emotions. Source: Lauri Nummenmaa, et al., "Bodily Maps of Emotions," *Proceedings of the National Academy of Sciences of the United States of America* 111, no. 2 (2013): 646–651.

fear with anxiety, fear showed less activation in the upper chest but more activation in the limbs and in the head, making it an activating emotion. However, a cluster analysis revealed that the emotion closest related to anxiety is not fear, but shame. The explanation might be that both anxiety and shame are nonbasic, more social emotions that require interpersonal awareness and representation skills.

But Hietanen and colleagues wanted to solve yet another puzzle: Do people with different cultural backgrounds also perceive emotions differently? To solve this puzzle, they compared a Western European group consisting of Swedish and Finnish people with a Taiwanese group. When comparing the Western European and East Asian samples, they did not find any statistically significant differences in their emotion-specific activation maps. Therefore, they concluded "that emotions are represented in the somatosensory system as culturally universal categorical somatotopic maps."[20]

The Finnish group of biomedical researchers conceptualized the markings on the body silhouettes as emotion-specific activation maps, with different colors representing decreased and increased activation of certain regions of the body. The visualization of the activation status of certain body/brain regions is well established in functional neuroimaging; this technique was even used in an attempt to identify and localize the four defining characteristics of sexual drives as delineated by Freud (their pressure, aim, object, and source).[21] As the terms *pressure* and *source* already indicate, the common underlying principle seems to be a notion of psychodynamically flowing energy that has been conceptualized many times over as water, steam, ether, or electricity—depending on which technology metaphor is *en vogue*. Indeed, the idea of catharsis (κάθαρσις), the purging or cleansing of (unwanted) emotions through an outlet (e.g., art) dates back to Aristotelian and Platonic thinking and is therefore deeply rooted in the self-identity of Western culture. The Chinese equivalent of this mysterious energy flowing in our bodies would be the concept of *Qì* (氣). *Qì* can best be understood as the basic component that fuels and composes life and all related processes: All organic lifeforms and emotions depend on *Qì*. *Qì* constitutes air, every breath, and even dignity, but also anxiety or justice. In the local context of rural areas, *Qì* sometimes even implies a sense of emotional judgment in terms of social recognition and sometimes simply emotions as such.[22] *Qì* also represents a link between all beings on earth. An interesting example for interspecies exchange of *Qì* with regard to anxiety is mentioned in one of the classical medical textbooks written by Chen Shiduo 陳士鐸 (1627–1707):

> When eating dog meat and beef, [the patient] suddenly suffered from heart pain. He wanted to vomit, but this was not possible, it urged him to diarrhea, but [this too] was not possible. These [were signs that] the poison was stuck in the heart and stomach. It could not [escape] upwards nor could it [escape] downwards. Normally it is appropriate to use a treatment method that induces vomiting. But there are also people who [cannot] vomit. [The meat] of dog and cattle is good for building up blood and essence, how can this contain poison? This can be explained by the fact that before they [are to] die, the dog and cattle were not healthy. Moreover, they are tied up immediately before they are slaughtered. This arouses their anger [lit. anger *Qì*], and so poison [of disease and anger] is stuck in the flesh between the heart and liver [of the animals]. The people know nothing of this and eat it. The place [between the heart and the liver where the poison gets stuck in the animals] corresponds exactly to the

place [of poisoning in humans]. Accordingly, when they eat it, the [poisoning] disease arises. 人有食牛犬之肉, 一時心痛, 吐不能, 欲瀉不可, 此毒結於心胃, 不升不降也。論理亦宜用吐法, 然亦有探吐之不應者。夫牛犬乃資補精血之物, 何以有毒? 此必牛、犬抱病將死未死之時, 又加束縛以激動其怒氣, 毒結於皮肉心肝之間, 人不知而食之, 適當其處, 故食而成病。[23]

Thus, animals facing slaughter accumulate harmful *Qi*, which is subsequently consumed by the person eating their meat. This ancient understanding from a 17th-century medical textbook still bears relevance for the present: Modern research confirms that animals about to be slaughtered indeed suffer from extreme levels of stress and anxiety, which deteriorates meat quality.[24]

Transforming *Qi* Flows: Curing Anxiety with Anger?

Apart from interspecies transmission, problems also arise when *Qi* is blocked or oppressed or when it stagnates. In this context, it is important to remember that, since ancient times, *Qi*-processes were topically linked to emotional processes. Even in contemporary China, patients seek remedy and advice in outpatient clinics for Chinese medicine, convinced that, for example, a chronic accumulation of *Qi* in their liver causes their pathological condition.[25] In an analogy to the Western concept of catharsis, a holding back of discharge, for instance, in the form of outbursts of anger, will lead to grave consequences, such as an imploding congestion. People should also beware of long-standing thinking, that this will lead to knotted thoughts in the chest, again causing *Qi* to accumulate and stagnate in the heart, which in turn will cause states of depression (*yù bìng* 鬱病). Thus, it is vital to treat and dissolve stagnation.[26] This conviction contrasts sharply with the Western perception of Chinese culture as a culture that suppresses emotions, or at least the expression of emotions.

Indeed, since ancient times, Chinese philosophers and political advisers raised concerns about emotions as potential threats to the normative order. This concept is nothing alien to Western philosophy, as it has been discussed in various forms since antiquity. In China, beginning as early as in the 12th century when the Confucian canon was compiled, philosophers conceptualized the equilibrium (*zhōng* 中) as ideal state. In this ideal state, emotions like pleasure, anger, sorrow, anxiety, and joy are not yet evoked (*wèi fā* 未發). In contrast to *zhōng* (中), emotions were ascribed a *yīn* (陰) nature that was associated with greed (*tān* 貪). Consequently, every member of society should work hard to prevent emotions from being evoked (*yǐ fā* 已發) by maintaining tranquility (*jìng* 靜) and avoiding activity (*dòng* 動). Only in the state of ideal equilibrium, heaven and earth attain the proper order and all things will flourish:[27]

> Before joy, anger, sorrow and cheerfulness develop (*wei fa* 未 發), one speaks of the equilibrium (*zhong* 中). When [these emotions] are already developed and balanced (*zongjie* 中 節), one speaks of harmony (*he* 和). The equilibrium (*zhong* 中) is the great foundation of the world, and harmony is its universal path. When equilibrium and harmony are realized to the highest degree, heaven and earth will attain their proper order and all things will flourish. 喜怒哀樂之未發, 謂之中; 發而皆中節, 謂之和。中也者, 天下之大本也; 和也者, 天下之達道也。致中和, 天地位焉, 万物育焉 (Zhu Xi 朱熹, Sishu zhongju jizhu, 18; and Zhu Xi 朱熹, Sishu zhongju jizhu, 18[28]).

Many times, the state of equilibrium is compared to still water, with a quiet mountain sea as a most commonly used metaphor. In this metaphor, emotions would be a sudden gust of wind that would cause the sea to overflow, leading to a catastrophe for the inhabitants of the valley below. Anger, fear, and anxiety can be seen as explosive emotions, clearly affecting the social space of communities. On a collective level, these emotions virtually seem to be made for triggering social change, or even sociopolitical and economic earthquakes on a global scale. The social connection between anger and anxiety is evident,[29] but they are of opposing character: while anxiety is seen as pressing down, anger is seen as moving upward.[30] In China, since the 12th century medical textbooks suggest the "induction of emotions" as therapeutic process for various emotional diseases and unbalances, and this method was also applied for centuries.[31] For example, it is advised to use "anger" and "joy" as powerful instruments for curing major depressive disorders.[32] Thus:

> If you want to treat this type of disease entirely with medication, this is actually not a method of treatment. However, if you want to treat without medication and [just wait] for it to recover on its own, this is not a therapeutic method either. In general, the resolution of the thinking/longing-depression disease can be achieved by induction of joy and next by induction of anger. This way (the stagnation) can be dissolved. 人之鬱病, 婦女最多, 而又苦最不能解, 倘有睏臥終日, 痴痴不語, 人以為呆病之將成也, 誰知是思想結於心, 中氣鬱而不舒乎? 此等之癥, 欲全恃藥餌, 本非治法, 然不恃藥餌, 聽其自愈, 亦非治法也。大約思想鬱癥, 得喜可解, 其次使之大怒, 則亦可解。[33]

Today, we witness a "psychoboom" (*xīnli rè* 心里热) for psychotherapy, while psychotherapeutic methodology is currently reshaped according to ancient knowledge and concepts. Once again, psychotherapists use anger as a powerful therapeutic tool for dissolving stagnation, depression, and long-lasting anxiety.[34] This therapeutic step-by-step approach of adjusting and balancing the *Qi* flow in the inner viscera (*Diao* 調) requires a close observation of how dimensions and directions are moving. As discontent and indignation cause an unbalanced *Qi* (氣不平) on one hand, and oppressed anger causes disastrous suffering on the other, it becomes apparent why Chinese medical experts have made transforming and manipulating *Qi* flows one of their main concerns. Of note, the concept of evoking (hidden) emotions (e.g., anger or guilt) is not foreign to psychotherapeutic approaches in Western culture—indeed, the discovery and processing of suppressed emotions is seen as a vital prerequisite for healing many psychological conditions.

Anxiety and the Caring Society

So far, it has become apparent that Chinese concepts of anxiety—while using terminology that may seem exotic to Westerners—are far from being alien or incompatible with classic philosophical or even modern biomedical Western concepts of clinical anxiety. On the contrary, contemporary and historical Chinese medical conceptualizations offer many points of reference and common ideas that could serve as a source of enrichment inviting Western philosophers and medical experts to think a little bit out of the box. A particular topic of Chinese conceptualization that could be of interest and potential value to Western thinking is the concept of unity. Take the example of anxiety: Here it is the emotional incongruity between two internal organs (heart and kidneys) that is seen as affecting, as spreading anxiety to the gall bladder. Anxiety causes the gall bladder to tremble, and this jolting movement provokes a condition like insomnia as the patient becomes afraid of, for instance, being haunted by spirits. In this context, the relationship between two organs embodies more than a metaphoric description that is built on similarity or illustrative character. Instead, the connection between the organs, the disease, and the patient is to be interpreted as *metonymy*: the link is based on some understood association or contiguity, and all participating entities are of equal interest. If only one sphere is mentioned explicitly (*in praesentia*), the other sphere (*in absentia*) is of equal and essential importance. This link between both physical realms (the inner and the outer) works not in a causal but in a temporal contiguity, and the relationship is seen as based on objective grounds and vicinity. Thus, the patient suffering from insomnia can be substituted by his bodily content (in this case, the gall bladder): The frightened gall bladder startles—and so does the patient. In a sense, the gall bladder causes a medical condition, but at the same time the condition (e.g., insomnia) also represents the causative agent (e.g., the gall bladder). Therefore, the body is more than a mere vessel for its inner organs; it is not a mere stage for the inner organ's soap opera. Instead, the inner and outer realms are contiguously linked with each other but also with the sociopolitical environment. For example, the medicinal textbooks from the 17th century also mention fear of failure and fear of loss. Thus, these and other descriptions not only offer insights into the knowledge about bodily sedimentations and physical processes but also into the sociopolitical conditions of these times. As a consequence, medical reports can be interpreted as indicators for the cultural, social, and political conditions and transformations of their respective time. Being aware of somatic processes becomes imperative not only for writing a world history of emotions but also for examining our own contemporary emotional transformation processes.

From around 1839 until 1949, China suffered from a long period of semi-imperialistic intervention and subjugation by Western powers (the so-called Century of Humiliation, *qūrǔde shìjì* 屈辱的世紀). As with many other Indigenous people on all continents of the world, Western powers justified their interventions by dehumanizing the inhabitants and devaluing their culture. Denying someone to have feelings, or at least to have the same amount of feelings, is a powerful tool with which to dehumanize another human being. Contemporaneous with their colonization efforts, Western observers started to describe Chinese people as being unable to "feel in appropriate manners," meaning that Chinese people were incapable to perceive emotions with the same intensity as Europeans.[35] Thus, emotional authenticity served as the base for conceptually establishing the dichotomy between East and West.

Unfortunately, the invention of this false dichotomy proved to be a full, long-lasting success as it still shapes the relationship with China on both individual and political levels. As late as 1986, researchers comparing Chinese to American children stated that Chinese children are "in general . . . inclined to be more restrained, and less impulsive, excitable, spontaneous, and natural than Americans."[36] For a critical reflection of the perception of Chinese emotionality, we had to wait until the early 21st century. Researchers in the fields of Indigenous and Cultural Psychology recognize the need to examine "knowledge, skills and beliefs people have about themselves and how they function in their familial, social, cultural and ecological context."[37] Still, Chinese culture is perceived or labeled as a culture not allowing the expression of feelings. As mentioned earlier, the opposite is true because the suppression of emotions is seen as causing severe imbalances in the flow of *Qi*. Just as in Western culture, public displays of emotions are seen as a threat to harmony and collective well-being, and therefore they need to be balanced. Needless to say, the numerous social, cultural, and political transformations and catastrophes in the long Chinese history triggered much anxiety.[38] Regime changes, wars, famines, and natural disasters have caused anxiety worldwide. With regard to China, economic and social transformation processes came in extreme, accelerated ways during the last century. This period caused increased social injustice, and people's perception of life purpose, individuality, and freedom slowly began to change.[39]

Conclusion

Traditionally, anxiety is associated more with the older generation. The first wave of attention to anxiety in China observed a role reversal: suddenly, it was the younger generation suffering from anxiety.[40] In addition, anxiety was not only affecting the poor, but also the rich and successful, leading to the phenomenon of "anxious wealth."[41] The rapid demographic changes also caused discomfort and frustration in the elder generation. Due to increased demands of their professional lives, the younger generation increasingly abandoned traditional values like "filial care" (*xiao* 孝). In 2013, the Chinese government introduced a law that made financial and social support for the parents and grandparents mandatory, but this did not help much as younger family members simply did not have time or space to take care of family members. This led to increased levels of insecurity, frustration, and disenchantment among both the elderly and the young. Increasing suicide rates among elderly people are a very unfortunate indication of this development.[42] Yet, if in the end everybody suffers from anxiety, the young and the old, the poor and the rich, winners and losers of societal transformation, then something does not seem to hold here. Maybe it is not age or gender, and not cultural, social, or economic transformation that are the driving forces behind anxiety. Perhaps it is yet another term that must be thrown into the equation, a term that is connected to all the aforementioned possible factors: *care*. Change does not necessarily lead to anxiety, but maybe the loss of traditional social communities has caused a deterioration of care systems, thereby affecting the young and the old, the rich and the poor alike.

NOTES

1. Nancy N. Chen, "Between Abundance and Insecurity. Securing Food and Medicine in an Age of Chinese Biotechnology," in *Bioinsecurity and Vulnerability, School for Advanced Research Advanced Seminar Series*, ed. Nancy N. Chen and Lesley A. Sharp (Santa Fe, NM: School for Advanced Research Press, 2014), 87–102.

2. Roberto Lewis-Fernández et al., "Culture and the Anxiety Disorders: Recommendations for DSM-V," *Depression and Anxiety* 27, no. 2 (2010): 212–229.

3. Lewis-Fernández et al., "Culture and the Anxiety Disorders," 224.

4. Sing Lee et al., "A Community Epidemiological Survey of Generalized Anxiety Disorder in Hong Kong," *Community Mental Health Journal* 43, no. 4 (2007): 305–319.

5. Laurence Roulleau-Berger, "Multiple Modernities, Inequalities and Intermediate Spaces," in *European and Chinese Sociologies. A New Dialogue*, ed. Laurence Roulleau-Berger and Li Peili (Leiden & Boston: Brill, 2012), 83–92.

6. Li Hanlin 李汉林, 组织 和制度 变迁的社会程。种拟议的综合分析 [The societal process of changing organizations and systems. Draft of a summary analysis]. 中国社会科学 [Chinese social sciences] 1 (2005): 94–108; and Yunxiang Yan, *The Individualization of Chinese Society* (Oxford: Berg, 2009).

7. Sun Liping 孙立平, 断裂—20 世纪 90 年代以来的中国社会 [Fractures: The Chinese society of the 1990s]. (Beijing: 会科学文献出版社 Scientific Literature Press, 2003).

8. See Andreas Heinz, Xudong Zhao, and Shuyan Liu, "Implications of the Association of Social Exclusion With Mental Health," *JAMA Psychiatry* 77, no. 2 (2020): 113–114; Zheng-Hong Mao and Xu-dong Zhao, "The Effects of Social Connections on Self-Rated Physical and Mental Health Among Internal Migrant and Local Adolescents in Shanghai, China," *BMC Public Health* 12, no. 1 (2012): 1–9; and Feng Wang et al., "Mental Health Among Left-Behind Children in Rural China in Relation to Parent-Child Communication," *International Journal of Environmental Research and Public Health* 16, no. 10 (2019): 1855.

9. For example, see Song Bai et al., "Anxiety in Residents in China: Prevalence and Risk Factors in a Multicenter Study," *Academic Medicine* 96, no. 5 (2021): 718–727; Xiaojing Guo, et al., "Meta-Analysis of the Prevalence of Anxiety Disorders in Mainland China from 2000 to 2015," *Scientific Reports* 6, no. 28033 (2016); Xin Ma et al., "Generalized Anxiety Disorder in China: Prevalence, Sociodemographic Correlates, Comorbidity, and Suicide Attempts," *Perspectives in Psychiatric Care* 45, no. 2 (2009): 119–127; and Wei Yu et al., "Generalized Anxiety Disorder in Urban China: Prevalence, Awareness, and Disease Burden," *Journal of Affective Disorders* 234 (2018): 89–96.

10. Ma Danmeng and Ren Qiuyu, "Depression and Anxiety on the Rise in China, Study Shows," *Sixth Tone*, February 25, 2019, https://www.sixthtone.com/news/1003598; and Liz Carter, "Why Anxiety Is on the Rise in China," *The Atlantic*, May 17, 2013, https://www.theatlantic.com/china/archive/2013/05/why-anxiety-is-on-the-rise-in-china/275967/.

11. Li Zhang, *Anxious China, Inner Revolution and Politics of Psychotherapy* (Oakland, CA: University of California Press, 2020), 2.

12. Yeen Huang and Ning Zhao, "Generalized Anxiety Disorder, Depressive Symptoms and Sleep Quality During COVID-19 Outbreak in China: A Web-Based Cross-Sectional Survey," *Psychiatry Research* 288 (2020): 112954; Junfeng Li et al., "Anxiety and Depression Among General Population in China at the Peak of the COVID-19 Epidemic," *World Psychiatry* 19, no. 2 (2020): 249–250; and Zhengjia Ren, Yuchu Zhou, and Yanhong Liu, "The Psychological Burden Experienced by Chinese Citizens During the COVID-19 Outbreak: Prevalence and Determinants," *BMC Public Health* 20, no. 1 (2020): 1617.

13. For example, see Kai Liu, "'It's OK to Feel Anxious.' How a Professor in China Faced Coronavirus Disruptions and Fears," *Science Magazine*, March 17, 2020, https://www.sciencemag

.org/careers/2020/03/it-s-ok-feel-anxious-how-professor-china-faced-coronavirus-disruptions
-and-fears; Angelika C. Messner, "Anger, Hate, Aggression," in *The Routledge History of Emotion in
the Modern World*, ed. Katie Barclay and Peter Stearns (London: Routledge, in press); Vivian Wang
and Javier C. Hernández, "China Long Avoided Discussing Mental Health. The Pandemic Changed
That," *The New York Times*, December 21, 2020, https://www.nytimes.com/2020/12/21/world/asia
/china-covid-mental-health.html; and Zhou Wenting, "Insomnia and Rise in Anxiety Emerge as
Big Problems," *China Daily*, April 3, 2020, https://www.chinadailyhk.com/article/126633.

14. Transition refers to the dynamic processes from collectively organized institutions toward
a privately and commercialized system. See Sun Liping 孙立平, "Transition Sociology Trends and
New Prospects," in *European and Chinese Sociologies, A New Dialogue*, ed. Laurence Roulleau-
Berger and Li Peili (Leiden: Brill, 2012), 75–81.

15. Nihongo Master, "Definition of 悶," 2017, https://www.nihongomaster.com/dictionary
/kanji/2701/%E6%82%B6.

16. Shide Cheng 程士德, Hongtu Wang 王洪图, and Zhaolin Lu 鲁兆麟, eds., 黄帝内经素问.
素問注釋匯粹 [Collection of Commentary on Su Wen], Vol. 1 (Beijing 人民卫生出版社 People's
Medical Publishing House, 1982).

17. Cheng, Wang, and Lu, eds., 黄帝内经素问. 素問注釋匯粹 [Collection of Commentary on
Su Wen].

18. Angelika C. Messner, *Zirkulierende Leidenschaft: Eine Geschichte der Gefühle im China
des 17. Jahrhunderts* (Köln, Weimar, Wien: Böhlau Verlag, 2016).

19. Laurie Nummenmaa et al., "Bodily Maps of Emotions," *Proceedings of the National Academy of Sciences of the United States of America* 111, no. 2 (2013): 646–651.

20. Nummenmaa et al., "Bodily Maps of Emotions," 646.

21. Serge Stoléru, "Reading the Freudian Theory of Sexual Drives from a Functional Neuroimaging Perspective," *Frontiers in Human Neuroscience* 8, no. 57 (2014).

22. Ying Xing 应星, "气"与抗争政治: 当代中国乡村社会稳定问题研究 ["Emotions" and con-
tentious politics in contemporary rural China]. (Beijing: 社会科学文献出版社 Social Science Academic Press, 2011).

23. Chen Shiduo 陳士鐸, "Bianzheng lu 辨証錄," in *Chen Shiduo yixue quan shu* 陳士鐸醫學
全書, ed. Liu Zhanghua 柳長華 et al., 691–1010 (Beijing: 中国中医药出版社 Chinese Medical Publishing House, 1999), 934.

24. Lutz Reidt, "Umgang mit Schlachttieren. Gestresstes Schwein schmeckt nicht gut,"
Deutschlandfunk (2017), https://www.deutschlandfunk.de/umgang-mit-schlachttieren-gestresstes
-schwein-schmeckt.724.de.html?dram:article_id=376999.

25. Yanhua Zhang, *Transforming Emotions with Chinese Medicine. An Ethnographic Account
from Contemporary China* (Albany, NY: State University of New York Press, 2007), 62–65.

26. Angelika C. Messner, "Soziale Ligaturen im Wandel. Fragmente einer Analyse sozialer
Ungleichheiten," in *Anders Altern. Sammelband der Vorträge des STUDIUM GENERALE der
Ruprecht-Karls-Universität Heidelberg*, ed. Óscar Loureda (Heidelberg: Heidelberg University
Publishing, 2017), 31–45.

27. Martin W. Huang, "*Desire and Fictional Narrative in Late Imperial China* (Cambridge,
MA: Harvard University Press, 2001), 28–29.

28. For a translation, see Wing-Tsit Chan, ed., *A Source Book in Chinese Philosophy* (Princeton, NJ: Princeton University Press, 1963), 98.

29. Messner, *Zirkulierende Leidenschaft: Eine Geschichte der Gefühle im China des 17*, 212.

30. Angelika C. Messner, "Aspects of Emotion in Late Imperial China," *Asiatische Studien/
Études Asiatiques* LXVI, no. 4 (2013): 893–913; and Messner, *Zirkulierende Leidenschaft: Eine Geschichte der Gefühle im China des 17*.

31. Angelika C. Messner, *Medizinische Diskurse zu Irresein in China (1600–1930), Münchener
Ostasiatische Studien* (Stuttgart: Franz Steiner, 2000), 162–171.

32. Hsiu-Fen Chen, "Emotional Therapy and Talking Cures in Late Imperial China," in *Psychiatry and Chinese History*, ed. Howard Chiang (London: Pickering & Chatto, 2014), 37–54.

33. Chen Shiduo 陳士鐸, "Bianzheng lu 辨証錄," 774.

34. Messner, "Soziale Ligaturen im Wandel. Fragmente einer Analyse sozialer Ungleichheiten," 31–45.

35. Angelika C. Messner, "Transforming Chinese Hearts, Minds, and Bodies in the Name of Progress, Civility, and Civilization," in *Civilizing Emotions: Concepts in Asia and Europe*, ed. Margrit Pernau, Helge Jordheim, and Angelika C. Messner (Oxford: Oxford University Press, 2015), 231–249.

36. Kuo-shu Yang, "Chinese Personality and its Change," in *The Psychology of the Chinese People*, ed. Michael Harris Bond, 106–170 (Oxford: Oxford University Press, 1986), 143.

37. Uichol Kim, Kuo-Shu Yang, and Kwang-Kwo Hwang, "Contributions to Indigenous and Cultural Psychology: Understanding People in Context," in *Indigenous and Cultural Psychology. Understanding People in Context*, ed. Uichol Kim, Kuo-Shu Yang, and Kwang-Kwo Hwang, 3–25 (New York: Springer, 2006), 4.

38. Messner, *Zirkulierende Leidenschaft: Eine Geschichte der Gefühle im China des 17. Jahrhunderts*, 187.

39. Mette Halskov Hansen and Cuiming Pang, "Idealizing Individual Choice: Work, Love and Family in the Eyes of Young, Rural Chinese," in *iChina. The Rise of the Individual in Modern Chinese Society*, ed. Mette Halskov Hansen and Rune Svarverud, 39–64 (Copenhagen: NIAS Press, 2011).

40. Carter, "Why Anxiety Is on the Rise in China."

41. Edwin Schmitt, "Anxious Wealth: Money and Morality among China's New Rich," *Asian Anthropology* 12, no. 2 (2013): 181–183.

42. Beifeng Chen 陈柏峰, 代际关系变动与老年人自杀—对湖北京山农村的实证研究 [Changes in intergenerational relationships and suicide among the elderly: An empirical study in Jingshan County, Hubei Province], 社会学研究 [Sociological research] 4 (2009): 1–21; Sing Lee, "Depression: Coming of Age in China," in *Deep China. The Moral Life of the Person. What Anthropology and Psychiatry Tell Us about China Today*, ed. Arthur Kleinman et al., 177–212 (Berkeley: University of California Press, 2011); and Fei Wu, "Suicide, a Modern Problem in China," in *Deep China. The Moral Life of the Person. What Anthropology and Psychiatry Tell Us about China Today*, ed. Arthur Kleinman et al., 213–236 (Berkeley: University of California Press, 2011).

PART FOUR

MIGRATION, LANGUAGE, AND CULTURE

Introduction

KAREN STRUVE

Global migration is an omnipresent and challenging phenomenon of all times. In 2019, more than 272 million people worldwide set out to leave their home countries on a long-term or permanent basis.[1] Their reasons to migrate are varied and almost always accompanied by worries or fears. These worries and fears usually increase during migration, because the abandoned homeland as well as the transit and the destination country are full of uncertainties and often concrete dangers. Although migration is always associated with anxieties, it cannot be argued that migration experiences are fundamentally anxiety experiences. Migrants associate the change of place with hopes and demonstrate the courage to take an often-difficult path. The emotional spectrum of their feelings is wide ranging, possibly extending from fears of death to despair, anger, and grief, to feelings of happiness in the best case. But, tragically in refugee contexts, there is no freedom from anxiety in the receiving countries, where migrants might find it difficult to maintain their identity, face social discrimination and exclusion, miss a community for sharing their experiences and stories, and feel marginalized in the public social spaces of school, work, or leisure. The World Health Organization has noted that the "prevalence of common mental disorders such as depression, anxiety, and post-traumatic stress disorder (PTSD) tends to be higher among migrants exposed to adversity and refugees than among host populations."[2]

Migrants often experience a politically hostile atmosphere in the country that accepts them. They encounter disturbing concerns of the host society, such as the usually factually unfounded fear of becoming a quantitative minority or of being culturally alienated. The Migration Fear Index of migration-related fears in German, French, British, and American newspapers clearly shows in which way so-called migration or refugee crises coined by discourses on migration, assimilation, or even human trafficking coincide with expressions of fear, panic, concerns, or even bombs or terror.[3]

This section is devoted to the relationship between migration contexts and their emotional dimensions. The chapters included show that crossing borders means not only changing one's place of residence but also crossing cultural spheres, confronting new and often unfamiliar political concepts, losing linguistic and cultural ways of life and being surrounded by new ones, living as a stranger among strangers, sharing space with unfamiliar people, coexisting, asserting oneself, recommuning, and responding to all this with a wide range of affective reactions.

In the first chapter of this section, Paul Mecheril and Monica van der Haagen-Wulff examine the crisis that is triggered by the migrant's transformation of *borders*. This results in disturbing the "natio-racial-culturally coded orders of societal belonging" by crossing both physical and cultural borders. Such transformations are accompanied by media portrayals of (apocalyptic, thanatological) experiences of fear—fear that "Europe will not survive" or that labor markets and economies will perish without migrant workers as the remedy. Moreover, the discourse behind these portrayals frequently reveal fear-coded concepts of alterity and identity whose positions of power must be preserved.

Regarding preservation, Emmanuel Kattan and Karen Struve then detect another discourse within the narratives of migrants: the fear of losing or being disconnected from the past. They pursue the question of how fictional texts not only repeat discourses of fear in terms of violence, fractures, and trauma, but also foster, support, and even transform (hi-)stories.

Next, Eva Daussà and Bàrbara Roviró focus in their analysis of language policy on the importance of valuing and preserving the migrants' heritage language(s), especially when these are regional varieties and lesser used than the widespread national languages. If no attention is paid to the particular multilingualism of migrants, this is likely to cause anxieties among them that counteract their successful integration into the host society. In their study, the authors identify the context of school as crucial and elaborate on aspects that can contribute to the collective and individual well-being of these heritage-language speakers.

Finally, Julie Mostov's chapter explores how anxiety over who belongs within "our" borders and the vulnerability of democratic spaces to infiltration and contamination turns us toward a hardening of borders, which, in turn, actually weakens and endangers the very democratic practices they are meant to protect. Anxiety about who counts results in a numbness to the inhumanity of containment, deportation, and death at one's borders and fear of agency in those who would cross these borders. As such, anxiety is intimately linked to mobility and immobility. An alternative to this outcome is to reimagine the open nature of democratic spaces.

NOTES

1. "The Number of International Migrants Reaches 272 Million, Continuing an Upward Trend in All World Regions, says UN," United Nations Department of Economic and Social Affairs, September 17, 2019, https://www.un.org/en/desa/number-international-migrants-reaches-272-million-continuing-upward-trend-all.

2. "Mental Health and Forced Displacement," World Health Organization, August 31, 2021, https://www.who.int/news-room/fact-sheets/detail/mental-health-and-forced-displacement.

3. "Migration Fears and EPU," Economic Policy Uncertainty (EPU), https://www.policy uncertainty.com/immigration_fear.html.

CHAPTER TWELVE

Crisis, Affect, and Migration

The Production of Legitimacy within Political Orders

PAUL MECHERIL AND

MONICA VAN DER HAAGEN-WULFF

If migration is a specific form of bodily border crossing, then it is fair to say that there have been movements across borders almost everywhere and in all historical eras.[1] The consequences of movements across borders can be examined and understood as a phenomenon in which new knowledge, experiences, languages, and perspectives are introduced into existing social constellations and as a result are rearranged and inevitably changed. Crossing borders, or the border-crossing movement of people (the movement of their languages, stories, memories, ways of life) mobilizes the function of borders. It also raises the question of their functionality and challenges the registers of the symbolic, legal, and moral legitimacy of borders. Migration in the form of crossing borders is however also concomitant with a reconfirmation of the already existing societal formations. The borders of nation states, for example, become particularly visible and affirmed in their legitimacy at the very moment of their crossing, and as the history of the Schengen Agreement[2] shows, even wholly rearranged. Crossing borders, put succinctly, both weakens and strengthens their legitimacy.

In this sense, the central sociotheoretical hallmark of this border-crossing mobility, defined as migration, consists in its ability to unsettle social relations and regulations. Perhaps it is useful to depart from the assumption that it is the phenomenon of *unsettlement* or agitation that turns mobility into migration in the first place. Applying this premise, analytical elements pertaining to a definition of migration would be won: the movement of people and their ways of living over significant borders, as a result of which natio-racial-culturally coded orders of belonging,[3] understood as patterns of iterative border-demarcation practices, become unsettled. This sense of unsettlement or agitation is a phenomenon that results from the structural logic of natio-racial-culturally coded orders of societal belonging and can be interpreted politically from two different perspectives when presented as a crisis—either as a threat or as a chance. The social significance of crossing borders is not simply given but rather generated in complex discursive processes in which social reality is affirmed, negotiated, and ultimately changed.

Migration should not only be conceived as a phenomenon involving movements of people across borders but also as a phenomenon of discourses, and to that extent as a phenomenon of hegemonic power relations. The term *discourse* is particularly meaningful here, because migration does not simply happen as the physical movement of bodies. Rather, phenomena arising from crossing borders are generated by political discourses, understood here as socially constructed systems of knowledge, affect, imagination, and understanding, that label and give meaning to these phenomena politically, aesthetically, and culturally.

The political interpretation of migration as crisis can effectively lead to changes in social regulation, by conceptual and interpretive modifications being made to the constitutive dimensions of social and political affiliation and belonging such as membership, efficacy, and connectedness.[4] The state of agitation, disturbance, or unsettlement and associated affects such as anxiety, fear, and anger, can likewise lead to a confirmation and endorsement of the given regulative order: here the signification of unsettlement as threat plays a functional role.

Europe Will Not Survive

Media headlines in 2018 quoting a senior diplomat of the Visegád Group (Poland, Czech Republic, Slovakia, and Hungary), warned that "Europe will Not Survive Another Refugee Crisis" and that in her opinion sealing the Southern and Eastern European borders was of highest priority.[5] Two years later, in full view of the humanitarian disaster of the refugee camps in Greece (Moria), in Bosnia (Lipa/Bihac), and increasingly the Canary Islands in Spain, the European asylum-crisis discourse hardens, demonstrated by German Federal Minister of the Interior Horst Seehofer's outspoken refusal to "go it alone again," referencing Germanys intake of Syrian refugees stranded in Hungary in 2015. In a TAZ newspaper article, he is quoted as saying: "The very great danger is that pull-effects are established, that means that all refugees become concentrated in one country. And we have all resolved, that 2015 must never be repeated [our translation]."[6] In another article of the same newspaper, it is reported that Seehofer and Merkel, although rivals in the Autumn 2015 so-called asylum crisis, had come to an agreement regarding migration. The new political position as reported in TAZ is that "German borders should never be open for asylum seekers if Europe doesn't take in its fair share. Thus, the new doctrine reads. It applies—regardless, of how many drown in the Mediterranean Sea, regardless, of whether the Moria camp burns down, regardless, of whether German major cities offer to take in refugees [our translation]."[7]

This emotionally charged rhetoric of a beleaguered Fortress Europe rising united to the threat of imminent invasion and overwhelmed through floods of asylum seekers is further demonstrated in the bitterly fought over political demands made by the German CDU, CSU, and SPD parties for a German asylum *Obergrenze*—"upper limit" of between 180,000 and 220,000 per annum[8] and demands to process asylum seekers *vor Ort*—"on-site" in third-party arrival countries.[9] According to this formula, the asylum intake in 2018 was at 165,000 and as such well below the bottom margin of the yearly limit. Nevertheless, these affect-driven demands of maintaining border control that entail keeping the masses of asylum seekers geographically contained outside the EU borders and numerically confined within an upper limit of possible entries, has since been translated into policy through the European Commission's newly proposed pact on migration and asylum, as presented in Brussels on September 23, 2020. The core elements decided upon by the commission propose a "compulsory solidarity mechanism" in times of crisis, more efficient border procedures to fast-track legal asylum as well as speeding up deportations of those without a claim to stay, stronger collaboration with third-party countries on-site, more legal border entries, and a united and resolute strategy to combat people smugglers.[10]

Although United Nations statistics indicate that migrants who come to Europe via the Mediterranean Sea have decreased steadily from its peak in 2016 at 373,652 persons to 86,649 persons in 2020, headlines such as the "Gateway To Europe: More and More Migrants Reach Spain" and the accompanying article incite a sense of dread through numerical asylum-arrival overwhelm.[11]

The most recent data from the Spanish internal affairs ministry reports that 41,861 persons reached the Spanish shores in 2020, with more than half arriving in the Canary Islands. Despite the pandemic, which until the summer had to a large extent brought the world to a standstill, Spain registered 32,531 more migrants than in the previous year—and the highest number in the entire EU. According to the International Organisation for Migration, 34,100 migrants were registered in Italy, 15,500 in Greece, and 94,177 in the EU overall. A similar trend could continue into 2021, even though the number of new arrivals in December had fallen slightly, after having reached 800 in November. The predominant number of migrants originally came from distant countries like Mali, Senegal, and the Ivory Coast. More recently, Moroccans are marginally in the majority. Increasing numbers are also coming to Spain from Algeria. More than 11,000 Algerians were registered according to the internet portal "El Confidencial"—which is unprecedented compared to previous years, and represents the second-largest group of new arrivals. Many are fleeing from Algeria due to the enduring political and economic crises resulting from oil prices that had been falling prior to the pandemic.[12] [Authors' translation]

As the preceding examples indicate, it is not uncommon for the manifold media representations and public statements about the sociopolitical significance of asylum and migration that have infiltrated the public consciousness to draw on the rhetoric of crisis and threat scenarios.[13] In this last example, the discourse of migration is seamlessly transformed into the rhetoric of threat through hyperbolic numeric superlatives and yearly comparisons, indicating a threatening increase and enduring upward trend of migration intake.

Furthermore, the numbers quoted stand in no relation to the larger migration context and overall intake capacity.[14] Although the Canary Islands are clearly struggling with this sudden and novel increase to its region, here, as stated above, the fact that the sum total of yearly migration over the Mediterranean Sea route to European ports has steadily decreased from its peak since 2016, does not get in the way of the threat scenario played out in the media report. The infiltrators are clearly marked and natio-racial-culturally differentiated and affectively assigned into two camps—those from faraway places such as Mali, Senegal, and the Ivory Coast, presumably sincere asylum seekers potentially fleeing from political persecution, war, famine, or environmental degradation, and those closer to home, Morocco and Algeria, now in the majority, clearly represented as economic refugees[15] due to the current economic downturn, and thus branded as bogus[16] or fake asylum seekers. The quoted article goes on to cite the average death toll from the Mediterranean Sea, which shows an equally alarming upward trend. The tenacity and determination perceived in those willing to risk everything in the sea crossing is highlighted in the article by citing the high death toll, which on the surface would seem to appeal to a sense of compassion and the need to provide a safe passage and haven; however, the subtext speaks to a sense of fear and dread of being at the mercy of such a determined force that will stop at nothing, not even the risk of self-destruction to gain access to the inner sanctum of Fortress Europe.

Coming back to the political strategy of a compulsory solidarity mechanism suggested by the EU Commission and concluding our first example of crisis representation in the media, clearly this statement is a contradiction in terms or put simply, an oxymoron. Solidarity is by definition inherently democratic, based on a free choice and personal conviction. According to Sabine Hark and Paula-Irene Villa, solidarity represents a political practice that enables an alternative position to a totalitarian worldview that homogenizes and relativizes the complexity of the world.[17] The new EU Commissions Immigration pact, outlined above, much like Gebhardt describes when analyzing the migration politics of the EU Dublin agreement, is based on the economic logic of fair and effective work distribution and is thus a thinly veiled form of pseudosolidarity, far from its humanitarian ideal.[18] If, thinking with Lauren Berlant, "maintaining solidarity requires skills for adjudicating incommensurate visions of a better good life,"[19] then the adjudication of the better life, in this instance, is not between the visions of the EU nations and those of the asylum seekers awaiting a better life at the margins, but rather the adjudication of which EU nations' vision of a good life gets to be unsettled more or less by the infiltration, from the outer margins into the inners sanctum, by the refugee. Thus, it is a kind of insider solidarity aimed at maintaining maximum privileges for and between European nation states rather than a commitment of solidarity and hospitality extended to those seeking refuge.

Looking at the flipside of what is called the migration crisis in our second type of media examples, a headline of the *Deutsche Welle* in December 2019, by Sabine Kinkartz reads "Germany Needs Immigrants: If Angela Merkel extends invitations to a 'Summit' in the chancellery, then the problem must be big. The shortage of skilled labour is indeed becoming critical. A new law should help."[20] The article states that according to a survey commissioned by the Chamber of Commerce and Industry, 430,000 refugees have found employment in Germany in the last four years, 40,000 among them as trainee apprentices, but that this number is well below the required amount to cover the demand for skilled personnel and the workers for the labor market. It is reported that every second business is affected by this shortage of skilled labor and that this represents the biggest risk to the German economy. The prognosis is bleak—by the year 2030, so many employees will enter retirement that 6 million potential workers will be missing. This deficit is already being felt in the trade and building sector where a current deficit of 250,000 to the labor force is documented.[21] The dependency of the German government on immigration from third-party countries due to an aging population is also confirmed by the results of a survey by Bertelsmann Stiftung carried out with the Institute for the Employment Market and Job Research at the Coburg Institute of Applied Science. The current immigration numbers and resulting rise in birth rates change nothing on that prognosis according to the results of this study. By 2060 Germany will need 260,000 immigrants, a number which the EU is far from being able to cover. According to this study, a yearly intake of 146,000 immigrants from non-EU countries will be required to meet demands.[22]

Using economic justifications, migration, in the medical allegory of diagnosis, quickly takes on the function of an antidote: migration as a remedy of the crisis. In the above scenario the numbers are stacked alarmingly in the opposite direction, this time not enough immigration represents the threat. The following example indicates, however, that immigration to Germany is, and has been since its formation as a nation state in 1871, a highly selective affair. An article in the *Epoch Times*, covering the aforementioned Skilled Migrant Summit (*Fachkräftegipfel*) in Berlin, December 2019, states the urgent need for Germany to recruit young skilled migrant workers from population-rich countries such as Brazil, India, and Vietnam. CDU health minister Jens Spahn, talking to a press conference, was adamant about the right to insist on clear-cut criteria for the immigration of foreign skilled workers. "Foreign help is sought that: 'fits with us: is motivated, well-qualified and prepared to share and live according to our values' Spahn told the newspapers of the *Funke Mediengruppe*. This being stated as, "exactly the kind of immigration that we want [our translation]."[23] As a result of this Summit the immigration act for skilled personnel (*Fachkräfteeinwanderungsgesetz*) was passed in Parliament on March 1, 2020.

Emphasizing the right to choose those who fit with us, in this case, clearly, young, preferably unattached, adaptable Christian Brazilians, Hindu Indians, and Buddhist Vietnamese; however, gauging from the absence of any proposed Islamic countries, clearly not Muslim migrants. The resulting implementation of laws that regulate this natio-racial-culturally coded selection process is not a new concept. In early February 2024, the Bundesrat changed its nationality law for dual citizenship to make it more attractive for highly qualified professionals and "well-integrated" residents to work in Germany. Simultaneously it passed a bill to simplify and speed up returns of those deemed without prospects of remaining permanently in Germany. The bill included increased police jurisdiction to search documents, data, and living arrangements of those considered a potential threat. SPD Federal Minister of the Interior and Community Nancy Faeser, in her introduction of the new bill, formulates it thus: "If you do not share our values, you cannot become German. We have made this crystal clear in the law. As a consequence, anyone with antisemitic or racist views cannot be naturalised. We live by the values of our constitution."[24] In the meantime, (far-)right wing parties such as the AfD have gained 17.3% of the vote and 77 seats in parliament, through predominantly anti-immigration rhetoric including warnings against "imported Antisemitism" from Muslim countries.[25] The instrumental double standard of this claim hardly warrants elaboration here.

In the preceding examples, we have outlined the contours of two diametrically opposing perspectives of a present moment—namely, the politically motivated media representation of the nation state staged as being in crisis, more specifically Europe's threat emanating from migration and conversely the threat to Europe from the lack thereof. The contradictory nature of their claims to a discourse and object of threat, and the legal resolutions chosen to counter this threat, tell us reams about the political playing field, the interests being actively pursued and protected, that are inherent to any given crisis and its discursive formation.

What type of crisis is presented in the media examples? Migration becomes interpolated as a danger and migrants of a particular type as dangerous. This potential danger and the affective moral panic that accompanies its iterative media dissemination does not only enable the legitimization of deportation, selective border closure, increased border securitization, and ultimately leaves those seeking asylum to die trying, but furthermore increases the legitimacy of translating into law the continued instrumentalization and inhumane treatment of migratory human capital. Stephen Castles et al. have termed this process the "asylum-migration nexus,"[26] which operates according to what Gutiérrez Rodríguez calls the "coloniality of migration,"[27] an expression she has adapted from Anibal Quijano's "Coloniality of Power," whereby contemporary racism in Europe generally and Germany in particular is expressed by the trope of the "refugee" and the role of the media in evoking a "refugee crisis" in political and public debates.

Crisis, Affects, and the Regulation of Social Order

Migration leads to the crisis of the given circumstances, at least when a particular interpretation exists and can generally be agreed upon through communication. In medical terms the word *crisis* connotes a state of uncertainty or limbo that is moving toward a turning point.[28] Since early modernity, the medical definition of *crisis* is carried over and applied to the realm of the social. In line with this analogy, societal and political conditions are occasionally compared to a feverish and critical condition that depends for its continuity on a decisive change one way or the other. Those who declare a crisis see themselves in the position to proclaim or respectively demand preventive, therapeutic, or immediate courses of action. Koselleck suggests that crises are cultural constructions that are thus intrinsically related to perceptions, contexts, and interests.[29] They point to the need for quick decision-making. Crisis diagnoses, especially when they concern "our present" are then often accompanied by an alarmist sensibility.

The successful staging of crises has since early modernity, as Jan Marco Sawilla points out,[30] made it possible to view the state as an organism that allows for action against a crisis to become legitimate; furthermore, the pressure to take action establishes a certain tolerance toward the failure of the countermeasures applied. Where the crisis is of the order of a social context, the crisis of a (local) present can be made credible for those who are significantly affected by this present, and this leads to the opening and questioning of the imaginary social context.[31] The disputes that now take place in this space opened by a crisis interpretation that has become credible can be understood as disputes about what can be lost in the future, what would be a significant loss, or about what is worth possessing in the present future; it is about the preservation of values and advantage, and ultimately about the idea of a proper social order. These political struggles and contentions come to an end when the political fight has temporarily been decided one way or the other, and the societal cohesion has been symbolically locked into place and thus regulated, so to speak. Whenever we are dealing with an imagined-crisis diagnosis based on the present, we are also always already dealing with an imaginary, a subjunctive imaginary (what-if imaginary), that is inherently addressed within the respective crisis diagnosis. In the crisis diagnosis, therefore, an imaginary

Us is always addressed, which is called into question by the crisis, and must be strengthened or weakened accordingly.

With every interpretation and assertion of a crisis, a specific need for the regulation of social relations that are understood to be in crisis is always perceived, and legitimacy is procured for it. This is done for instance by regulating natio-racial-culturally coded orders of belonging through enabling and/or restricting concepts of membership, efficacy, and connectedness. Every social order does not just simply exist, rather it is performatively (re-)produced. The need for regulation and, in particular, the diagnosis of a crisis together with the various arguments over its validity, are important moments of the (re-)constitution of political and social orders. It is now the validated crisis diagnosis that legitimates, makes plausible, and thus gives birth to new regulative principles. In this example, the EU political decisions are legitimated by the threat posed to European border control. The regulation of natio-racial-culturally coded orders of belonging is thus related to the fact that a certain crisis of the present is set as a given, a certain description of the crisis is hegemonically enforced, corresponding solutions to the crisis are discussed, certain options for solutions are understood as legitimate solutions, and in the process an Us is invoked.

In these regulatory processes affect has a particular role to play. In the literature on affect and emotion, both within the field of psychology and the social sciences in general, there are a myriad of different definitions. Paul and Anne Kleinginna found 90 different definitions alone for the term *emotion*, depending on the area of expertise, perspective, interest, and language in which it was being used.[32] We understand affect as an exceptionally generic term that incorporates a variety of different bodily and emotional states ranging from frequently changing conscious feelings and emotions to long-lasting conscious or unconscious moods or emotional states.

Although affect is mostly felt and expressed nonverbally, affects are generated through a whole range of socioculturally inscribed affective scripts and are thus always a matter of interpretation. Borrowing from Sarah Ahmed, the assumption is that affect is always culturally and politically constructed and coded.[33] Affects are more than just expressions of monadic individuals but are rather of multiple contextualized and emergent individuals. Relevant contexts in relation to this are societal discourses and practices that always have a historical dimension. Only by contextualizing this affect logic[34] does it become possible to understand the origin and genealogy of one's own and others' affects and the process of meaning formation within the dominant societal discourse.

Long neglected in political and philosophical social theory, there has been a tradition of affect (or more precisely, affectivity) being understood as dichotomous or pejorative to, thus undermining rationality, reason, maturity, and enlightenment, among others. In this view, affect in politics or the social sciences more generally is associated with a regression to the uncivilized, barbaric, and animalistic of society. The affective turn in the analysis of the political has meant recognizing the affective as a constitutional dimension of all political processes. The question is thus not whether affect is relevant at all but rather what part it plays in the political processes. The Affective Studies research group in Berlin bases its foundational thinking on Baruch Spinoza's ideas on *affectio* interpreted through Gilles Deleuze,[35] as a "dynamic relational ontology" of beings and matter in time and space and the resulting impact, impression, and traces left on those engaged in the encounters of different modes.[36] Spinoza uses the term *affectus* to mean affections that "either increase or diminish the power—agentive capacities or *potentia*—of the entities in question."[37] In other words, "affect is inextricable from an approach to power, understood as relations of reciprocal efficaciousness."[38] As such it is an effective analytical tool to examine the interconnection between affect, power (-structures), and subjectivity.

Differing from early affect theory as exemplified by Massumi[39] or Sedgwick and Frank,[40] who positioned themselves as a radical break with poststructuralist theories founded on discourse and language-based approaches to cultural articulation, and similar to the Affective Society's approach, we do not depart from thinking of the affective as a purely prelingual, and prediscursive phenomenon. The affective, rather, is transmitted and articulated through discursive and material structures and furthermore reproduces these, yet it is not fully realized nor completely defined by these discursive and material structures. This perspective views affective arrangements as located and productive in sociohistorical contexts rather than purely examining a unified field of prepersonal free-floating affective intensities disconnected to the material machinic conditions within time and space.[41] Applying this post-structuralist analysis, the manifestation of an individual's affective *potentia*, which Slaby and Mühlhoff also liken to Bourdieu's concept of *habitus* or Butler's *performativity*, can be examined through an analysis of the institutional structures together with the intersectional, for instance, racialized and gendered affective interrelations that occur within these settings and thereby make visible concomitant hegemonic routines and power structures.[42]

To summarize the above and place it in the context of our current investigation—namely, the role of affect in producing the legitimacy of a political order in relation to discourses of migration and crisis—we would need to ask for ways of examining the microsocial presuppositions involved in the processes of affecting and being affected that are common for the subjectivities that engage in these discourses, power structures, and movements.[43] It would also entail looking at what these interactions produce on a political, structural, and institutional level, for instance, in terms of the implementation of policies and laws. Put another way, affect theory according to this definition does not grant affect or emotion explanatory power as such; rather it is an investigation into what affect theorist Ben Anderson explains as "modes of enquiry that discern the geo-historically specific apparatuses, encounters, and conditions through which affective life becomes organised."[44]

For Lauren Berlant, in line with this thinking, a politics of feeling requires shifting the focus from a subjective sensory perception of power to an understanding of affect as active agents and tools of politics. This understanding makes transparent that affect can be used as a way of governing, a way of establishing and maintaining a hegemony, "for instance, how the nation-state is also constituted through feelings."[45] Berlant speaks of affect metaphorically as the "noise of the reproduction of life," which defines power relationships in the everyday and speaks about ambient citizenship as the "place where the question emerges of whose noise matters, and how" and the need to ask questions regarding affects such as: "whose anger is deemed honourable and whose is deemed a threat; whose sentimentality is a sign of moral virtue and whose a sign of weakness that needs to get regulated" and that the "adjudication of the noise is especially what happens in a democracy when groups speak as minor, refusing to delegate attention to 'representative' authority: some noise is sanctioned and invited to dilate, while some noise calls out the police."[46] Affective politics, as has become clear in the four years of the Trump presidency and other nation states shifting increasingly to the right, have been used to mobilize the spread of racism, antisemitism, and white patriarchal supremacy. As such, "a political grammar of feeling is not connected to a naïve optimism, but instead it argues for a critical engagement with affect in (neo-) liberal times and for scrutinizing where and what kind of emotionalization is at work."[47]

Sarah Ahmed's work on the cultural politics of emotion[48] and racism in institutional diversity structures[49] examine the interrelationship of affect, race, and structural materiality and is of particular relevance as an analytical category for examining issues of migration and migration policy. Ahmed effectively shows how affect, as in Spinoza's *potentia*, "sticks" to bodies, thus enhancing the movement of some and decreasing or disabling the movement of others. The discursive and institutional operations constitute the material and psychosocial spaces within which bodies negotiate their capacity to move, be heard, and express agency. The freedom of movement and the ability to articulate affect manifest as fear, anger, and threat, which then translate into concrete actions either in the form of immigration laws and border policy from inside the EU border or in the successful acquisition of asylum status from outside the EU border, as exemplified in the previously mentioned media examples, is not equally distributed.

Affects such as fear and anger, but also the affective state of indifference toward the suffering of others,[50] is born out of crisis narratives that effectively serve to ratify a given crisis as real and therewith stabilize its hegemonic legitimacy. Through the interplay of these affects, the evident nature of the crisis is always coconstituted with a societal Us that is experiencing the crisis. Affects become the means of imaginatively securing an Us. This safeguarding is then particularly necessary when the Us is allegedly under threat, through the uncomfortable messages and meanings of migration for instance.

A particular type of affect and affective way of speaking in the European public sphere is tied to racist differentiations between a natio-racial-culturally coded Us and the dangerous, backward Them (Not Us), which furthermore serves to strengthen this differentiation and can be described and understood as a practice of Othering/Selfing with recourse to staged threat scenarios and scenes. [51] In this context, *othering*, a term coined by postcolonial theorist Gayatri Chakravorty Spivak[52] and analytically developed by Edward Said's work on orientalism, can be understood as a double process; the others are constructed by means of specific knowledge production practices that legitimate the establishment of colonial dominance, and, likewise, it is this hegemonic (political, economic, cultural) intention that makes these epistemic practices appear "plausible" and "useful" and naturally "dominant."[53]

Thus, we are dealing here with two sides of a coin: the imagination of the other and the process of securing material and symbolic privileges. The staged affect scenarios that we are witnessing today—the intensity with which, on the one hand, a sense of threat is felt, and on the other, the ever-growing danger of becoming a victim of racist incidents, which are then largely ignored or de-thematized in wider society—can only be understood if we are clear that what is at issue here is a battle over sovereignty and positions of privilege, and that this battle requires pictures and imagined constructions of the other.

Three ideal typical distinct moments of affect can be distinguished as follows:

(a) With the fear of and the anger against the other, it becomes possible to repudiate the legitimate, but uncomfortable and not necessarily explicitly for-mulated, apparent demands of others. A paradoxical anger about the suffering of others is currently etched into many people's voices, postures, and faces. The logic of this affect can be explained with reference to the type of anti-Semitism that was particularly relevant to Germany in the second half of the 20th century and that is called "secondary anti-Semitism," a hatred against Jews, not despite, but because of Auschwitz. The Israeli psychoanalyst Zvi Rex sarcastically encapsulates it thus: "The Germans will never forgive the Jews for Auschwitz."[54] Following this logic: We, who are geopolitically privileged, can-not forgive the asylum seekers and refugees, the waste of the world order,[55] the "disposable populations,"[56] a World Order that was in no small measure created by Western protagonists and instances, and from which the West prof-ited immeasurably. We do not forgive the refugees that they suffer and that with their suffering they invade our living quarters and suburbs and literally get under our skin. That is why they must be demonized, degraded, and ulti-mately dehumanized.[57]

The demonization of the other serves in the maintenance of a hegemonic global order. Within this global order, the prosperity of a privileged minority is established and maintained at the cost of the global Other: the European fishing industry; global waste management; mobile telephones, which could not function without mined coltan from the Congo; people living in African countries rich in mineral resources live in bitter poverty not least because of national wage-labor politics that are massively influenced by transnational corporations, both legally and illegally; ecological devastation; and the list goes on.

The West's preservation of an "imperial life-style"[58] necessitates the demon-ization of those whose bodily presence and associated narrative potential (they too have stories to tell about the world order) is hard to bear for the global privileged minority because it points to the intolerable nature of the global situation from which this privileged minority continues to profit. Cap-italism (potentially) not only loses its necessary outside upon which it relies for its continued production through an inbuilt destructive mechanism of continuous expansion and totalization,[59] rather capitalism paradoxically sets up the premise that the shadow beings of those appearing from the periphery manage to enter the interior and in so doing make conscious the inside/outside, center/periphery divide. One method used to avoid having to take global inequality and one's own responsibility to act into account is the demonization and symbolic and factual repatriation of the others to the outside realm, where, all the better if directed by their own free will, they belong.

(b) With the fear of and the anger against the Other, it becomes possible to silence and thus avoid addressing the historical, political, and economic responsibility that Europe has in creating the current global circumstances, which must be understood both as a reality from which Europeans continue to profit in no small measure and as an influence causing global population movements. The fundamental potential for and concrete crises of a natio-racial-culturally coded Us are potentially lessened by setting the stage for a threat from the outside, through the coming of something or someone from outside. The construction of a "threatened Other" goes hand in hand with that of a "threatened Us." The generation of threat makes it possible "to align bodies with and against others."[60] The waste of the world order reminds us that Europe's prosperity, from a global perspective of existing privilege, needs to be questioned, not so much factually but ethically. The demonizing of the Other functions to avoid the ethical question and thus to preserve individual privileges and the current global order that support them. This means deflecting all direct and indirect questioning of this order, for instance, by discrediting the couriers of the message of inequality in the world, from which Europe is nourished.

(c) With the fear of and the anger against the Other, it becomes possible to enshrine and renew the positive, almost sacred, self-image of Europe. The extent to which asylum seekers, North Africans, and Muslims are spoken about in a derogatory manner in Germany and Europe, the intensity with which the Other is constructed and staged as sexually dangerous, can only be explained if we are very clear that there is something to lose—namely, the status of material privilege and its unquestioned entitlement and the idea of a justifiable, reasoned supremacy of a natio-racial-culturally coded Us. Psychoanalytically speaking, media representations of the fantasized, constructed ("Arabic," "North-African," "Muslim") other can be understood as an attempt to fight that which cannot be accepted within oneself by projecting it onto the abject other (e.g., I as a European man complain so relentlessly about the chauvinism of the allegedly Muslim man by projecting onto and fighting out on his body that which I cannot accept within myself). This kind of affect is currently so intensely felt and performed in European societies because contained within it is the desire to preserve the self based on an idealized sacred image of Europe. Europe is contradictory; Europe is the place and project of barbarity, of slavery, the Shoah, the ecological-economic exploitation of the world, of colonialism. Yet Europe is also the place and project of enlightenment, of human rights, and the pursuit of a good life for all. Europe is clearly contradictory.[61]

However, this contradiction is dissipated and reappropriated in the process of speaking about others. The self-aggrandizement of Europe is a hallmark and an integral part of the European Project and makes visible (typical of "grand narratives," particularly those with a pronounced sense of superiority) Europe's constitutive vulnerability and susceptibility to crises. For several reasons, Europe currently finds itself in a fundamental crisis. Europe, in denial of the more than 30,000 dead in the Mediterranean Sea, who lost their lives as a direct result of European border politics, stages itself as a place of the chosen good, of civilized values, as the cradle of gender equality and, in light of a growing social inequality, duplicitously as a place of social justice. For this political staging, the Others are needed—their ugliness, their dangerousness, their savagery. Measured against the "moral panic" ignited by the phantasmagorical picture of the natio-racial-culturally coded "floating signifier" Muslim other, his sexuality and physical intensity, the construction of which goes back in history well before September 11, 2001, and invoked ever since, Europe secures its advantage.[62] Europe's civility requires the savagery of the Others; Europe's self-imago of holy innocence requires the debased sexuality of the Other.

This phenomenon becomes possible not least because natio-racial-culturally coded distinctions carry within them a religious moment. It is the sacred and thus affective dimension of natio-racial-culturally coded contexts of belonging that can be powerfully mobilized due to their religiosity. Emile Durkheim traced religion back to the concept of community by introducing as the basis of all religions a fundamental differentiation between the sacred and the profane, whereby he ultimately understood the sacred as symbolizing community itself. [63] Whether this interpretation does justice to an understanding of the sacred as such remains open for interpretation; however, in this instance, Durkheim's religious reflection's lead us on a theoretical path that allows us to understand the sacred as a symbolizing modus of affective natio-racial-cultural forms of belonging.

Natio-racial-culturally coded contexts are imagined spaces with a territorial reference. The nation state, for example, can be conceived as a political imagination with the goal of expressing "the will" and defending the interests of a nation living in a specific territory.[64] In order to achieve this goal, it is first and foremost necessary to create "a will" in general and second to believe in it. According to the Israeli historian and political scientist Shmuel Eisenstadt, an attempt is made in modern nation states to overcome the tension between the profane and the sacred world. [65] The nation state is "in no way only a secular formation, rather, it takes on the spiritual demands of a religion, complete with accompanying obligations which the individual now has in relation to the state as a whole."[66] Natio-racial-culturally coded practices of belonging allow for a considerable degree of meaning making that incorporates elements of the sacred and, as such, depends on this sacred element. For this very reason, the occasional recourse to the religious takes place in order to strengthen such natio-racial-culturally imagined derivatives such as "culture/civilisation," "occident," and "Europe"; or by means of the religious to confirm these constructions, "It is significant that the immediate 'reaction' to the visibility of Islam in Europe has less to do with the strengthening of a culture of Christianity and more to do with a culture of political nationalism."[67]

There seem to be at least two operative modes of creating affective bonds between individuals to an imagined, anonymous, grand collective. First, the connections are presented as noncontingent. Second, those who participate in this collective and are able to physiologically and emotionally mark themselves as belonging to this grand collective are rewarded with the increase of an affective *potentia*, manifested as higher self-worth through a participation in an imagined nonprofane reality.

The bond with and attachment to a natio-racial-culturally coded context lives from assumptions on the level of social familiarity and proximity that allow past experiences (one's own but also mediated experiences) to be projected into the future such that they appear dependable and trustworthy. The imagined natio-racial-culturally coded Us is thus a fantasized Us, that contains predominantly positive features. This regressive fantasy places natio-racial-cultural embeddedness in a reference frame of previous, fundamentally asymmetrical relations, in which one's own needs have been satisfied and a deep sense of safety achieved. When this regressive, phantasmagorical moment becomes the affective focus and natio-racial-cultural coded constructions of Us are mobilized by an ever-increasing regression, then the psychological ground is made fertile that "millions of people" are ready "not so much to kill" for such constructions as nations, the occident, or Europe, but "are willing to die for such limited imaginings."[68]

Closing Reflections or Love Matters

Borrowing from Martha Nussbaum's book, *Political Emotions: Why Love Matters for Justice*, the mechanism of crisis management outlined in this paper is symptomatic of a form of narcissism that sees others, in this case, asylum seekers and migrants, as lesser beings, mere slaves, without agency and desires of their own. She asks whether narcissism might ever be overcome in good societies toward "the direction of a stable concern for others" and argues that the real problem is the emotional combination of narcissism and helplessness that is resented and at the very core of "where 'radical evil' originates" and that it "is exercised in the tendency to subordinate other people to one's own needs."[69]

According to Nussbaum's hypothesis, it is not the asylum seeker or migrant's humanity per se that is resented and denied, but rather "it is the helplessness that we feel, on account of bodies that are vulnerable and often powerless."[70] What is at stake, both on a personal and a societal level, is the need to come to grips with the frustration of one's own or society's sense of need and pain in the face of the external independent Other. Nussbaum, quoting Donald Winnicott, states that it is the "[I]ncomplete adaptation to need" that "makes objects real, that is to say hated as well as loved."[71] She elaborates that it is the infant's narcissistic stance that fully resists this reality since perfect adaptation is needed for full omnipotence. Applying this logic to the European border politics, it is the perfect adaptation, as in full control of the European outer borders and the disciplinary placement of the asylum seekers and migrants within the structural confines of a racially selective *Obergrenze* and geographic placing *vor-Ort* outside European borders and in service and subservient to the European will that is the narcissistically inspired outcome of this omnipotent imaginary.

How, then, is it possible to overcome Eurocentric grand narratives of modernity? An omnipotent imaginary that has historically left so much devastation in its path is now being witnessed once again in the asylum crisis at Europe's gates, replete with the time-tested, racist, political mechanisms to cement desired political orders and thus power. Not in answer to this question (single answers and general theories being part of the problem), but rather as a way of thinking toward what might be possible, we leave this paper with a few final reflections about what we consider the urgent necessity for a rebuilding of heart and with it the possibility of actively imagining a future world that is less structured by violence and injustice.

We suggest two possible movements, one outward into the world and the other inward into the body. Nussbaum, following Winnicott and reflecting on ways to bear the tension of an incomplete adaptation, suggests cultivating a generous, erotic, outward-seeing movement of the mind toward the world that is intelligent, emotional, and curious. It would be a kind of seeing that views the objects in the world with wonder and love as a way to propel "the infant" beyond the frozen state of narcissism.[72] Deleuze, drawing on Spinoza, advocates an inward movement away from a radically individualistic omnipotent imaginary toward an embodied and connecting form of trans-subjectivity.[73] This being the condition of possibility for a complex emergent unity that is more affectively potential and expresses each individual in terms of those aspects they share in common.[74] It is exercised through an affirmative containment of the other, or more aptly, a mutual containment that occurs through interrelational affectivity (meaning bodies, as Spinoza insists) that are not separate from minds nor I from (an)Other, affecting and being affected within time and place. This implies that harming others/them results in harming ourselves/us and brings with it a loss of positivity, the ability to interrelate, and as such a loss of *potentia*. With this gone, we also lose the ability to be free.[75] The acceptance, as opposed to their narcissistic negation, of our human limits, vulnerabilities, mutual dependency, and common human bondage can turn the tide of negativity toward a transformative process of achieving freedom of understanding to the state of inter-being and as such dispels the divisive omnipotent power grab. It is complex and complicated, but in the end, it is a choice: Do we stay alone in the confines of our separate contained selves, subjugating others to our will or conversely being subjugated? Or do we dare to take in the other, to be the other, and as such stand up together for one another?

NOTES

1. Stephen Castles, "International Migration at the Beginning of the Twenty-First Century: Global Trends and Issues," *International Social Science Journal* 165, no. 52 (2000), 269–281.

2. Ruben Zaiotti, *Cultures of Border Control: Schengen and the Evolution of European Frontiers* (Chicago: University of Chicago Press, 2011).

3. In our perspective, the basic analytical category of migration research is the relationship of individuals and groups to natio-racial-culturally coded orders of belonging, as well as in the transformation of this relationship; Paul Mecheril et al., "Migrationsforschung als Kritik? Eine Annäherung an ein epistemisches Anliegen in 57 Schritten," in *Migrationsforschung als Kritik?*,

eds. Paul Mecheril et al. (in Volume I and II) (Wiesbaden: Springer VS, 2013), 7–55. The expression natio-racial-cultural ("natio-ethno-kulturell," see Paul Mecheril, *Prekäre Verhältnisse: über natio-ethno-kulturelle* (Mehrfach-) Zugehörigke*it* (Münster; München: Waxmann, 2003), 118–251) refers on the one hand to the fact that the concepts of nation, ethnicity, race, and culture are often used in a diffuse and undifferentiated way, both in research and everyday communication. On the other hand, this term indicates the fact that concepts of nation, ethnicity, race, and culture are manifested formally in laws and regulations, materially through border controls and identity documents, and also socially through symbolic practices that generate rather blurred meanings and outcomes that are subsequently used politically. For more detail, see Paul Mecheril, "Orders of Belonging and Education: Migration Pedagogy as Criticism," in *Migration. Changing Concepts, Critical Approaches*, eds. Doris Bachmann-Medick and Jens Kugele [Berlin: De Gruyter, 2018], 121–138).

4. Mecheril, "Orders of Belonging and Education: Migration Pedagogy as Criticism."

5. Stefanie Bolzen and Hannelore Crolly, "Streit in Brüssel: 'Eine zweite Flüchtlingskrise überlebt die EU nicht,'" 2017, https://www.welt.de/politik/ausland/article171609163/Eine-zweite -Fluechtlingskrise-ueberlebt-die-EU-nicht.html.

6. TAZ and DPA and AFP, "Bundesinnenminister Seehofer zu Moria: 'Humanitäre Notlage,'" in taz.de (04.02.2021), https://taz.de/Bundesinnenminister-Seehofer-zu-Moria/!5713668/.

7. Stefan Reinecke, "Deutsche Politik nach Brand in Moria: Wir wollen das nicht schaffen," in taz.de (11.09.2020), https://taz.de/Deutsche-Politik-nach-Brand-in-Moria/!5713727/.

8. Manuel Bewarder, "Deutschland Obergrenze," in *Die Welt*, April 7, 2019.

9. Friedrich Merz, then presidential candidate for the CDU, was outspoken about his opposition to taking in asylum seekers from the Greek and Bosnian refugee camps. He stated in a press conference: "The entire European Union has, above all, the obligation to help asylum seekers in the Balkan countries or the Greek Islands, on site," and that "This human catastrophe is not solved, however, when we say: All of you come to Germany. This route is no longer open." Redaktionsnetzwerk Deutschland, "Merz gegen Aufnahme von Flüchtlingen aus Bosnien und Griechenland," https://www.rnd.de/politik/merz-gegen-aufnahme-von-fluchtlingen-aus-bosnien -und-griechenland-RNAZXTJOXYP7YXJHL4VFQEJEQE.html.

10. Summarized from the European Commission Press release: "A fresh start on migration: Building confidence and striking a new balance between responsibility and solidarity," September 23, 2020, https://ec.europa.eu/commission/presscorner/api/files/document/print/en/iP_20 _1706_EN.pdf.

11. Hans-Christian Rössle, "Tor Nach Europa: Immer mehr Migranten erreichen Spanien," *faz.net*, January 1, 2021, https://www.faz.net/aktuell/politik/ausland/tor-nach-europa-immer -mehr-migranten-erreichen-spanien-17131963.html.

12. Rössle, "Tor Nach Europa."

13. See also Heidrun Friese, *Flüchtlinge: Opfer—Bedrohung—Helden: Zur politischen Imagination des Fremden* (Bielefeld: transcript, 2017), Zygmunt Bauman, *Strangers at Our Door* (Cambridge: Polity Press, 2016).

14. Statista, "Stimmen sie der Aussage, die Anzahl der aufgenommenen Flüchtlinge sei eine Bedrohung für den Wohlstand in Deutschland voll und ganz zu, eher zu, eher nicht zu oder gar nicht zu?" July 2017-January 2018, https://de.statista.com/statistik/daten/studie /915635/umfrage/umfrage-zur-bedrohung-des-wohlstands-durch-fluechtlinge-nach-herkunfts gruppen/.

15. The term *economic refugee* operates according to a double mechanism: first, the insinuation of economic interest as the only motive for migration, and second the vilification and scandalization of this economic motivation, which stands in direct contradiction to the fact that the capitalist system encourages all individuals to align their actions according to economic interests (*homo economicus*).

16. The term *bogus asylum seeker* has discursively replaced the earlier term *exile* and wholly undermines the right to sanctuary, contained in its original meaning, and based on economic hardship caused by war, famine, environmental degradation, but also global economic forces that cause severe poverty and suffering; Encarnación Gutiérrez Rodríguez, "The Coloniality of Migration and the 'Refugee Crisis': On the Asylum-Migration Nexus, the Transatlantic White European Settler Colonialism-Migration and Racial Capitalism," in *Refuge* 34, no. 1 (2018), 16–28.

17. Cited in Mareike Gebhardt, "The Populist Moment: Affective Orders, Protest, and Politics of Belonging," *Distinktion: Journal of Social Theory*, (2019), 55.

18. Gebhardt, "The Populist Moment," 55.

19. Lauren Berlant, *Cruel Optimism* (Durham: Duke University Press, 2011), 228.

20. Sabine Kinkarz, "Deutschland braucht Einwanderer," *Deutsche Welle*, December 16, 2019, accessed October 14, 2022, https://www.dw.com/de/deutschland-braucht-einwanderer /a-51700947.

21. Kinkarz, "Deutschland braucht Einwanderer."

22. "Fachkräfte dringend gesucht: Deutschland braucht laut Studie Zuwanderung," February 2, 2021, accessed October 14, 2022, https://www.n-tv.de/wirtschaft/Deutschland-braucht-laut -Studie-Zuwanderung-article20852455.html.

23. Epoch Times, "Fachkräftegipfel geplant: Anwerbung ausländischer Fachkräfte in Brasilien, Indien und Vietnam," in epochtimes.de (04.03.2021), https://www.epochtimes.de/politik /deutschland/fachkraeftegipfel-geplant-anwerbung-auslaendischer-fachkraefte-in-brasilien -indien-und-vietnam-a3098978.html.

24. "Legal Prerequisites Established to Manage Migration," Federal Ministry of the Interior and Community, February 2, 2024, https://www.bmi.bund.de/SharedDocs/kurzmeldungen/EN /2024/02/02_manage_migration.html.

25. Deutscher Bundestag, "Distribution of Seats in the 20th German Bundestag," accessed May 24, 2024, https://www.bundestag.de/en/parliament/plenary/distributionofseats; and Deutscher Bundestag, "AfD Calls for Measures against 'Imported Anti-Semitism,'" September 11, 2023, https://www.bundestag.de/presse/hib/kurzmeldungen-976448.

26. Stephen Castles et al., "Global Perspectives on Forced Migration," *Asian and Pacific Migration Journal* 15, no. 1 (2006), 7–28.

27. Gutiérrez Rodríguez. "The Coloniality of Migration", 16–28.

28. Reinhart Koselleck, "Krise," in *Geschichtliche Grundbegriffe: Historisches Lexikon zur politisch-sozialen Sprache in Deutschland*, Vol. 3, eds. Otto Brunner and Werner Conze and Reinhart Koselleck (Stuttgart: Klett-Cotta, 1982), 617–650.

29. Koselleck, "Krise," 617–650.

30. Jan M. Sawilla, "Entschieden unter Zeitdruck? Zur Krisensemantik in der französischen Publizistik zwischen Religionskriegen, Fronde und Französischer Revolution," in Die Krise der Frühen Neuzeit, eds. Rudolf Schlögl and Philip R. Hoffmann-Rehnitz and Eva Wiebel (Göttingen: V&R, 2016), 333–368.

31. Hegemony theorists (for instance: Louis Althusser, Cornelius Castoriadis, Ernesto Laclau and Chantal Mouffe, and Claude Lefort) understand "society" not as an unquestioned unity with a given identity, but rather depart from the premise that, in particular, nationalistically inspired societies are based on self-conceptions and imaginations that are continually (re-)produced in order to emphasize the continuity, coherence, identity and unity in opposition to difference and inconsistencies.

32. Cited in Luc Ciompi, "Affektlogik, affektive Kommunikation und Pädagogik: Eine Wissenschaftliche Neuorientierung," in *Literatur und Forschungsreport—Weiterbildung des Deutschen Instituts Für Erwachsenenbildung zum Thema Gehirn und Lernen*, eds. Ekkehard Nuissl, Cristina Schiersmann, and Horst Siebert (Bielefeld: wbv, 2003), 62–70.

33. Sara Ahmed, *The Cultural Politics of Emotion* (Edinburgh: Edinburgh University Press, 2014).

34. Paul Mecheril and Monica van der Haagen-Wulff, "Bedroht, Angstvoll, Wütend: Affektlogik der Migrationsgesellschaft," in *Die Dämonisierung der Anderen: Rassismuskritik der Gegenwart*, eds. Paul Mecheril and María do Mar Castro Varela (Bielefeld, transcript, 2016), 119–143.

35. Gilles Deleuze, *Spinoza: Practical Philosophy* (San Francisco: City Lights Books 1988).

36. Jan Slaby and Rainer Mühlhoff, "Affect," in *Affective Societies: Key Concepts*, eds. Jan Slaby and Christian von Scheve (London and New York: Routledge, 2019), 29.

37. Baruch Spinoza, "Ethics," in *The Collected Works of Spinoza* (Vol.1.), ed. and trans. Edwin Curley (Princeton University Press, 1985). Original work published in 1677.

38. Slaby and Mühlhoff, "Affect," 27.

39. Brian Massumi, "The Autonomy of Affect," *Cultural Critique* 31 (1995), 83–109.

40. Eve K. Sedgwick and Adam Frank, "Shame in the Cybernetic Fold: Rereading Silvan Thomkins," *Critical Inquiry* 21, no. 2 (1995), 496–552.

41. Slaby and Mühlhoff, "Affect," 34.

42. Slaby and Mühlhoff, "Affect," 34.

43. Laura Kemmer et al., "On Right-Wing Movements, Spheres, and Resonances: An Interview with Ben Anderson and Rainer Mühlhoff," *Distinktion: Journal of Social Theory* 20, no. 1 (2018), 25–41.

44. Laura Kemmer et al., "On Right-Wing Movements."

45. Brigitte Bargetz, "Mapping Effect. Challenges of (Un)Timely Politics," in *Timing of Affect: Episthologies, Aesthetics, Politics*, eds. Marie-Luise Angerer, Bernd Bösel, and Michaela Ott (Zurich: Diaphanes, 2014), 300.

46. Berlant, *Cruel Optimism*, 230.

47. Bargetz, "Mapping Effect," 301.

48. Ahmed, *The Cultural Politics of Emotion*.

49. Sara Ahmed, *On Being Included: Racism and Diversity in Institutional Life* (Durham: Duke University Press, 2012).

50. Bauman, *Strangers at Our Door*.

51. This passage is taken from Paul Mecheril and Monica van der Haagen-Wulff, "Migration, Europe, and Staged Affect-Scenarios," in *Europe Now*, 2018, https://www.europenowjournal.org /2018/07/01/migration-europe-and-staged-affect-scenarios/.

52. Donna Landry and Gerald MacLean, *The Spivak Reader* (London and New York: Routledge, 1996).

53. The term *Othering* was coined by Gayatri Chakravorty Spivak, borrowing from Lacan theoretical framework in which subjectivization and identity formation is negotiated through a constant "mirror dynamic." According to Spivak, colonized subjects can only be recognized as such through the dominant discursive practices of the colonial center, and indeed in a dependent relationship with it. Colonizing practices create subjects. Another perspective focuses on exactly those discursive practices that designate some as "others," and in so doing, creates a collective identity. This perspective has become widely known and influential, largely on account of Edward Said's works on the construction of the "Orient" as an antagonistic foil to the "Occident." The mechanisms and the efficacy of these practices can only be understood, according to Said, in the context of European imperialism, and thereby as the legitimation and stabilization practices of claims to dominance in relation to the constructed "other"; Edward W. Said, *Orientalism* (New York: Pantheon Books, 1978).

54. Gessler, *Sekundärer Antisemitismus*, 2006.

55. Zygmunt Bauman, *Wasted Lives: Modernity and its Outcasts* (Cambridge: Polity Press, 2004).

56. Étienne Balibar, *We, the People of Europe? Reflections on Transnational Citizenship* (Princeton: Princeton University Press, 2004).

57. We assume that dehumanization is also a narcissistic strategy aimed at avoiding feelings of helplessness and pain due to the presence of others' suffering; we return to this idea at the end of this essay.

58. Ulrich Brand and Markus Wissen, "Sozial-ökologische Krise und imperiale Lebensweise. Zu Krise und Kontinuität kapitalistischer Naturverhältnisse," in *VielfachKrise. Im finanzdominierten Kapitalismus*, eds. Alex Demirović et.al. (Hamburg: VSA, 2011), 79–94.

59. Klaus Dörre, "Landnahme. Triebkräfte, Wirkungen und Grenzen kapitalistischer Wachstumsdynamik," in *Die globale Einhegung. Krise, ursprüngliche Akkumulation und Landnahmen im Kapitalismus*, ed. Maria Backhouse et al. (Münster: Westfälisches Dampfboot 2013), 112–140.

60. Ahmed, *The Cultural Politics of Emotion*, 72.

61. Nikita Dhawan, "Doch wieder! Die Selbst-Barbarisierung Europas," in *Die Dämonisierung der Anderen: Rassismuskritik der Gegenwart*, eds. Paul Mecheril and María do Mar Castro Varela (Bielefeld, transcript, 2016), 73–97.

62. Stuart Hall et al., *Policing the Crisis: Mugging, The State, Law & Order* (London: Red Globe Press, 2013). Stuart Hall et al., in their book introduce the notion of a "floating signifier" when analyzing media representations of the black Caribbean man in the Thatcher era whereby he becomes a "floating signifier" for racial fantasies manifest as sexual and existential anxieties and fears of the white population. The way of dealing with this anxiety was to increase the social control with the introduction of racial profiling and increased policing. The term *moral panic* first coined by Stanley Cohen was used in this text to describe social impact of these racist fantasies about inferior, animalistic, criminal racialized others; Stanley Cohen, "Whose Side Were We On? The Undeclared Politics of Moral Panic Theory," in *Crime Media Culture* 7, no. 3 (2011), 237–244.

63. Émile Durkheim, *The Elementary Forms of the New Religious Life* (London: Routledge, 1984).

64. Rogers Brubaker, *Citizenship and Nationhood in France and Germany* (Cambridge: Harvard University Press, 1992).

65. Shemuel N. Eisenstadt and Brigitte Schluchter, *Die Vielfalt der Moderne* (Weilerswist: Velbrück Wissenschaft, 2000).

66. Hubert Knoblauch, *Populäre Religion: Auf dem Weg zu einer spirituellen Gesellschaft* (Frankfurt a. M.: Campus, 2009).

67. Knoblauch, *Populäre Religion*, 37.

68. Benedict Anderson, *Imagined Communities: Reflections on the Origin and Spread of Nationalism* (London: Verso, 1991), 7.

69. Martha C. Nussbaum, *Political Emotions: Why Love Matters for Justice* (Cambridge: Harvard University Press, 2013), 172.

70. Nussbaum, *Political Emotions*, 172.

71. Nussbaum, *Political Emotions*, 172.

72. Nussbaum, *Political Emotions*, 174.

73. Rossi Braidotti, "Affirmation, Pain and Empowerment," *Journal of Women's Studies* 14 no. 3 (2006), 7–36.

74. See Deleuze, *Spinoza*, 49–51.

75. Braidotti, "Affirmation, Pain and Empowerment," 17.

CHAPTER THIRTEEN

Narrative Anxiety

An Examination of Fractured Memory Through the Lens of Contemporary Francophone Literature

EMMANUEL KATTAN AND
KAREN STRUVE

Over the last few years, numerous studies have revealed a growing sense of anxiety and insecurity within French society. According to a February 2020 Sciences Po Cevipof poll, 41% of French people do not feel confident about their future.[1] A full 56% believe that France should protect itself from the rest of the world, and 72% believe that their way of life is threatened. Many objective fears help explain this incapacity to envisage the future with confidence: the continuing impact of the global COVID-19 pandemic and threats of future public health crises; the fear of a looming recession and the economic insecurity it will bring; the increasingly dramatic impact of climate change; and the rise of populism and violent political movements.

One creative laboratory for anxiety is literature. In this context, literature serves as a field for experimenting with anxiety: for the Goncourt Prize winner Leïla Slimani, for example, fear is even the vanishing point for her writing: " 'J'écris sur ce qui me fait le plus peur' [I write about what scares me the most]."[2] At the same time, francophone literature, film, and series show that feelings of restlessness and insecurity, often leading to paralyzing panic attacks and anxiety disorders are all too common today. And this does not only appear in the realm of traditional anxiety literature in the tradition of H. P. Lovecraft[3] or in other forms of the thriller and horror genres. Anxiety also manifests itself in the literary processing of sociopolitical discourses, which in literature leads to particularly dazzling insights, when authors turn their gaze inward and analyze in great detail their relationship with society. This narrated or narrative anxiety is found in many areas and genres of literature. Michel Houellebecq might be one of the most famous anxiety detectors: fear of technology, artificial intelligence, and biotechnology (*Les Particules élémentaires*[4]); loneliness despite omnipresent communication, fear of being held back by anti-authoritarian 68er parents—especially mothers (*Extension du domaine de la lutte*[5]); fear of physical closeness and sexual frustration; fear of losing patriarchal structures and privileges; and more and more importantly, fear of the other. In *Soumission* Houellebecq expresses his fear of the (racially marked) foreigners in France.[6]

This leads us to another source of anxiety, which may be more difficult to measure, but is nonetheless real and subject of many literary texts: the growing feeling, among many sectors of the French population, that their collective identity and their sense of rootedness in the past is under threat. This concern is apparent in the proliferation of debates focusing on French history, especially the memory of the Vichy regime, the Algerian War, and the slave trade. Over the last 30 years, the collective memory of specific groups within French society has gained increasing recognition in the public space. The advent of memorial laws, the creation of official commemorations, monuments, and museums, as well as the reevaluation of history textbooks has led to the acknowledgment of historical narratives that had previously been excluded from national history. At the same time, the emergence of group-based historical narratives generated a competition among different communities, leading to what historian Benjamin Stora called "memorial communitarianism."[7]

It is also visible in what Amin Maalouf called 15 years ago the "exclusion machine" France has become. Fear of almost everything is its fuel:

> Son carburant, la peur. Peur de l'Europe, soudain;—encore un "nous" qui s'est transformé insidieusement en "eux"! Peur des Anglosaxons. Peur de l'islam. Peur de l'Asie qui s'élance. Peur de l'Afrique qui piétine. Peur des jeunes. Peur des banlieues. Peur de la violence, de la vache folle, de la grippe aviaire . . . Peur et honte de son passé, au point d'enterrer ses dossiers et de ne plus oser célébrer ses victoires. Ceux qui chérissent la France et qui se sont nourris de son Histoire, ceux qui y sont nés comme ceux qui l'ont choisie, ne peuvent que souffrir au spectacle d'une société tremblante et honteuse qui n'ose plus se regarder dans le miroir du temps.[8]

Maalouf denounces the xenophobic use of the word *francophone* based on the affective constructions of alterity along cultural, social, spatial, and political difference. But Maalouf refers to another point that is crucial for the analyses of francophone literature: the fear of the francophone other goes hand in hand with the fear of the past and of history. And this past cannot be kept outside any longer. Francophone narratives reflecting colonial power dynamics are no external additions to a French historiography of anxiety narratives. In other words, francophone narratives may be strange, but they are no strangers. They are part of French culture, society, and literature. Francophone authors do not write from the margins but from the very center. The issue, then, is no longer whether one should be "against francophone literature,"[9] but whether and how a new kind of "Francophonie" can be written?

For many French citizens, it has become increasingly challenging to relate to a unifying, national historical narrative. The collective rituals and memories they identify with only tell a fragmented story. The single narrative that fed French imagination and helped France find its place in the world is increasingly splintered. The construction of France as a holistic "imagined community,"[10] as Benedict Anderson would put it, becomes highly problematic because, on the one hand, the members of the modern French community suffer from anonymity, isolation, and self-alienation; on the other hand, postcolonial France has to integrate various, different, and sometimes even contradictory and conflicting narratives of memory and identity. The fragmentation of national memory is reflected in France's sometimes fractious relationship with its former colonies, which today form part of the loose grouping of countries called the Francophonie.

Two dynamics are at play here: first, the Republican narrative, which imposed a dominant vision of the past since the French Revolution, is now being called into question by collective narratives attempting to come to terms with a history of violence and silence. Second, new or renewed (counter-)narratives of belonging, in France and in the wider Francophonie (Algeria, sub-Saharan Africa, or the Antilles), are attempting to reconstruct broken links with the past and chart new pathways of identity.

This is where literature comes into play. Fictional narratives play a significant role in this effort and provide useful templates that can help us understand and deal with the splintering of French national memory. Indeed, to what extent can novels from the Francophonie provide insights about the rehabilitation of the collective memory of minority groups and their place in the contemporary historical landscape? Can fiction provide us with fresh perspectives that can help redraw the map of fragmented memories and rediscover or even reinvent connections among them? In what way do fictional

texts not only repeat or mimetically reflect discourses of fear in terms of violence, fractures, and trauma but also foster, support, and even transform (hi-)
stories? Are the ghosts of the past in the form of whispering ancestors, warning
voices, or impressive hallucinations objects of fear or consoling advisers and
wise archivists of experiences? Do they cause or help to mourn a lost but
"present past?"

We propose to seek answers to these questions through works of contemporary fiction that expose fractured memories and offer clues about
threading them back into a more complex, multilayered human history. An
analysis of loss, absence, and forgetting in these works will enable us to examine to what extent they can reconnect fractured memories—not through the
invention of new national myths but through the creation of individual narratives that offer us an opportunity to question our place within collective
memories and reinterpret our own lives.

Narrative Anxiety from a Francophone Perspective: Frightening Fractures

A central feature of francophone contemporary literature is the effort to
deal with what we would call "historiographical fractures" (*fractures histo-
riographiques*): the cultural-historical fractures in postcolonial historiography (unlike Vergès et al. who prefer speaking of ruptures instead of fractures[11];
historiographical fractures are closer to Guilluy's French fractures[12]). Since the
decolonization of the francophone colonies in the 1960s, the explosive question of a common (literary) historiography has arisen for writers from the
Francophonie but also in France. In francophone literatures, veritable counter-
histories were initially developed in which, from a personal as well as a collective point of view, one's own marginalization is narrated (e.g., Assia Djebar's
novel, *La disparition de la langue française* (*The Disappearance of the French
Language*).[13] Beyond marginalization, these works reflect a quest for identity,
an effort to tell one's own story using both the spoken and the written word
(a very important feature of Antillean literature[14]), and a determination to pass
on one's own myths and legends while maintaining close ties with French-
Western literary traditions.

The concept of fractures aims at something that, at the heart of the text, has
to do with the emotional-affective charge and the essence of literature: What
emotional engagement with these fractures can literary texts develop? In
French and Francophone literature, one can find a whole spectrum of emotional involvement: pain, grief, powerlessness, and above all, fear and anxiety.[15]

At the same time, literary texts make it possible to clothe this fear of the loss of one's own history—both in the forgetting indigenous history and in the invisibility within the French national history—in linguistic images and narrative procedures.

Literary texts in particular can, first, portray a whole range of emotional shades of fear, from latent feelings of insecurity to fear for pure survival, and translate them into language. Second, literary texts can help shape and modify the literary historiography of France by rewriting canonical texts, for example, from Césaire's *Une tempête*[16] to Daoud's *Meursault, contre-enquête*.[17] They can tell new stories from their own perspectives. In recent contemporary literature, this has the effect of telling stories from the marginalized position of the periphery and in genealogy as the (former) colonized, in the sense of a *writing back*.[18]

However, especially in recent francophone literature, this also has the effect of sensitively calling into question the principle of national literary historiography. This is reflected, for example, in the debate about French world literature,[19] which was initiated in the 2000s after francophone literatures increasingly won the major literary prizes in France. These debates testify that neither French history nor French literary history can be told hexagonally and eurocentrically. But the debates also demonstrate that the integration of stories from colonial post-memory[20] and emotional experiences from (post-)migration into the (hi-)story of France does not happen harmoniously and without conflict.

This very conflictual relation between France and its strangers and France's refugee policy is at the center of Sinha's novel *Assommons les pauvres!* (*Slay the Poor!*).[21] In her novel, refugees spill onto the seashore like abhorrent jellyfish. And the Bengali-French author Sinha caused quite a stir in France because a literary voice objected to France's integration policies and, at the same time, the novel expressed the fears of migrants and their experience of everyday racism. The semantics of fear in French and francophone contemporary literature unfold in a spectrum ranging from dull unease (malaise) to suffocating panic. In Sinha's novel *Slay the Poor!*, these feelings are also expressed by the main character, a nameless woman working as an interpreter at the integration office in Paris. She describes a certain resigned discontent and aversion to those people who come to France as asylum seekers:

> *je pense encore à ces gens-là qui envahissaient les mers comme des méduses mal-aimées et se jetaient sur les rives étrangères* [I still think of those people who invaded the seas like unloved jellyfish and threw themselves on foreign shores].[22]

Finally, the fears of others break into her dreams, in which the young woman then literally threatens to drown in the murmurs, whispers, and screams of people.

Rather, the literary texts in particular reveal a struggle for interpretive sovereignty over collective and subjective history. The texts narrate the anxieties that accompany these fractures by first making visible the omissions and erasures of counter-histories in the archive of French history and narrating the histories violently excluded and repressed from collective memory: under the countless literary texts one might quote, for example, the forgotten slaves of Tromelin in the 18th century[23] or Daeninckx's novel about the massacre in 1961 in Paris;[24] the texts of the writers of the Antilles like Edouard Glissant, whose literature is concerned with the (im-)possibility to narrate genesis, which he calls a "di-genesis" ["di-genèse"],[25] or Daoud's counternarrative of the ones who are killed in silence in Camus's pretexte.[26]

What is very revealing and due to postcolonial perspective of the deconstruction of power relations,[27] is that both sides of the colonial relation have to deal with fear: Narrative Anxiety makes the fears of the repressed visible as well as the fears of the violent colonial power, which initiated the repression and tabooed the history of violence out of fear of its own guilt.

Second, fiction addresses the fear of fractures by telling their own corrective, alternative, critical stories that don't minimize fear with stable self-images and narratives but rather by holding in abeyance in literature the ambivalence of self-empowerment and powerlessness, fear and resistance, like in Wilfried N'Sondé's novel *Le silence des esprits* (*The Silence of the Spirits*), a novel about an illegal person and a Parisian woman who share their demons in the safe space of her apartment.[28]

The perspective, however, on literary constructions of fear is even more interesting on a third level and will be illustrated in the following by means of exemplary analyses. The hypothesis is that literature can articulate both individual and cultural, collective historical experience through the feeling of fear in the echo chamber of francophone literature. Narrative anxiety is in this sense not a purely subjective experience; rather, it is culturally coded and thus conventionalized, or even politicized in Ahmed's terms,[29] especially in the postcolonial perspective. It is precisely the moment of fear that dynamizes the historiographical fractures and deconstructs colonial dichotomies.

A recent and particularly celebrated attempt to tell the postcolonial story of France and Morocco as an *entangled history* (going back to Mintz[30]) is the current (still unfinished) trilogy *Le pays des autres* by Leïla Slimani.[31] This is about a family history that begins with the story of grandparents, a Moroccan farmer and a middle-class young Frenchwoman, who lead a meager life in Morocco in the 1940s. Slimani recounts the couple's multiple experiences of exclusion (in Morocco and later in France), their worries and fears but also their tenacity, and many protagonists' multiperspective views of life in the French-Moroccan colonial situation. Slimani tells a rather classical situation of cultural conflict. While the plot focuses on the life stories of the individual characters (e.g., with the Moroccan neighbors, in catholic French school) and delves into the history of Moroccan independence and its impact on the family saga, at the emotional level it is the moments of violence and fear that make the love story between Amine and Mathilde a multilayered, grueling story of power negotiations. The feelings of fear (of Morocco as unfamiliar land to Mathilde, of the Moroccans who see in Amine the enemy who fought for France in World War II, of the problematic legacy of colonial history in general) lead on the one hand to a kind of postcolonial melancholia, as Paul Gilroy would put it,[32]and on the other hand to a constant struggle with the present situation of the protagonists.

Debt and Memory

Many fictional narratives from the Francophonie offer valuable insights into the problematic transmission of past events, conflicts about interpretations of history, and anxiety about remembrance, which these conflicts generate. At a theoretical level, fictional accounts have a strong power of explanation: through the destinies of fictional characters, they enable us to visualize the emergence of divergent interpretations of the past and to envisage in their complexity the struggles of individuals as they strive to reconcile these narratives.

But much more intriguing is the power of fictional accounts to transform the reader's own relationship with the past. At a practical level, fictional narratives pave the way for this kind of transformation in three ways: First, fictional narratives help resurrect forgotten historical figures or individuals whose lives have been smothered under the weight of dominant representations of history. Second, they illustrate the relationship of debt that binds today's generations with the past and the need to restore human dignity to those whose stories were forgotten or distorted. Finally, they provide readers with a pathway to experience the past not simply as a succession of events but, to borrow an idea expressed by Walter Benjamin, as a *jetztzeit*—a "now-time," a past still rife with possibilities, a present still in the making. [33]

Resurrecting the "Forgotten"

When Guadeloupean writer Maryse Condé became interested in the history of the Salem trials, what caught her attention was the story of Tituba, the first woman accused of witchcraft during the 1692 trials. Little is known about Tituba. Born in South America, she lived in Barbados before coming to the United States as an enslaved woman. Her master, the Puritan minister Samuel Parris, forced her to confess to witchcraft and to denounce others. Tituba was jailed in Boston and, following the trials, sold again into slavery. "To whom? Such is the intentional or unintentional racism of the historians that we shall never know," says Condé.[34] In the face of this lack of interest in the destiny of Tituba, Maryse Condé sets out to fill in the blanks and restore to the enslaved woman the dignity of a narrative.

This process of rehabilitation through fiction operates at three levels: First, Condé builds long stretches of narrative to give life to aspects of Tituba's destiny that were ignored by historians. In assembling the imaginary building blocks of Tituba's life, Condé did not aspire to historical accuracy or even plausibility. Her objective was to restore the entire narrative arch of a fragmentary life, whose individual tenor and unique perspective on the world had not been deemed worthy of historical interest.

At a second level, Condé attempts to reconstruct the character of Tituba by reclaiming the narrative that slavery denied her. In doing so, Condé's *I, Tituba* articulates a unique form of anxiety toward the past: an anxiety born, not from an uncertainty about past events, but from the incompleteness of a life cut off from its roots. Indeed, slavery, as Condé explains, is not only the violation of physical freedom, but it is also the erasure of one's past.

If slavery denies human beings their humanity by annihilating their past and their stories, even after they have died, then rebuilding their narrative, however imaginary it may be, can be a way of restoring this humanity, postmortem. This is the task that Maryse Condé embarks on with her novel, *I, Tituba*.

Finally, Condé uses witchcraft to create a third pathway toward the rehabilitation of Tituba. Communicating with the "invisibles" provides witches with the capacity to connect with the past, unearthing the stories of ancestors that have long been forgotten or suppressed by the writers of history. By collecting stories and testimonies from her mother, her teacher, and other dead souls, and transmitting them to her contemporaries, Tituba becomes a bridge between the past and the present. She is a guardian of memory.

This response to what could be called "transmission anxiety" illustrates the close connection between story building and emancipation. Here, the powers of the witch resemble those of the writer: the first uses necromancy to knit back together the present and the past; the second uses imagination to claim back forgotten stories and provide a template for the narrative unity of human life. Condé's *I, Tituba* can be read as a celebration of the emancipating power of storytelling: communicating with the dead allows Tituba to inscribe her destiny in the long line of women, witches, and slaves striving to become the authors of their own lives.

Narrative and Debt

In the constellation of Patrick Modiano's work, *Dora Bruder*, published in 1997, occupies a unique position.[35] Neither novel nor biography, the book mobilizes fiction to bring to life the story of a teenager about whom very little is known. Dora Bruder was born on February 25, 1926, in the XIIth arrondissement in Paris. Her father, Ernest Bruder, was a Jew from Vienna. Her mother, Cécile, was Hungarian. During France's Occupation, in 1941, Dora, a rebellious teenager, was sent to a boarding school, Saint-Coeur-de-Marie. She escaped twice. She was arrested and then deported to Auschwitz on September 18, 1942.

Based on a wanted notice he finds in a 1941 newspaper, author Patrick Modiano sets out to rebuild, piece by piece, the life of Dora Bruder, based on scraps of information he is able to gather. The result of his inquiry is disappointing. Most of Dora Bruder's life remains clouded in mystery. But beyond Dora's brief and tragic life, it is Modiano's own narrative that is compelling: his description about how he painstakingly researches every little detail about Dora Bruder's life, about her parents, and about her family history. Revisiting the neighborhood where she lived (and where he, himself, used to live), Modiano engages in an elaborate literary detective work, searching for clues about the people who knew Dora, those who might have shared her room in Tourelles, or those who may have been on the same train when she was deported to Drancy, then to Auschwitz.

Modiano's inquiry is all about fact gathering and yet it delivers very little by way of facts. It does little to enrich our understanding of the Occupation. Rather, *Dora Bruder* should be understood as the fulfillment of a debt.

What is the nature of this responsibility? First, it does not appear that Modiano is fulfilling the duty of a witness. He never knew Dora Bruder, nor did he witness the Occupation (he was born a month before the end of the war). Second, could *Dora Bruder* be construed as a response to a "civic duty to remember"? Could Modiano's book be conceived as a cautionary tale, a warning against the banality of persecution and the constant danger that discriminatory or racist policies represent?

We would argue, however, that such a reading would be reductive. In the last 30 years in France, a conception of the duty to remember as a prophylactic against historical violence has become increasingly popular in education, media, and political circles. But to view Modiano's inquiry as aiming to warn future generations against the repetition of tyranny and intolerance is both problematic and simplistic. It is simplistic because it reduces a complex, multilayered, multidimensional narrative to a unitary, utilitarian function. It is also problematic because it presupposes that knowledge of past crimes can somehow better prepare an individual to take a stand against similar crimes in the future. In other words, evoking the abject policies of Vichy France, the persecution of Jews by the Nazis, and their consequences on the destinies of individuals, could instill the resolution to fight against new instances of state violence and persecution today. While it is certainly true that accurate and detailed historical knowledge can enhance an individual's understanding of contemporary politics and provide them with arguments to engage in a political cause, the resolution to take a stand against injustice is not correlated with knowledge or awareness of past persecutions, as sociologists Sarah Gensburger and Sandrine Lefranc demonstrated.[36]

If Modiano's sense of debt does not derive from his position as a witness or from a civic duty to remember, what is it founded on? In his collection of essays, *The Drowned and the Saved*, Primo Levi articulates his duty toward the past as a debt toward the dead.[37] This duty, in his case, is closely linked to his responsibility as a witness. As a survivor, he is called upon to be the voice of the disappeared. Modiano, while he is not a witness, feels a unique responsibility toward Dora Bruder (although the nature of their connection is not immediately clear). If his narrative fulfills an "injunction to remember," it is, primarily, a debt toward the dead.

By virtue of an imagined kinship with Dora, Modiano feels a sense of inescapable responsibility, as if he had been chosen to preserve the memory of the teenage girl. Indeed, Modiano feels as though he is the only remaining link between the past and the present. *Dora Bruder* casts the notion of the injunction to remember in a different light and helps us rethink anxiety about the past and the fractured transmission of memory. Fulfilling our debt toward the past is not about ambitious speeches and declarations; it is not about bravely taking a stand against lying politicians, demagogues, and powerful manipulators. Rather, it is about opposing the erasure of time.

At the end of the book, Modiano states that all that remains of Dora is her secret—how she spent her time during her two escapes in the winter and spring of 1942. Faced with the enigma of Dora Bruder's life, Modiano decides that he should not try to imagine what she did during that time. Against the novelist's instinct, which would be to fill in the blanks to create a rich narrative (as Maryse Condé does in her novel *I, Tituba*), Modiano resists the temptation of drawing from his imagination to add flesh to the bones of Dora's story. He decides to honor the teenager, not by elucidating the mystery of her ultimate days on earth but by acknowledging that Dora had a secret and that this secret was part of what made her human.

Narrative Anxiety and Messianic Time

Fiction creates the illusion of life through a variety of technical devices: detailed descriptions of places that transport the reader into a carefully constructed universe; interior monologues that reveal a character's complex psychological profile; and dialogues that reproduce the depth and complexity of human interactions. Fiction also creates the illusion of possibility. Even though the narrative is fixed and the destiny of the characters is sealed, the novel transports us to a position in time when all alternatives seem open, when the heroine or the hero has yet to choose which path to follow. Fiction introduces the principle of uncertainty in our relationship with the past. It resurrects situations when the future is still open, when each moment is still pregnant with possibilities.

This relationship with a past that remains undecided was articulated by Walter Benjamin in his "Theses on the Philosophy of History."[38] Benjamin contrasts the mechanical conception of time, which is measured by clocks and divided in equal units that flow in regular patterns, with messianic time—a moment that interrupts the march of history and carries the potential for radical change. Benjamin calls this moment *jetztzeit*—now-time—which, "as a model of messianic time, comprises the entire history of mankind in a tremendous abbreviation . . ."[39]

Messianic time connects the present to revolutionary moments in the past—half-fulfilled historical events whose potential in the fight for the oppressed was significant but ended up unexploited. Together, they form what Benjamin calls "constellations:" past and present connected, not through links of causality but through a common meaning, a joint aspiration for freedom. Messianic time offers historical actors the opportunity to leap into the past and, as Michael Löwy explains in his reading of the "Theses," seize a forgotten event (e.g., an aborted revolution) and resuscitate its potential for radical change. Such reigniting of past possibilities is illustrated, for example, by the rediscovery in the 1970s of texts of Olympe de Gouges, "the author of pamphlets denouncing slavery and of the 'Declaration of the Rights of Woman' (1791)."[40] Olympe de Gouge was executed during the Terror, but her work was unearthed during the feminist movement of the 1970s and her ideas helped conceptualize and energize demands for equality and justice.

The Power of Narratives

Benjamin wrote from the perspective of the "historical materialist," who attempts to thread together moments that carried radical potential for change and renewed hope in the struggle for the oppressed. We would like to put forward the hypothesis that fiction can simulate in our consciousness a comparable reopening of possibilities. Narratives have the power to unseal a moment that seems frozen in the past. By breathing life into a character, they allow us to go back to the moment when, right before he or she made their decision, the future laid open, ripe with possibilities.

Such a moment, burgeoning with historical possibilities, is described vividly by Québec author Pierre Samson in his novel *Le Mammouth*.[41] Samson's starting point is a little-known fact in Québec history: In 1933, a Ukrainian immigrant named Nikita Zynchuck is killed by a policeman in Montreal. This event takes place at a time of high political tension, in a city where revolutionary dreams, communist ideas, and fascist ideology rivaled in the public arena. Immigrants, destitute individuals, and the unemployed lived cheek by jowl, struggling to make a living, while demagogues jostled for their political support. In this explosive context, the assassination of Zynchuck (whose nickname is "le mammouth") almost triggers a revolution. Samson's large cast of characters all strive for equality and social justice in a struggle that often echoes today's social movements and calls to resist.

Samson's work illustrates the power of fiction to revisit the past and seek out disregarded moments of history to breathe new life into the potential for radical change that they harbored. Samson's narrative is a work of literature, of course, and, as such, should not be characterized as a social or political tool. However, it reveals a singular property of fictional narratives: that of reinjecting into the past the power of possibility. Fiction introduces principles of uncertainty and undecidedness into a sealed and uniform past, revisiting each moment and releasing the dormant possibilities it contains. Samson's novel focuses on one of these now-times, these moments of hope when historical continuity is interrupted and the universal struggle against oppression comes into focus. We come to recognize that this aborted revolution forms a constellation with all other messianic moments in which the "fight for the oppressed past" arose,[42] a realization that resonates strongly with the dedication of Samson's book: "To all those who resist."

This reading of Samson's work helps articulate the idea that stories are experiences that carry the potential of repairing our relationship with the past. They achieve this not by restoring a lost unity, but by reinjecting into the past a sense of promise and possibility. Indeed, the past is made up, not only of facts and events but also of possibilities never realized, choices not made, avenues left unexplored. Fiction restores the power of the possible.

There are several ways in which narratives can help envisage the possibility of reconciliation with the past. Fiction can rehabilitate forgotten historical characters (Maryse Condé); it can provide a template to memorialize the dead and help us recognize the debt we owe them (Patrick Modiano and Kamel Daoud); and it can reignite the possibilities that the victors of history have denied (Walter Benjamin and Pierre Samson).

These narratives provide different pathways toward addressing the challenges of a fractured history and the anxiety that arises from it. Fiction offers a potential avenue toward reconciliation, not by recreating a unitary vision of the past, but by giving expression to the forgotten voices of history. Fiction can recapture the potential for change contained in key moments of the past that have been left by the wayside by dominant national narratives. The antidote to narrative anxiety is not certainty nor is it confidence in the future. Rather, it lies in the power of fiction. While history enables us to make sense of causal chains of events based on testimonies, archives, and artifacts, fiction shines a light on the interstices between causes and effects—the unvisited, unexplored moments where choices are made and new ideas are ushered in.

NOTES

1. "En quoi les Français ont-ils confiance aujourd'hui?" Sciences Po Cevipof, Vague 11, February 2020, https://www.sciencespo.fr/cevipof/sites/sciencespo.fr.cevipof/files/OpinionWay%20 pour%20le%20CEVIPOF-Barome%cc%80tre%20de%20la%20confiance%20en%20politique%20 -%20vague11%20-%20Comparaison-1.pdf.

2. Célia Héron, "Leïla Slimani: 'J'écris sur ce qui me fait le plus peur,'" *Le Temps*, March 15, 2019, https://www.letemps.ch/societe/leila-slimani-jecris-me-plus-peur.

3. Howard Phillips Lovecraft, *Supernatural Horror in Literature* (New York: Dover Publications, 1973).

4. Michel Houellebecq, *Les particules élémentaires* (Paris: Flammarion, 1998).

5. Michel Houellebecq, *Extension du domaine de la lutte* (Paris: Nadeau, 1994). The "generation of 68" in France is coined by the student protest movement for freedom, emancipation, sexual liberty, and critical analysis of the Holocaust.

6. Michel Houellebecq, *Soumission* (Paris: Flammarion, 2015). In his latest novel, the fear of the disappearance of a self-confident, politically powerful, and masculine French identity is in the spotlight of a dystopian novel. Michel Houellebecq, *Anéantir* (Paris: Flammarion, 2022).

7. Benjamin Stora and Thierry Leclère, *La guerre des mémoires: la France face à son passé colonial*, L'Aube poche essai: L'urgence de comprendre (La Tour d'Aigues: Aube, 2007).

8. Amin Maalouf, "Contre 'la littérature francophone,'" *Le Monde*, March 9, 2006, https://www.lemonde.fr/livres/article/2006/03/09/contre-la-litterature-francophone_748933_3260.html.

9. Maalouf, "Contre 'la littérature francophone.'"

10. Benedict Anderson, *Imagined Communities: Reflections on the Origin and Spread of Nationalism* (London: Verso, 2016).

11. Françoise Vergès et al., *Ruptures postcoloniales. Les nouveaux visages de la société française* (Paris: La Découverte, 2010).

12. Christophe Guilluy, *Fractures françaises* (Paris: Bourin, 2010).

13. Assia Djebar, *La disparition de la langue française* (Paris: Michel, 2003).

14. Ralph Ludwig, *Écrire la "parole de nuit:" la nouvelle littérature antillaise; nouvelles, poèmes et réflexions poétiques* (Paris: Gallimard, 1994); Ralph Ludwig, *L'Errance et le Rire. Un nouveau souffle de la littérature antillaise* (Paris: Gallimard, 2022), 15, 19.

15. For pragmatic reasons of space, we do not discuss the conceptual difference between fear and anxiety according to our literary analyses. For theoretical considerations, cf. the introduction of this companion.

16. Aime Césaire, *Une tempête: d'après "la Tempête" de Shakespeare; adaptation pour un théâtre nègre* (Paris: Éd. du Seuil, 1969).

17. Kamel Daoud, *Meursault, contre-enquête* (Arles: Actes Sud, 2014).

18. Bill Ashcroft, Gareth Griffiths, and Helen Tiffin, *The Empire Writes Back: Theory and Practice in Post-Colonial Literatures* (London: Routledge, 1989).

19. Michel Le Bris und Eva Almassy, *Pour une littérature-monde* (Paris: Gallimard, 2007).

20. Marianne Hirsch, *Family Frames: Photography, Narrative, and Postmemory* (Cambridge: Harvard University Press, 2012).

21. Shumona Sinha, *Assommons les pauvres!* (Paris: Éditions de l'Olivier, 2011).

22. Sinha, *Assommons les pauvres!*, 9.

23. Sylvain Savoia, *The Forgotten Slaves of Tromelin* (Europe Comics, 2016), https://www.izneo.com/en/graphic-novel/dokumentation/the-forgotten-slaves-of-tromelin-12120/the-forgotten-slaves-of-tromelin-20293.

24. Didier Daeninckx, *Meurtres pour mémoire* (Paris: Gallimard, 2011).

25. Édouard Glissant, *Traité du tout-monde* (Paris: Gallimard, 1997).

26. Daoud, *Meursault.*

27. Homi K. Bhabha, *The Location of Culture* (London: Routledge, 2010).

28. Wilfried N'Sondé, *Le silence des esprits* (Arles: Actes Sud, 2010).

29. Sara Ahmed, *The Cultural Politics of Emotion* (Edinburgh: Edinburgh University Press, 2004).

30. Sidney Wilfred Mintz, *Sweetness and Power: The Place of Sugar in Modern History* (New York: Sifton, 1985).

31. Leïla Slimani, *Le pays des autres* (Paris: Gallimard, 2020); and Leïla Slimani, *Regardez-nous danser. Le pays des autres, 2* (Paris: Gallimard, 2022).

32. Paul Gilroy, *Postcolonial Melancholia* (New York: Columbia University Press, 2005).

33. Walter Benjamin, "Theses on the Philosophy of History," in *Illuminations*, trans. Harry Zohn (New York: Schocken Books, 1968), 263.

34. Maryse Condé, *I, Tituba: Black Witch of Salem* (Charlottesville: University of Virginia Press, 1992), 183.

35. Patrick Modiano, *Dora Bruder* (Paris: Gallimard, 1997).

36. Sarah Gensburger und Sandrine Lefranc, *Beyond Memory: Can We Really Learn from the Past?* trans. Katharine Throssell (Cham, Switzerland: Palgrave Macmillan, 2020).

37. Primo Levi, *The Drowned and the Saved*, trans. Raymond Rosenthal (New York: Simon & Schuster, 2017).

38. Benjamin, "Theses on the Philosophy of History."

39. Benjamin, "Theses on the Philosophy of History," 263.

40. Michael Löwy, *Fire Alarm: Reading Walter Benjamin's "On the Concept of History,"* trans. Chris Turner (London: Verso, 2016), 99.

41. Pierre Samson, *Le Mammouth* (Montréal: Héliotrope, 2019).

42. Benjamin, "Theses on the Philosophy of History," 263.

CHAPTER FOURTEEN

Multilingual Anxiety in Migration Contexts

EVA J. DAUSSÀ AND
BÀRBARA ROVIRÓ

When people are expected to perform in a language in which they feel insecure, they experience an elevated degree of fear, apprehension, and anxiety.[1] This linguistic insecurity can be traced to the language in question being a foreign language, a stigmatized variety of their own language, or a family heritage language without widespread public presence and educational support. Or one might be frowned upon because of showing grammatical and pragmatic signs of belonging to a distinctive multilingual repertoire.

In this chapter, we explore the linguistic dimension of anxiety culture in the context of migration, focusing on the importance of valuing and maintaining one's heritage language(s), especially when these languages are not powerful state languages but minority varieties. We specifically delve into the importance of supporting them in the domain of schooling. Language can be a contributing factor to the anxiety of the individual or the community, and in the case of a minority language, it may be the target of cultural mocking and other forms of aggressions. We then propose ways in which such anxiety can be addressed by examining the other side of the coin: how language can contribute to the subjective well-being of a person or a whole community, and how we could, in a relatively straightforward way, modify our linguistic practices within the school to increase subjective happiness and reduce collective and individual anxiety.

The Linguistic Needs of a Diverse Community and the Real Goal and Path of Integration

The diffuse nature of migration since the end of the 20th century has impacted the cultural and linguistic diversity in societies all over the world. The paradigm of *multiculturalism* (built on so-called *ethnic minorities*[2]) has been complemented by the notion of *superdiversity*, which tries to capture the variety among the individual members of this population with regard to nationalities, languages, religions, ethnicities, migration patterns and trajectories, and motivations and desires toward labor and cultural participation.[3] The characteristics of migrant groups in a given territory are increasingly unpredictable, and those who could claim historical or traditional local anchorage in their linguistic and culture practices are also becoming less recognizable, as new generations of these diverse populations take hold of territories and change their reality.

This exerts a strenuous pressure especially on those groups that, smaller in nature or minoritized in their sociolinguistic context, are historically the first to face the threat of dissolution into more dominant ones. In the linguistic arena, scholars have for a long time been warning about the disappearance of linguistic diversity,[4] with languages spoken by a small number of people rapidly going extinct, and even those of medium size that are not supported by a propitious government (or even worse, that are continuously challenged by a hostile one) having a higher chance of falling into the abyss of oblivion.[5] Sadly, and to make things worse, when migration puts a language, itself endangered in its original territory, into contact with a local minoritized one, instead of recognizing a common precarity, they are often constructed as being in linguistic competition with each other. On occasion, however, solidarity emerges between them, and the proposal emerges of supporting one another in the struggle for survival, a possibility that seems to depend on the standing of the particular languages at play.[6]

Policy responses to this relatively newly acknowledged superdiversity brought about by massive migratory movements have moved from the key constructs of *assimilation* and *adaptation* of migrants to their new environment, to the kinder *integration* of migrants[7] (and other subculture groups) and the richness that they bear, with the goal of building a more *sustainable* and harmonious community directed to increase the *well-being* of all members.

In the process of integration, learning the local language is proposed as the key element,[8] with the goal of participation in social life without being burdened by the language barrier. Moreover, this would allow differences in lifestyle or cultural habits to be explained and negotiated in and through a common language. However, this model of integration posits a one-sided effort in which an *outsider* becomes part of the group by a unilateral effort of personal adaptation to their new environment by learning the hegemonic language.

What is forgotten, as Bloemaert already pointed out, is that "the endpoint of integration, and the usefulness of language therein, consists of happiness: a range of experience of adequacy and satisfaction in highly diverse social milieux."[9] Integration is not a singular process but a multiple one, and integration in one milieu[10] does not guarantee integration in another—not even linguistically, since it is well known that different spaces within a single community use different registers, or even languages, especially in multilingual societies. In this sense, passing a standard language exam, the ultimate proof of integration demanded from immigrants to officialize their status and become eligible for a job, might not offer much in terms of a satisfying interaction with their neighbors, their sense of belonging, or their positive, constructive participation in their common affairs—all of which are essential components in their perceived feelings of well-being.

Moreover, at the more intimate level, individuals might desire not only to maintain their cultural and linguistic richness for themselves and their longstanding connections but also to share it with the people newly important in their lives: colleagues, neighbors, friends, partners, and their own children. Especially in the latter case, this goal is difficult to achieve without a sound support from their environment—for as the saying goes, it takes a village to raise a child. In other words, while learning the hegemonic language surely promotes productive communication and social cohesion, it alone does not meet all the individual's needs; for that, it is also necessary to adopt a holistic approach in which the totality of the linguistic repertoire of the individual (and their family) is considered and emotional (side-)effects have to be taken into account.

In sum, in the construction of an inclusive, equality-based society, it is crucial to achieve a harmonic interplay between the needs of the whole community and those of multilingual individuals and their families, regardless of the size and official status of their respective languages, their historical and sociological standing, or the way they came to be in that particular territory.

This is especially delicate in places with a long-standing struggle for the survival of a local minoritized language that is not only struggling to hold its ground vis-à-vis state or globally promoted languages but which also has relatively suddenly received a plethora of new languages through migration. Following Modood's two-way integration model,[11] Lanz, Daussà & Pera[12] propose that the most cost-effective and promising security strategy to achieve sustained social peace in these situations is to promote the acquisition of the minoritized language among the immigrant population at the same time that an agenda of respect and support for immigrant heritage languages is firmly adopted, a process that requires a coordinated collaboration between government, school, and the individuals themselves. Beyond issues of social justice, moreover, we would like to propose that what is really at stake is the life satisfaction of citizens both as individuals and as community members and, eventually, their well-being—which in turn promotes the concord and peaceful existence of the community at large.

In addition, the situation of minority languages is made more complicated by the popularization of new media and technological forms of communication and information circulation, as well as the globalization of markets not only for material goods but also for cultural ones. It is intuitively still the case that the survival of these languages should better not be left to the forces of the market, which rarely favor the smaller (or weaker) group. But even in the callous environment dominated by the supremacy of economic interests, in some cases new technologies can contribute positively to the lives of minority languages. For example, an otherwise endangered language can find an unexpected boost for its survival in the breathing space that these new technologies provide,[13] as well as in its commodification for its symbolic associations with cultural or boutique tourism;[14] likewise, the same effect can be achieved if it is maintained and transmitted in diasporic populations that would have otherwise typically shifted to the language of their new surroundings.[15]

To better understand the beneficial or adverse effects of societal language maintenance support, we must consider the spheres in which language plays a central role and which are typically targeted by linguistic policies: the family, the school, and the community.

The Family

Research documenting the desire of parents to raise their children to be proficient in all the languages naturally provided by their environment is abundant.[16] In discussing multilingual upbringing, a usual starting point is the finding that parenting styles affect children's development, for example, on academic outcomes.[17] Beyond academic success, the effect of maintaining high proficiency in a family, or heritage, language has been found to also have positive effects on the family dynamics and the healthy social development of teenagers and young adults, because of its role in facilitating communication inside the family during a potentially stressful life stage such as adolescence.[18] Thus, in one study teenagers who were supported in their multilingualism at school reported a stronger feeling of school and community belonging, which resulted in lower rates of antisocial behavior.[19] Supporting family multilingualism, even in societies with a marked monolingual hegemony, is fundamental in promoting a healthy acceptance of one's whole self. Multilingual youth, in particular, who are subject to considerable pressure to fit in, notably engage in a constant dance between two (or more) constructed selves as they strive to present themselves as perfectly adjusted members of the different cultures that coexist with relative impermeability to each other when going from family to school or the streets.[20]

Other findings seem to confirm that when students are recognized, valued, and supported in their multilingualism (and especially if they are supported in the development of their linguistic skills in all their languages), they show not only better relationships with their families,[21] but also a higher level of self-perception as a native speaker[22] and an increase of self-acceptance as a multicultural person.[23] In addition, not supporting children in developing full competence of both family and societal language has been found to correlate with worse relationships with their parents, higher incidences of confrontational attitudes toward school and society (e.g., increasing the incidence of joining violent street gangs in one study in Los Angeles), while promoting what De Houwer calls *harmonious bilingualism*[24] (i.e., the full development of all languages in the child's environment) was correlated with more identification with society, more and better communication within and between families and teachers, and a higher degree of positive impact in the community.

In research about heritage language maintenance, we often find that families tend to make efforts to maintain those languages associated with positive values. Some studies indicate that beyond the instrumental (economic and professional), and the role in maintaining (transnational) networks, it is so-called personal values that eventually determine intergenerational transmission, especially in the case of smaller languages with little or no international presence in the immediate community or in the global scale. Thus, for example, Daussà[25] reports that the Catalan diasporic population of New York City has a higher transmission of Catalan, their family-anchored language, than a comparable Galician diasporic population (which favors Spanish) has of Galician, and parental motivations can be traced to higher values of Catalan (as compared to Galician) in the dimensions of emotional attachment, symbolic construction of identity, everyday sense of pleasure linked to the linguistic practices, and historical or heritage significance—all of which are identifiable markers of subjective well-being. Furthermore, in her study of Korean Americans, Cho[26] finds that those who had managed to develop their heritage language in addition to English (the societal language supported by formal education) had a number of sociocultural advantages as well as personal benefits, such as a more stable ethnic identity; a greater understanding and knowledge of the cultural values, ethics, and manners of their elders; a stronger connection to their community; and even better psychological and physical health. The author concludes that such benefits provided a personal gain that eventually contributed positively to the betterment of society at large.

It might appear then that parents are thus happier when they can transmit their linguistic inheritance to their children. In addition, it seems that children are happier too, but the picture might not be so clear. DeWaele and Sevinc[27] find that first- and second-generation Turkish immigrants in the Netherlands typically experienced majority language anxiety (that is, anxiety regarding the language supported by school and official agents, in their case, Dutch), while second- and predominantly third-generation immigrants suffered from heritage language anxiety (that is, anxiety toward the language of some of their ancestors). However, it might be the case that the anxiety is created by the school (and society at large) not only failing to support their heritage language but in fact projecting negative prejudices and values related to the cultural ideas around those who speak it. It would be interesting to see whether those feelings of anxiety linked to the heritage language would also be present in a society in which individual multilingualism, especially one that comes about by family transmission, is positively valued regardless of the constellation of languages involved. Presumably, such documented anxiety could be turned into the kind of positive emotions that contribute to the well-being of the Catalan Americans reviewed above.

In sum, the evidence would seem to point toward an abundance of beneficial effects when family-inherited multilingualism is supported, as well as the existence of negative effects when it is not. It is thus a straightforward conclusion that an agenda geared toward increasing the support of individual and family multilingualism would increase the level of well-being and happiness (and even the physical health) of the population, thus decreasing its anxiety. However, one of the difficult decisions migrant parents are confronted with as their children enter education systems in the host country is which kind of language support their children should receive. When choosing multilingual (or multilingual-friendly) programs for their children's education to preserve their heritage languages, parents' anxieties will most notably center around ensuring their children's language proficiency in the hegemonic language of the community.[28]

The School

Not all languages present in society, or even in the classroom, have a place in schools. That this circumstance is largely taken for granted by the community, as well as by schools and even by the speakers of those absent languages themselves, cannot leave one untouched in view of the negative consequences it has. We examine this situation from three different perspectives: that of the administration, that of the educators, and (again) that of the students and their families.

School administrations face numerous challenges: social heterogeneity, linguistic-cultural diversity, artificial intelligence, digitalization, climate change, and political developments, to name a few. All these aspects are accompanied by several problems, most of which call for political decisions. As far as dealing with linguistic diversity in the classroom is concerned, administrations always seem to drive remedial strategies that are not always fully developed in collaboration with the actors on the ground. This has consequences for the acceptance of such measures, which are often perceived as top-down decisions by teachers and other stakeholders. Another serious factor is that the necessary measures consume financial resources and require planning efforts that are not always measurably fruitful.

Unfortunately, positions on migration policies are among the most polemic issues both in election campaigns (where they usually do little to increase the electorate) and in legislative initiatives in so-called host-societies (in Europe, the United States, Canada, etc.), because the gap between wishful theory and lived practice seems vast. As a result, these top-down politically based measures, which must be implemented by administrations, are always given little publicity and, in turn, do not play a leading role toward avoiding societal polemics. In this context, the way diversity is dealt with in schools is but a reflection of public culture, in that it presents an inclusive discourse characterized by popular maxims that are seldom backed by actual implementation strategies.[29]

The main school agents who could decide the role of heritage languages in the classroom and effectively implement the policies around them are teachers, which explains the wealth of existing studies examining their attitudes and practices. For example, Lee and Oxelson conclude that there is a "need for all educators to better understand the critical role and functions of heritage languages in the personal, academic, and social trajectories of language minority students."[30] The fact that teachers' attitudes toward heritage languages are important for the classroom climate in this respect cannot be denied. Whether teachers hold a positive view toward maintaining and fully developing the heritage languages of their students is likely to be critical to whether students feel accepted and valued in the classroom for their linguistic-cultural differences, the consequences of which we already mentioned. In addition, the attitude of the teacher shapes the attitudes of the rest of the student body. Against this backdrop, it is striking to learn from the aforementioned study by Lee and Oxelson that teachers who have not received training as language educators or the dynamics of multilingualism in general, tend to have a negative or indifferent attitude toward supporting heritage languages and cultures, and they do not see any role to be played by themselves or schools in this regard.

Indeed, studies indicate that teachers find it difficult to incorporate the classroom's linguistic diversity in their teaching; lacking specific training, they are left to act on common sense.[31] In practice, this leads to teachers agonizing over how to react to pupils who use a language unfamiliar to them in their classrooms, and they often resort to restricting the use of any languages other than the one used at the school.[32] In most cases, teachers justify their decisions on outdated theories grounded in the traditional immersion approach to multilingual acquisition where the different languages are kept strictly separated. A few cite more sophisticated theories, such as Cummins's Interdependence hypothesis,[33] which also assumes separate linguistic systems, but which feed each other. However, it has been pointed out that with this prevailing strict separation between the languages of home and school in immersive school systems, potential learning resources are wasted and developmental possibilities are thwarted.[34] As García and Kleyn show,[35] more modern approaches to multilingualism, such as the *translanguaging* one (i.e., when the whole linguistic repertoire of the student is mobilized regardless of conventional language boundaries or the linguistic affiliations of the languages at hand), can have scaffolding effects in the learning process and result in higher eventual levels of all languages involved.

Teachers seem also convinced that ignoring or compartmentalizing the linguistic and cultural diversity in their classrooms through an ideal of homogenization is the best way to achieve common ground and harmony within the group. Yet, even in the absence of a diversity brought about by migration, "the completely homogeneous classroom is a myth: each child brings their unique background, personal history, learning styles and personality with him or her."[36]

Despite these documented practices and attitudes, there is an increased awareness of the unavoidable reality of the linguistically diverse classroom on the part of teachers, as well as a growing willingness to integrate it in their teaching in an explicit manner. Training in this direction demands two things: First, teachers need to be aware of the specific languages they are confronted with. Second, teachers need specialized training in the workings of multilingual education, including methodologies and resources that effectively incorporate heritage languages into their teaching, which need not include them mastering such languages themselves. Furthermore, students as well as teachers need to be backed by the school administrators' positive willingness to embrace linguistic diversity, through conversations and guidelines on ways in which this linguistic diversity can be taken into account in the totality of the school context in a way that is appreciative and not exposing or discriminating. This might mean the promotion of structural measures that encourage overworked teachers to embark in additional effort, by providing facilitations such as staff support for formative workshops during work hours, free access to resources, communication platforms between school and home, visits to successful pioneering programs, participation in research projects, and such. Only then would teachers see their investment justified to further educate themselves in the field of diversity management and be encouraged to put innovative methods into practice.

This may be particularly important where minoritized heritage languages are present, for they are at greater risk of denial or displacement from the school context due to being unfamiliar to the teachers, who are more likely to support well-established state languages with a recognized instrumental and social value. As a rule, diasporic communities of minoritized languages tend to be small, and so their opportunities to enact this otherness in everyday life within the wider community might be fewer. It is therefore not surprising that speakers of minoritized heritage languages feel a greater sense of anxiety, because they suffer more invisibility and find it difficult to draw on their full personality and cultural richness.[37]

In addition to heritage languages brought to the classroom by the students, school multilingualism is relevant when it comes to teaching curricular foreign languages, or languages that are not recognized as being historically or traditionally rooted in a given territory, yet have an established place in the educational programs of the school. These so-called L2 languages, or additional languages, are selected on the basis of their social, economic, or cultural value in the society the school belongs to. They tend to form a recurrent limited set, with English, for example, being a prominent member because of its current status as undisputed global language. Since school curricula hardly offer the space to include many other foreign languages, the choices offered at schools may be perceived as rather random and limiting by multilingual children. This can lead to motivational problems among students, most of whom do not find their own heritage language in the offerings and do not understand why they should instead learn another one that does not feel as relatable. This implied declassification of their own heritage languages, especially among students with minoritized languages or nonstandardized varieties, might also lead to insecurities and identification problems, which in turn may cause anxiety. The resulting tensions can have a negative impact on learning readiness, self-perception and self-esteem, and social integration,[38] which also naturally increase anxiety among the students.

In sum, research and teachers themselves report on the benefits of explicitly accommodating and supporting students who are fluent in languages other than those used in the school and included in the school curricula—or rather, the negative effects of not doing so. Supporting multilingualism has the potential to make a decisive contribution to reducing anxiety among both teachers and students—or at least, to reduce the school-related anxiety in this environment. In turn, greater identification with the school and an increased sense of belonging and appreciation that extends beyond the school grounds is likely to impact the entire community, which can go a long way toward alleviating collective anxiety.

The Community

In multilingual communities where several historically rooted languages coexist, there is hardly ever a perfectly balanced equilibrium between them. Often the situation causes one or more of the languages to be in a minoritized position—that is, with less power or representation compared to other one(s), due to social constructs and not to their respective number of users. As a result, when it comes to observing language dynamics in multilingual communities where several (official) languages coexist, the survival of local minoritized languages comes into focus. Because linguistic vitality depends not only on speakers avoiding language shift but also on increasing the number of its users, in a context of heavy immigration, a key issue becomes the language choice of the newcomers (called *new speakers*), who will decide which of the available languages to learn for a variety of subjective and objective reasons. In some cases, the balance is so precarious (e.g., when a minoritized language is struggling for survival in the context of a hegemonic language with global recognition) that the language that succeeds in winning over the new speakers will have a decisive role in whether the minoritized language will find new vital strength through migration flows, or whether it will find itself in an even more precarious situation that is likely to seal its fate in as little as one generation.[39]

This may be particularly relevant in the case of minoritized heritage languages without a firm historically rooted presence in the host culture or without official recognition. As a rule, these groups of speakers tend to be smaller, and so the opportunities to effectively incorporate this otherness into everyday life are fewer. These speakers of minoritized heritage languages feel a greater sense of anxiety, because they are in a perennial situation of not being able to live by their full personality and cultural expertise. Paradoxically, while in most cases heritage languages will experience severe displacement or even elimination from social use, sometimes languages with high market value might be overrepresented in specific areas, such as, for example, gastronomy (Spanish, Italian, Japanese, etc.) or advertising (English).[40] In some cases, marginal presence of an anachronistic multilingualism can be preserved if they feed the nostalgia for a bygone era and a sense of historical continuity with the past, for example, in case of the so-called ghost signs. It is unclear whether commodifying one's heritage language in this specialized form alleviates the individual's anxiety caused by the lack of normalized inclusion in the social tapestry, or whether it increases the feeling of racialization and exoticism toward not only the language per se, but those who speak it.

Anxiety Culture and the Other Side of the Coin: Happiness and Well-Being

Measures targeting the happiness or well-being of a community as subjectively reported have been proposed by the Organization for Economic Co-Operation and Development's (OECD) in their initiative of measuring subjective well-being. The OECD, an international organization that provides a forum where governments work together to share experiences and seek solutions to common problems, has developed a framework that acts as an analytic and diagnostic tool to assess the well-being of people and communities based on three indexes: material conditions, quality of life, and sustainability of well-being over time.[41] Reports started in 2011 and are released biannually. Other measurements of well-being have been proposed, such as the dimension of spirituality (developed by Center of Bhutanese Studies and GNH Research in Bhutan), or an array of objective and subjective qualities,[42] but none of them incorporate the component of language.

Likewise, in studies of migration, a prevalent perspective points out the economic circumstances that either led to migration or occur as its outcome. However, Lovo[43] shows that the motivations of migrants are not solely economic but are connected to quality of life. Thus, migrants hope that their migration, in addition to increasing their income, would enhance their well-being and life satisfaction.[44] Indeed, research indicates that migrants tend to move to happier countries[45] and experience an increase in their well-being after migrating.[46] Nevertheless, there is a tendency to measure their increased happiness in terms of economic prosperity rather than in terms of their community integration and societal participation, although the two might indeed be connected.[47] Research repeatedly shows that happiness is an important factor in migration, because it plays a role in an immigrant's choice of destination[48] in the sense that people tend to migrate to countries where well-being indicators (such as equality, human rights, social rights, etc.) are higher than in their home countries.[49] Educational prosperity is also an important factor in migratory contexts, with studies showing that children of migrants get a better education in their host country than they would get in their parent's original one,[50] and children of migrants might achieve higher occupation status than both first-generation migrants and their family members left behind. Finally, some evidence shows that the benefits of migration are two-way, as the receiving society might also experience positive effects of a more ethnically diversified community.[51] These results are far from generalizable, and in some cases higher diversity is correlated with lower life satisfaction.[52]

The outcomes of migration are not always conducive to a higher sense of well-being. Specifically concerning language, we saw that it can be a focus of anxiety. Since outcomes vary in different contexts, it is likely that the policies and practices are an important factor. For example, Koopmans[53] found that, within the EU, countries with low naturalization rates and less multicultural policies performed better in terms of migration outcomes than countries with high naturalization and more multicultural policies.

In sum, there is a link between migration and well-being, and the relationship can be influenced by language diversity management. Taking well-being as the telltale sign of a diminished personal and collective anxiety, how can we promote the growth of the former to combat the latter?

In multilingual contexts the social and school invisibility of heritage and other minoritized languages and its relegation to the private sphere leaves speakers of minoritized heritage languages at a higher risk of suffering from linguistic anxiety. This often leads to the abandonment of minorized (heritage) languages by interrupting their natural transmission and happens more often when the minorized languages in the countries of origin are already in sharp decline and barely stabilized.[54] The tension field where minority languages and majority languages are in competition creates an anxious atmosphere where individuals need to draw on special skills that they do not automatically possess. Conversely, identification with one's own heritage language, community appreciation, and the possibility to use this richness productively can help to reduce such tension.

An inclusive turn in education can be achieved by a prioritization of the holistic well-being of all school stakeholders, a commitment to the principle of educational equity, and a comprehensive acknowledgment and support of the existing linguistic-cultural diversity. Following these maxims, heritage languages take on a new role to be filled individually by teachers and students. If this succeeds in eliminating or at least relativizing the strict separation between home and school by allowing them to fully incorporate their own linguistic-cultural competencies, it is foreseeable that the persistent individual anxiety will thus be contained.

Conclusion

In an agenda geared toward supporting the existing individual, family, and community, multilingualism would increase the level of well-being and happiness and even the health of the population—thus decreasing its anxiety.

To maintain the abundance of beneficial effects when family-inherited multilingualism is supported and to avoid the negative effects when it is not, parents should be able to promote the heritage languages in the core family and in doing so improve the sociocultural competences of their children. The evidence shows that only mentally strong and healthy children will be able to succeed in school and society later on and will not have to hide or lose their linguistic-cultural background. Thereby heritage languages must be given a place in the school. Special attention should be paid so that already existing power constellations are not maintained and transferred to the school, for example, if only powerful and well-established national languages were implemented in the curricula as learning subjects, thereby replicating and continuing the discrimination of students with minorized heritage languages. Likewise, languages included in the curricula should be carefully selected and coordinated to avoid the very real danger of local ghettoization in schools, in which families with the same heritage language send their children to certain schools where their own family language would be offered as a subject.

To counteract all the risks listed here and to enable students to live an anxiety-free and hopeful existence, new paths must be taken, and teachers and administrators must be supported in their efforts with access to training and research participation. For example, promising proposals centered on the practices of bilingualism rather than on the languages themselves, such as described in García and Kleyn,[55] should be given attention and earnest trial in different contexts.

We should prepare teachers for facing diversity in the classroom, especially the heritage languages of the students, in a way that enables them not only to acknowledge and understand their students but to incorporate their reality into the classroom in a productive and appreciative way. There is solid hope that this can reduce individual and collective anxiety in this field of tension around the maintenance and care of heritage (and other minoritized) languages. Moreover, satisfied school graduates with strong linguistic and cultural self-awareness can make an enriching and productive contribution to the society to which they feel they belong. Finally, this society will be made up of members who, even if not primarily multilingual, have a greater sensitivity and appreciation for heritage languages.

NOTES

1. Robert C. Gardner and Peter D. McIntyre, "On the Measurement of Affective Variables in Second Language Learning," in *Language Learning. A Journal of Research in Language Studies* 43, no. 2 (1993), 157–194; Jean-Marc Dewaele and Yeşim Sevinc, "Heritage Language Anxiety and Majority Language Anxiety among Turkish Immigrants in the Netherlands," *International Journal of Bilingualism* 22, no. 2 (2016), 159–179.

2. See, for example, Tariq Modood, *Multiculturalism* (Cambridge: Polity Press 2013).

3. Steven Vertovec, "Super-Diversity and Its Implications," *Ethnic and Racial Studies* 30, no. 6 (2007), 1024–1054; Steven Vertovec, "Introduction: Depicting Diversity," *Diversities* 12, no. 1

(2010), 1–3; Jan Blommaert, "The Long Language-Ideological Debate in Belgium," *Journal of Multicultural Discourses* 6, no. 3 (2011), 241–256.

4. See, for example, David Crystal, *English as a Second Language* (New York: Cambridge University Press 2003).

5. F. Xavier Vila Moreno, ed., "Challenges and Opportunities for Medium-Sized Language Communities in the 21st Century: A (Preliminary) Synthesis," in *Survival and Development of Language Communities. Prospects and Challenges* (Bristol: Multilingual Matters 2012), 179–200.

6. Guus Extra and Ludo Verhoeven, eds., "Immigrant minority groups and immigrant minority languages in Europe," in *Bilingualism and Migration* (Berlin, New York: de Gruyter 2011), 3–28; Ingrid Gogolin, "Linguistic and Cultural Diversity in Europe: A Challenge for Educational Research and Practice," *European Educational Research Journal* 1, no. 1 (2002), 123–138; Guus Extra and Kutlay Yağmur, eds., "Urban Multilingualism in Europe. Immigrant Minority Languages at Home and School," *Journal of Pragmatics* 43, no. 5 (2011), 1173–1184, https://doi.org/10.1016/j.pragma.2010.10.007; Guus Extra and Durk Gorter, eds., "The Constellation of Languages in Europe: An Inclusive Approach," in *Multilingual Europe: Facts and Policies* (Berlin, New York: De Gruyter Mouton 2008), 3–62; and Tilman Lanz, Eva J. Daussà, and Renée Pera-Ros, "Two-way Integration of Heritage and Minoritized Speakers: Voices from Catalonia," in *Der Einfluss der Migration auf Sprach- und Kulturräume/The Impact of Migration on Language and Culture Areas*, ed. Ulrich Hoinkes and Matthias L. G. Meyer (Hamburg: Peter Lang 2020), 179–206.

7. Jan Blommaert, *Ethnography, Superdiversity and Linguistic Landscapes. Chronicles of Complexity* (Bristol: Multilingual Matters 2013); Tariq Modood and Nasar Meer, "Interculturalism, Multiculturalism or Both?" *Politics Insight* 3, no. 1 (2012), 30–33.

8. Blommaert, *Ethnography, Superdiversity and Linguistic Landscapes.*

9. Blommaert, *Ethnography, Superdiversity and Linguistic Landscapes.*

10. Pierre Bourdieu, *La Distinction: Critique sociale du jugement* (Paris: Minuit 1979).

11. Modood and Meer, "Interculturalism, Multiculturalism or Both?"

12. Lanz, Daussà, and Pera, "Two-way Integration of Heritage and Minoritized Speakers."

13. Guillem Belmar and Maggie Glass, "Virtual Communities as Breathing Spaces for Minority Languages: Re-Framing Minority Language Use," *Social Media* 14 (2019).

14. Monica Heller, ad Joan Pujolar, and Alexandre Duchene, "Linguistic Commodification in Tourism," *Journal of Sociolinguistics*, 18, no. 4 (2014), 539–566.

15. Eva J. Daussà, "Minority Language Families in Diaspora: Language Transmission among Catalans and Galicians in New York City," *Catalan Review* 35, no. 1 (2021), 23–47; Jan Blommaert, "Chronotopes, Scales and Complexity in the Study of Language in Society," *Annual Review of Anthropology* 44 (2015), 105–116.

16. Elisabeth Lanza, "Multilingualism and the Family," in *Handbook of Multilingualism and Multilingual Communication*, ed. Peter Auer & Li Wei (Berlin: Mouton de Gruyer 2007) 45–67; Kendall A. King and Lynn Wright Fogle, "Family Language Policy and Bilingual Parenting," *Language Teaching* 46 (2013), 172–194; Xiao Lan Curdt-Christiansen, "Family Language Policy: Sociopolitical Reality versus Linguistic Continuity," *Language Policy* 12 (2013), 1–6; Elisabeth Lanza and Li Wei, "Multilingual Encounters in Transcultural Families," *Journal of Multilingual and Multicultural Development* 37, no. 7 (2016), 653–654.

17. Christopher Spera, "A Review of the Relationship Among Parenting Practices, Parenting Styles, and Adolescent School Achievement," *Educational Psychology Review* 17, no. 2 (2005), 125–146; Ofelia García and Joanne Kleifgen, eds., *Educating Emergent Bilinguals: Policies, Programs, and Practices for English Language Learners* (New York: Teachers College Press 2010); Virgina P. Collier and Wayne P. Thomas, "Validating the Power of Bilingual Schooling: Thirty-Two Years of Large-Scale, Longitudinal Research," *Annual Review of Applied Linguistics* 37 (2017), 1–15; Zi Wang, "Addressing Migrants' Well-Being during COVID-19: An Analysis of Chinese Communities' Heritage Language Schools in Germany," *Migration Studies* 9, no. 3, (2020/2021).

18. Melinda Dooly, "How Aware are They? Research into Teachers' Attitudes about Linguistic Diversity," *Language Awareness* 14, no. 2–3 (2005), 97–111; Jim Cummins, "BICS and CALP: Empirical and Theoretical Status of the Distinction," in *Encyclopedia of Language and Education,* ed. Nancy H. Hornberger (Boston: Springer 2008), 487–499; Gogolin, "Linguistic and Cultural Diversity in Europe"; Heejung Park et al., "Transactional Associations between Supportive Family Climate and Young Children's Heritage Language Proficiency in Immigrant Families," *International Journal of Behavioral Development* 36, no. 3 (2012), 226–236; Annick de Houwer, "Harmonious Bilingual Development: Young Families' Well-Being in Language Contact Situations," *International Journal of Bilingualism* 19, no. 2 (2015), 169–184.

19. Vivian Tseng and Andrew J. Fuligni, "Parent-adolescent Language Use and Relationships among Immigrant Families with East Asian, Filipino and Latin American Backgrounds," *Journal of Marriage and the Family* 62, no. 2 (2004), 465–476.

20. Elli P. Schachter, "'When Possible, Make a U-Turn': Reflecting on 'the Narrative Turn,' Meaning, Morality and Identity," *Narrative Inquiry* 22, no. 1 (2012), 186–193.

21. Lily Wong Fillmore, "Loss of Family Languages: Should Educators Be Concerned?" *Theory Into Practice* 39, no. 4 (2000), 203–210; Grace Cho, "The Role of Heritage Language in Social Interactions and Relationships: Reflections from a Language Minority Group," *Bilingual Research Journal* 24, no. 4 (2000), 369–384; Alejandro Portes and Lingxin Hao, "The Price of Uniformity: Language, Family and Personality Adjustment in the Immigrant Second Generation," *Ethnic and Racial Studies* 25, no. 6 (2002), 889–912.

22. Ellen Bialystok, *Bilingualism in Development* (Cambridge: Cambridge University Press 2001); Aneta Pavlenko, A. ed., *Bilingual Minds: Emotional Experience, Expression, and Representation* (Bristol, Blue Ridge Summit: Multilingual Matters 2006); Adrian Blackledge and Aneta Pavlenko, "Negotiation of Identities in Multilingual Contexts," *International Journal of Bilingualism* 5, no. 3 (2004), 243–257.

23. Cho, "The Role of Heritage Language."

24. De Houwer, "Harmonious Bilingual Development."

25. Daussà, "Minority Language Families in Diaspora."

26. Cho, "The Role of Heritage Language."

27. Sevinç and Dewaele, "Heritage Language Anxiety and Majority Language Anxiety."

28. Bàrbara Roviró and Patricia Martínez Álvarez, "Do our Concepts of Bilingual Education Match the Anxieties of Migrants?" *EuropeNow,* July 2, 2018, https://www.europenowjournal.org /2018/07/01/do-our-concepts-of-bilingual-education-match-the-anxieties-of-migrants/.

29. Mechtild Gomolla, *Schulentwicklung in der Einwanderungsgesellschaft. Strategien gegen institutionelle Diskriminierung in Deutschland, England und in der Schweiz* (Münster: Waxmann 2005).

30. Jin Sook Lee and Eva Oxelson, "'It's Not My Job': K–12 Teacher Attitudes Toward Students' Heritage Language Maintenance," *Bilingual Research Journal* 30, no. 2 (2006), 453–477.

31. Jim Cummins, "BICS and CALP: Empirical and Theoretical Status of the Distinction," in *Encyclopedia of Language and Education,* ed. Nancy H. Hornberger (Boston: Springer 2008), 487–499.

32. Gogolin, "Linguistic and Cultural Diversity in Europe."

33. Jim Cummins, "Total Immersion or Bilingual Education? Findings of International Research on Promoting Immigrant Children's Achievement in the Primary School," in *Chancenungleichheit in der Grundschule,* ed. Jörg Ramseger and Matthea Wagener (Wiesbaden: VS Verlag für Sozialwissenschaften 2008), 46–55.

34. Gogolin, "Linguistic and Cultural Diversity in Europe."

35. O. García and T. Kleyn, eds., *Translanguaging with Multilingual Students Learning from Classroom Moments* (New York: Routledge, 2016).

36. Dooly, "How Aware are They?"

37. Fillmore, "Loss of Family Languages," 203–210.

38. Martínez Álvarez and Roviró, "Do our Concepts of Bilingual Education Match the Anxieties of Migrants?."

39. O'Rourke, Pujolar, and Ramallo, "Linguistic Commodification in Tourism."

40. Jan Blommaert, "The Long Language-Ideological Debate in Belgium," *Journal of Multicultural Discourses* 6, no. 3 (2011), 241–256.

41. OECD, *How's Life? Measuring Well-Being* (Paris: OECD, 2011); :OECD, *Guidelines on Measuring Subjective Well-Being* (Paris: OECD, 2013).

42. Ruut Veenhoven, "The Four Qualities of Life," *Journal of Happiness Studies* 1, no. 1 (2000), 1–39.

43. Stefania Lovo, "Potential Migration and Subjective Well-Being in Europe," *IZA Journal of Migration* 3, no. 1 (2014), 1–18.

44. Milena Nikolova and Carol Graham, "In Transit: The Well-Being of Migrants from Transition and Post-Transition Countries," *Journal of Economic Behavior & Organization* 112 (2015), 164–186.

45. Arthur Grimes and Dennis Wesselbaum, "Moving Towards Happiness?" *International Migration* 57, no. 3 (2019), 20–40.

46. Nikolova and Graham, "In Transit."

47. Alpaslan Akay, Olivier Bargain, and Klaus F. Zimmermann, "Home Sweet Home? Macroeconomic Conditions in Home Countries and the Well-Being of Migrants," *Journal of Human Resources* 52, no. 2 (2017), 351–373.

48. Martijn Hendriks and David Bartram, "Bringing Happiness into the Study of Migration and Its Consequences: What, Why, and How?" *Journal of Immigrant & Refugee Studies* 17, no. 3 (2019), 279–298.

49. Grimes and Wesselbaum, "Moving Towards Happiness?"

50. Carolina V. Zuccotti, Harry B. G. Ganzeboom, and Ayse Guveli, "Has Migration Been Beneficial for Migrants and Their Children? Comparing Social Mobility of Turks in Western Europe, Turks in Turkey, and Western European Natives," *International Migration Review* 51, no. 1 (2017), 97–126.

51. Akay et al., "Home Sweet Home?"

52. Simonetta Longhi, "Cultural Diversity and Subjective Well-Being," *IZA Journal of Migration* 3, no. 1 (2014), 1–19.

53. Ruud Koopmans, "Trade-Offs between Equality and Difference: Immigrant Integration, Multiculturalism and the Welfare State in Cross-National Perspective," *Journal of Ethnic and Migration Studies* 36, no. 1 (2010), 1–26.

54. Daussà, "Minority Language Families in Diaspora."

55. García and Kleyn, *Translanguaging with Multilingual Students Learning from Classroom Moments.*

CHAPTER FIFTEEN

Anxiety and Mobility/Immobility

Democracy and Authoritarian Closures

JULIE MOSTOV

Every day in the news, we are witnessing the increasing exposure of people to statelessness, blocked mobility, forced migration, and denial of political, civil, and basic human rights. Armed conflicts, state-base violence, expulsion, denials of citizenship, and economic and ecological crises are driving growing numbers of people from their homes, while ruthless policies and practices of border management, surveillance, and refugee and asylum control expose these people to enormous risks, harrowing travels, death at sea, imprisonment, and deportation.[1] Our failures to prevent or to respond to these contemporary tragedies of mobility and immobility (or our highly selective responses to them) reflect power politics sowing fear, ignorance, and unwillingness (or inability) to grasp new political and social imaginaries in the face of current global challenges. The consequences are not only traumatic for migrants but also for denizens of countries engaged in the hardening of borders and for the very democratic processes of social choice that the movement of peoples across borders is purported to threaten.

Anxiety about the fragility of democracy calls for hard border protections, but this link between closure and democracy actually feeds the dangerous slide to authoritarian populism that we are seeing today. This linkage sets the stage for repeated questions about who truly belongs and brings the process of establishing external hard borders inside the polity, casting suspicion on unacceptable or dangerous members within. Competing authoritarian leaders proclaim themselves as uniquely qualified to define and defend the national interest, severing notions of difference from democracy and, eventually, democratic values from national interests.[2] In such scenarios from Hungary, France, and Italy to Israel, India, and the United States, the nation's survival (or greatness) is set in contrast to democratic values and institutions.

By privileging closure as a necessary characteristic of viable political space and securing hard borders in defense of imagined, primordial national values, we put the rights of exclusive membership at odds with human rights and weaken both the egalitarian and liberatory aspects of democracy. Closure not only weakens the capacity of citizens to resist the accumulation of power in the hands of authoritarian/populist leaders and their attacks on media freedoms, voting rights, and judicial checks, but also normalizes fear of agency among the increasingly dangerous "Others." The cold resignation of citizens to the plight of those contained on the other side of the border or languishing in containment camps is supported by such assumptions about the vulnerability of democracy to openness.

The weakening of "our" democratic agency (however constrained it may be) increases our fear of it in others. Thus, our rejection of refugees who appear to be exercising agency, or the criminalization and demonization of "economic refugees."[3] The only acceptable refugees are now truly "innocent" and desperate asylum seekers or helpless children of certain religions, racial, ethnonational profiles, as opposed to the Others, those infiltrators making choices about survival.

While the war in Ukraine produced celebrated examples of humanitarian aid to the refugees streaming out of the country in the face of bombardment and armed conflict, it also produced examples of selective acceptance of suitable asylum seekers.[4] Anxiety understandably felt by many of the people living in the states neighboring Ukraine, particularly, former members of the Soviet Union, strengthened their resolve to provide safe harbor to those fleeing. This, in contrast to the unwillingness to recognize the same desperation in the plight of Syrian refugees or non-white international students among those fleeing Ukraine, speaks to the issue of who belongs/or deserves entry in the face of anxiety over demographic challenges or the "face" of our national spaces.

Migrants who threaten notions of belonging emerge as suspect groups who want to exploit the system and drain the resources of an Others' national space.[5] The border becomes a "complex system of machinery" characterized by "selective and variable permeability,"[6] sites for classifying (sortable, disposable) people and defining or denying their legal status. The seeming fragility of national space and border regimes generates new demarcations and mechanisms of classifying, separating, and degrading.[7]

Instead of the expected flourishing of democratic spaces (symbolized by the fall of the Berlin Wall), we have been experiencing a de-democratization in the face of economic challenges from global capital, new cross-border technologies, and major political disruptions linked to shrinking arenas of state sovereignty.[8] The proliferation of walls, technologies of surveillance, criminalization of others, expansion of borders within (and outside of) national spaces with extended mechanisms of patrolling, and increasing militarization are now needed to protect us against the invasion of democratic space. In the face of contemporary economic challenges, power shifts, and polarized political responses to changing demographic landscapes, we have given in to securitizing pressures to close and harden borders. These responses have given way to the construction of power relations around fixed definitions of difference and institutionalized practices of violence, including forced immobility or containment. We have accepted the logic of undemocratic practices to protect our democratic way of life. We have begun to question our earlier commitments to democracy itself, hence, the rise of theories and practices of "illiberal democracy" or the ease with which some political blocks trample on voting rights of others.

Anxiety about disappearing state sovereignty has, in other words, led us to refortify the borders of the national state, which, in turn, has led to new campaigns to preserve an imagined idealized original culture, national language, and way of life, together with calls for demographic revival grounded in racial/ethnicized biases and the need to control the female body and reproduction (and guard against the hypersexuality of the dangerous male Other). Such campaigns are accompanied by a rejection of difference and a narrowing of political space with pressure to conform, renewed displays of loyalty and patriotism, and a weakening of the electorate and its capacities and responsibilities for choices—a turn away from robust exercises of citizenship in favor of the crowd.

The gendered nature of the politics of national identity, in particular, cautions against the use of national or ethnonational bonds as building blocks of democracy. The desire to naturalize national boundaries and ethnic differences makes recourse to gendered roles in the reproduction of the nation particularly effective. As women have a special duty to reproduce the nation and ward off the threat of demographic tragedy, control of women's sexuality is tightly linked to control of national space and the transgressing of symbolic and physical borders. But, as we have seen, practices in the name of the nation in which Others are treated with hostility eventually undermine everyone's sense of security.[9] Relationships of sameness reaffirmed by institutional seg- regation and public exclusion support internal hierarchies of belonging and anxiety about one's own standing in the group. This anxiety tears at core val- ues of a democratic society, re-creating the lines of citizen and foreigner within.

The result is an enfeebled citizenry, which is vulnerable to autocratic lead- ers. We are seeing this in the current political landscape of the United States and Europe (for example, Italy, Hungary, and Austria) in India, Israel, and many other countries, some of which, claim to be democracies, but whose leaders currently appear to be more concerned about accumulating and maintaining their own power and asserting the illiberal voices of national closure.

The widespread loss of credible information from public offices and the ubiquity of the phrase *fake news* from Belgrade to Washington, DC, reflect this weakening of checks on abuses of power. Voters' rejection of democratic in- stitutions and embrace of the promises of populist leaders are not caused per se by the hardening of borders but by the politics of fear, blaming, and national belonging that accompanies this closure. Acquiescence by those across the political spectrum to significant limits on migration and mobility in the name of democracy contributes to democracy's weakening.

Democrats are wary of opening borders to large numbers of immigrants or asylum seekers because of the assumed negative effect of these newcomers on employment, social welfare, and already existing inequalities requiring re- distribution of resources and national solidarity in the provision of public goods. Others less concerned about equality within the polity see any open- ing as a prelude to flooding the nation space with others who do not share our values and eventually forcing us to include them in majoritarian politics. This, more than any violations of norms, is what threatens our democracy.

Flooding worries are contradicted by the need for immigrant labor to meet market conditions in the face of aging and diminishing labor forces in many countries. While some countries, such as Jordan or Bangladesh, are severely strained by heavy numbers of refugees from neighboring countries, many in Europe could benefit from new immigrants. As in the United States, the real need for immigrant labor is played down by a politics of national identity that gives into fear, xenophobia, and ignorance and that associates Otherness and border crossing with replacement and criminality.

The powerful narrative of threat to well-being and national culture is particularly useful to authoritarian closure and would-be populist leaders who climb to power and seek to maintain it relying on an identification of sameness and belonging among followers and inciting suspicion of those who might not be properly loyal or who might be susceptible to the contamination of Others. Their reliance on us versus them carries the seeds of a kind of exclusive belonging and the perils of infiltration or weakening of the national body. This leads, as noted, to a path of proscribed gendered roles. The reproduction of the Us is too crucial to leave unregulated, and gendered bodies are too vulnerable to violation and occupation to go without vigilance, that is, without surveillance and demographic policing. Proper gender roles are essential to the nationalist narratives of authoritarian imaginaries fueled by resentment at the demeaning roles left to beleaguered members of the "should-be dominant" groups/people by condescending elites or corrupt politicians, who have played into the hands of internal Others or been soft on immigrants, refugees, or asylum seekers. These gendered roles are often noted in feminist critiques of right-wing nationalism, but the relationship between gender and demographic anxiety is understudied in the increasingly pervasive literature on recent turns to populism and authoritarian closure.[10] While recognizing the hypermasculinity of populist leaders and their rhetoric, the gendered nature of this turn is often qualified by noting the increasing number of women engaged in or among the leadership of current populist parties.[11] This misses the important point about how anxiety over demographic change plays upon gendered notions of nation and supports authoritarian closure.

Theorists generally associate populism with the energized "ordinary" people who have been ignored and demeaned by an elitist few, who have gained control of society in their own interests (often by bringing in or valorizing religious or ethnic others/enemies/minorities) at the cost of the people and even the Nation. The "authentic" people rally under a charismatic leader who claims to be in a unique position to define and defend the interests of the people and to recover the values that support the people's prominence in the nation and restore the Nation to its glorious past.[12] Anti-immigration policies and religious or ethnic bigotry play a critical role in populist strategies, together with an imaginary of violation, occupation, and displacement by the dangerous, criminalized, and devious Others threatening the "assumed" majority, its rule, and its social, economic, and political standing.[13] Indeed, populists thrive on demonstrating their protection of Us against the dangerous Others and those elites who are ready to sacrifice us for them. This may speak to unemployed workers against immigrants; women fearful of losing privileged protections of race, class, or ethnicity; members of ethnonational, racial, or religious groups who are pitted against one another for the minimal benefits of inclusion; privileged communities afraid of the lawlessness of those demanding their basic rights; and members of self-proclaimed religious majorities threatened by those who believe differently. The desire to naturalize national boundaries and ethnic/racial differences makes recourse to gendered roles in the reproduction of the nation particularly effective.[14] As women have a special duty to reproduce the nation and ward off the threat of demographic tragedy, control of women's sexuality is tightly linked to control of national space and the transgressing of symbolic and physical borders. Hence continual or renewed attacks on reproductive rights. Women's role in reproducing the nation and upholding its values makes them the object of suspicion and surveillance: Our women can be seduced by the dangerous male Other or refuse their proper roles by failing to reproduce or doing so willingly with the Other; the Other's women threaten the demographic balance by increasing their own numbers. This narrative may be obscured in populist party appeals to women's equality in the workplace or at the ballot box, even in party politics, but the demographic threat of diminishing racial or ethnic group numbers and standing sneaks its way back in more or less vocal ways into narratives of threat and immigration policies. Gendered bodies become the object of control, from direct attacks on abortion rights, to racialized reproductive incentives and patriarchal narratives that stigmatize the Other's gendered practices, to family separations and decisions around deserving asylum seekers.

In gendered narratives of the nation, the Other's males are depicted as either hypersexualized predators of Our women or impotent or effeminate failures, unable to protect their women or fulfill other accepted male roles.[15] At the same time, male migrants who risk life and limb for their families are characterized as deeply embedded in patriarchal cultures and, thus, likely to be abusive toward their submissive women. The only migrants deemed deserving of possible asylum are those women whose situation is so dire that they are at the mercy of the receiving hosts, who look to save them from both their men and their culture. This sets up relationships that continue to build inequality and discrimination into contemporary society. Their women remain a collective symbol of backwardness to be saved through possible assimilation (and incorporation into the economy—often in the private sector or care chain). Their men remain collective threats to the Us through their entry into the labor market, dilution of the majority culture, and threat to Our safety as criminals, rapists, and terrorists, as well as threats to their own women. Cases of domestic violence or gender-based violence among the majority nation are never examples of accepted violent social norms, just individual cases of unfortunate behavior.[16] The simplistic dichotomy of Us versus Them aligns with these gendered narratives and reaffirms the ways in which populist parties may recognize the protection of women's (or even gay) rights in their public denigration of the masculine Other while ignoring these rights, even undermining their realization in everyday life.[17]

Populists like Trump, Orban, Salvini, and Modi gain the attention of their adoring crowds by promising to restrict who is eligible to be part of the demos (for example, Hungary's acceptance of only Christian immigrants or India's restriction of Muslims' citizenship rights), and emboldening their followers with narratives of return to a once great homogenous nation of like-minded men.[18] It is only in a polity of such men that ordinary people can count on the outcomes of voting to support their privilege (even minimal as it is over others), their expectations of recognition, and control over their lives as breadwinners and heads of households. This masculine imaginary is embodied in the leaders' financial and personal success, rhetorical style, and performative practices. This imaginary resonates with men by affirming their own gendered sense of self in the face of a reality that augers defeat and by promising to expel those who have emasculated them. This masculine imaginary can appeal to women who gain a place at the table through it, who themselves feel threatened in their precarious position as women (earlier denied the franchise and often questioned as capable of political judgment). They thus may rise in their standing over racial or ethnic Others by confirming their belonging to the would-be dominant nation. By virtue of this belonging, they demonstrate their fitness as part of the demos. But it is still a position of precarity, entrenched at a cost to others.

Anxiety engendered by the uncertainty of democracy and exacerbated by fear of reduced standing leads to closure: closed borders, immigration restrictions, citizenship restrictions. Attempts to protect the homogeneity of the demos or to define it in terms of ethnonational belonging and racial superiority or purity produce a range of exclusionary practices, including ethnic cleansing and deportation[19] as well as a constant questioning of the loyalty of those already within. This linkage between closure and democracy, in turn, feeds the harshness of asylum policies and increasingly establishes external hard borders inside the polity, casting suspicion on unacceptable or dangerous members within the polity. When the crowd begins to see cracks in the Us and looks for scapegoats for its demise, racial or ethnic Others are there to blame and to root out potential traitors.

A Response to Authoritarian Closure?

Is a democratic alternative that is open to current flows of migrants possible to imagine in a climate so fueled by anxiety over loss of privilege and fear of replacement? Could a softening of national borders be an alternative that would address the inhumanity of current refugee and immigration policies and the weakening of democratic practice? The stark contrast of human vulnerability and immobility juxtaposed against cross-border flows of global culture and information as well as capital and viruses, challenges us to question the crippling effect of such incongruence and to consider bold new transnational architectures of mobility. This would mean not only addressing the arguments that link the uncertainty of democracy to the need for closure and harsh immigration policies but also producing alternative scenarios that link strengthened democratic protections with openness and softer borders. Such an alternative soft border approach would need to interrogate the reasons for fixing boundaries and reveal the coercive power of de- and re-territorializing processes. Perhaps, this seems unimaginable at a time of death and destruction over border incursions and military occupations, like what we are seeing in Ukraine. But the enormous temptation to stake claims to territory, to redefine or challenge national space, or change national borders maintains the ongoing likelihood of violent conflict. Whether armies or desperate refugees, the potential of border crossing under the current linkage of democracy with closure exacerbates violence and encourages authoritarian politics and autocrats. Hard borders and hierarchies of mobility significantly limit our ability to change this.

An alternative would need to redefine political space to deflate the power of closure with a landscape of interdependence and cooperation, providing a framework within which to recast our attempts to respond to contemporary migration tragedies. Strengthening border patrols and building longer, higher walls or even improving rescue operations and health care in refugee centers will not make a sustainable difference. Humanitarian responses are necessary in the short term, but they do not address the deep trauma of displacement or humiliation; they do not create the conditions for social cooperation in our increasingly interconnected economies and ecologies and fractured geopolitical spaces. We cannot address deep insecurities created by globalizing trends and flows of capital, arms, drugs, weapons, and disease by trying to create national preserves, or continually accepting the cautionary tales of safety in closure. Accepting elaborate procedures for managing hard borders, offering refuge to a lucky few and prolonging the nightmare of uncertainty for hundreds of thousands more accepts the dehumanizing patterns of separating, classifying, and reifying space, individuals, and groups and, at the same time, undermines the democratic ethos in our societies.

We could shift our political imaginary by expanding the spaces for practices of inclusion and democratic "acts of citizenship,"[20] recognizing the richness of diverse mobile actors. We could reimagine border zones as spaces for the exercise of transnational citizenship that embraces rather than fears mobility, in which the personhood of migrants is recognized and valorized; where the agency involved in fleeing danger and finding a way to safe haven or opportunities to improve one's life chances is appreciated as a vital part of citizenship and a desirable characteristic of social cooperation.

In such an alternative account, the border could become a space of multiple and overlapping associations, removing the insecurity/anxiety of being undocumented or unauthorized or holding limited visas, the fear of being exposed to violence and the humiliation of being treated as disposable or at the mercy of the kindness of others (at and inside national borders). It would end the morally arbitrary boundary-setting authority of hard border exclusion. While hard border regimes linked to national identity and national citizenship are designed to protect borders and citizens within, we have noted that these exclusionary practices at the border have a tendency to move inward, replicating the boundary-setting practices of the nation-state over the bodies of diverse individuals (now suspect inhabitants) within. This reiteration of difference and insecurity unravels the fabric of our complex societies and undermines democratic and integrative processes in everyday life. We are not safer in the 21st century, nor more likely to treat each other well, when we strive toward homogenous communities within hard borders. Alternative practices of social choice and responsibility-sharing that recognize the status of citizen in all of us, in contrast, are more likely to enhance our bonds of social solidarity and trust as well as place democratic checks on the abuse of power.

This would mean recognizing the fluidity and malleability of softened borders and the negotiability of movement across these borders and within them. It requires understanding democratic social choice delinked from national or territorial belonging. This would deflate the power of our anxiety of belonging in the voices and politics of populists and autocratic politicians who are winning at the ballot box by vowing to stop immigration.

NOTES

1. Zygmut Bauman, *Strangers at our Door* (Cambridge, UK: Polity Press, 2016).

2. Hungary's Victor Orban is one of the clearest examples, touting his "illiberal democracy."

3. Karolina Szmagalska-Follis, "What is an Economic Migrant? Europe's New Borders and the Politics of Classification," in *Citizenship, Borders, and Human Needs* ed. Rogers M. Smith (Philadelphia: University of Pennsylvania Press, 2011), 117.

4. Chris Keulemans, "Pitanje doma" (The Issue of Home), *Pescanika*, June 6, 2022.

5. Szmagalska-Follis, "What is an Economic Migrant?," 118.

6. Szmagalska-Follis, "What is an Economic Migrant?," 121, 127–128.

7. Cynthis Bejarano, Maria Cristina Morales, and Said Saddiki, "Understanding Conquest through a Border Lens: A Comparative Analysis of the Mexico-US and Morocco-Spain Regions," in *Beyond Walls and Cages: Prisons, Borders, and Global Crisis*, eds. Jenna M. Lyod et al. (Athens: University of Georgia Press, 2012), 27–41.

8. Étienne Balibar, "Reinventing the Stranger: Walls All over the World, and How to Tear Them Down," in *Symplokë* 25, no.1–2, Passports (2017), 25–41. See also Wendy Brown, *Walled States, Waning Sovereignty* (New York: Zone Books, 2010); and Charles Tilly, "Inequality, Democratization, and De-Democratization," *Sociological Theory* 21, no. 1 (January 2003), 37–43.

9. Nenad Miscevic, *Nationalism and Beyond: Introducing Moral Debates about Values* (Budapest: CEU Press, 2001), 107–121. Moreover, limiting resources or right treatment to one's compatriots "corrodes" the community's sense of justice. See Daniel Weinstock, "National Partiality: Confronting the Institutions," *The Monist* 82, no. 3 (1999), 533; and Kok-Chor Tan, *Justice without Borders: Cosmopolitanism, Nationalism, and Patriotism* (Cambridge, UK: Cambridge University Press, 2004), 155.

10. Sahar Abi-Hassan, "Populism and Gender," in *The Oxford Handbook of Populism*, eds. Cristóbal Rovira Kaltwasser et al. (Oxford: Oxford University Press 2017), 426–444.

11. Sara R. Farris, *In the Name of Women's Rights: The Rise of Femonationalism* (Durham: Duke University Press 2017); Johanna Kantola and Emanuela Lombardo, "Populism and Feminist Politics: The Cases of Finland and Spain," *European Journal of Political Research* 58 (2019), 1108–1128.

12. Jean Cohen, "Populism and the Politics of Resentment," *Jus Cogens: A Critical Journal of the Philosophy of Law and Politics* 1, no. 1 (2019), 5–39; Nadia Urbinati, "The Political Theory of Populism," *Annual Review of Political Science* 22 (2019), 111–127.

13. Cristina Beltrán, *Cruelty as Citizenship: How Migrant Suffering Sustains White Democracy* (Minneapolis: University of Minnesota Press, 2020).

14. Julie Mostov, *Soft Borders: Rethinking Sovereignty and Democracy* (New York: Palgrave Macmillan 2008); Jacqueline Stevens, *Reproducing the State* (Princeton: Princeton University Press 1999).

15. Dibyesh Anand, *Hindu Nationalism in India and the Politics of Fear* (New York: Palgrave Macmillan 2011), 49–81; Mostov, *Soft Borders*.

16. Lila Abu-Lughod, "Do Muslim Women Really Need Saving? Anthropological Reflections on Cultural Relativism and Its Others," *American Anthropologist* 104 (2002), 783–790; Julie Mostov, "'Our Women'/'Their Women': Symbolic Boundaries, Territorial Borders, and Violence in the Balkans," *Peace and Change* 20, no. 4 (1994), 515–529.

17. Sara R. Farris, *In the Name of Women's Rights: The Rise of Femonationalism* (Durham: Duke University Press, 2017).

18. Marion Löffler, Luyte Russell, and Kathleen Stark, "Political Masculinities and Populism," *NORMA* 15, no. 1 (2020), 1–9.

19. Rhoda E. Howard-Hassmann and Margaret Walsh-Roberts, *The Human Right to Citizenship: A Slippery Concept* (Philadelphia: University of Pennsylvania Press, 2015).

20. Balibar, "Reinventing the Stranger," 39–41.

PART FIVE

TECHNOLOGY

Introduction

ULRICH HOINKES

This part, devoted to the topic of anxiety culture and technology, builds a bridge to the initial theoretical considerations on the role of anxiety in our societies. The contributions gathered in this part clearly show that from a Western, sometimes Eurocentric, point of view, we give anxiety a central place in our experience of reality as a constitutive element of modernity. While doing so we apply a concept of anxiety that no longer conceives of it as a consequence of what happens to us as a shared fate, but rather as the defining sensation of the free, self-determined human being in the sole responsibility for one's self and one's own kind.

A look at the technological development that has shaped our modern societies since the 19th century shows us that the addiction to progress has always provoked individual and societal fears associated with technological achievements. As part of the anxiety culture, scientists such as Albert Einstein, Jay Wright Forrester, or Stephen Hawking have always warned of the negative effects of our technological progress. It is tragic that these warnings so far have found little resonance in philosophical thought. The concentration of our thinking on the human being oscillates between the positive valuation as humanism and the negative valuation as anthropocentrism in more recent times. Slowly the realization is gaining ground that only the respectful treatment of the whole of nature, and not only of the *Conditio Humana*, is able to secure a future perspective of existence for our world.

How desperate the break between (human) nature and technology ultimately is can be seen in the public discussion since the middle of the 20th century at the latest. Consider the influential voice of the German-Jewish philosopher Ernst Bloch, who wrote his great work *Das Prinzip Hoffnung* (The Principle of Hope) in exile in the United States during the Second World War, in which he emphasizes the irreconcilability of nature and technology as long as the latter is not completely reconceived in the sense of a "second nature": "Our present technology stands in nature like an occupying army in enemy territory, and it knows nothing of the interior; the matter of the thing is transcendent to it."[1]

With this view, Bloch not only shapes a zeitgeist but he also raises a philosophical-historical question that gains importance in the postwar period: What contribution does technology make to our future? What motivates it? Is it capable of giving us sufficient confidence in a healthy and good further development of our world? The pervasiveness of these questions inevitably throws us back to the connection between technology and fear. The relevant discussion, however, is only just beginning, especially since recent technological developments with internet-based communication, automation, and artificial intelligence have brought far more drastic changes on the scene than were imaginable in Bloch's time.

Four contributions in this section deal with the aforementioned essential questions. Raphaël Liogier sketches a particular view of modernity which, in his opinion, is based on nihilistic fears and in which industrialism has established itself as a materialistic cult since the 19th century. In its consequence a kind of anti-ontology, technology-fixated industrialism in modernity, which as an epoch is characterized by a humanistic concept, thwarts its successful realization ("hijacking modernity") from the very beginning by repressing the essential fear of emptiness in society.

Karena Kalmbach opens a different perspective in her contribution. She turns the question of the impact of technology on human anxiety around and posits that anxiety is the driving force in the development of new technologies. This essential fact is often eclipsed by the discussion of a fear of technology (e.g., nuclear fear). In contrast, Kalmbach formulates the provocative thesis that modern technologies can also be interpreted as "coagulated fears of apocalyptic thinking."

A similarly critical and also ambivalent explanation of man's relationship to technology is given by Christine Blaettler in her chapter, which examines the intellectual perception of this relationship in an examination of the Prometheus myth in the history of ideas. In doing so, the author concentrates on the contribution that technology makes to the cultural development of man and raises the question whether man still controls the technologies he has created or whether he ultimately must submit to them. In the sense of the reference to Prometheus, the tragic idea that technological progress can be perceived as sacrilege against a divine order also plays a role.

The final chapter of this section, written by Markus Lemmens and Iris Wieczorek, is an examination of the political and economic understanding of technology and innovation in recent times, comparing the policies of Germany and Japan. Here, differences in the national configuration of our global anxiety culture become apparent. However, both countries deal with the problem of how far the acceptance of technological development can be promoted through policy making in order to reduce fears of new technologies and at the same time present them as problem-solving approaches. The authors reveal different emphases: While Germany, with its High-Tech Strategy, focuses more traditionally on securing economic growth through new technologies, the Japanese concept of Society 5.0, in conjunction with most of the world's industrialized nations, attempts to strengthen the view of the benefits of technological development in social discourse (creating economic, social and public value) and thus provides an important impetus for overcoming fears and anxieties about the future by means of technological innovation.

NOTES

1. Ernst Bloch, *Das Prinzip Hoffnung* (Frankfurt: Suhrkamp, 1973), 814. Translation is my own.

CHAPTER SIXTEEN

Anxiety Culture as Fuel for Industrialism

RAPHAËL LIOGIER

This chapter defends the idea that modernity, by freeing people from the traditional framework of existence, that is, from the framing and transmission of a unique and uncriticizable tradition, has at the same time released a charge of intolerable anguish (which I call the anguish of the void) that has provoked a process of collective reaction that can be divided into two major cycles.[1] The first cycle, which began in the 19th century, is that of the repression of the anguish of the void and is divided into three phases: conquering materialism (from the 19th century onward), neoliberalism (from the 1950s onward), and correlationism[2] (this last phase is the one that begins with the generalization of the internet and the progressive transformation of individuals into statistical profiles). The general culture of this first cycle is *schyzohumanism*, a way of making oneself believe collectively in the existence of immaterial principles (freedom, equality, democracy, conscience, happiness, etc.) while not believing in them intimately (remaining intimately materialist and nihilist).[3] The second and final cycle is the return of the repressed. It became slowly dominant at the beginning of the 21st century, when schyzohumanism—torn between the exhibition of political, ethical, humanitarian, and humanist discourses and the violent material realities of taming through marketing, of financial inequality, and of procedural generalization—could no longer contain the anguish of the void. This then translates into the conspicuous anxiety of loss of identity (fueled by the idea that everything is fake, inauthentic, that the political scene itself is just an inconsistent set with politicians who have become actors who do not believe in their own role). *Identitarianism* is the return of the anguish of the void that was repressed during the first cycle. Identitarianism becomes the general culture of the second and last cycle, which is reflected, for example, in the development of populism in the political field (the anguish of the loss of oneself which leads to the search for a charismatic leader who is the only authentic one). At this stage, the idea of progress (and modernity as a whole) is called into question in favor of projections of going backward, of returning to protective and reassuring traditions (what I call retro-utopias). The two cycles do not strictly follow each other: there are critical periods of identitarianism within the schyzohumanist cycle (e.g., in 1930s Europe), and there will probably be critical periods of schyzohumanism within the current identitarian cycle. In any case, neither culture (schyzohumanist and identitarian) is totally absent when the other is dominant, because they condition each other.[4]

In fact, this overall process (including the two cycles of dealing with the anguish of the void), which is a reaction against the modern promise of freedom, constitutes an anti-ontology (a system of negation of being) that I call *industrialism*. My thesis is that industrialism is the original hijacking of modernity while it appears as its consequence in authors like Heidegger, Arendt, Anders, or Jonas (and numerous others). In this sense, industrialism, which involves the tendency to produce a formatted, impersonal, consumerist, bureaucratic, inegalitarian, colonialist, predatory, inhuman society, is not the fatal consequence of modernity but in fact manifests the inability to accept modernity. Industrialism is a nihilistic regime (the first nihilistic regime in history), which feeds on anxiety culture. So, it is not necessary to get rid of modernity to get out of industrialism and overcome the anxiety culture that has become endemic, but rather it is necessary to return to the meaning of modernity and reflect on the reasons for our inability, after nearly three centuries, to become truly modern.

The Unconscious Choice of Determinism over Freedom

According to Jean-Paul Sartre, the knowledge of freedom provokes a kind of vertigo in the face of the infinite responsibility it entails. Once perceived, this knowledge cannot be forgotten. It is difficult to assume the uncertainty, the vertigo of emptiness that is inherent in freedom. [5] Modern humans know, however, that we can no longer turn back the clock, just as one can no longer return to childhood and spontaneously believe in Father Christmas. The deterministic dogma of materialism, which became dominant in Europe in the nineteenth century, allows us to suppress the awareness of this freedom, to no longer feel the vertigo above the void that it implies, but also to no longer have to admit the responsibility that it confers. An entirely deterministic world is a world of irresponsibility, which, under the pretext of scientism, allows us to believe in a destiny drawn from all eternity as in traditional societies. Under the guise of ultra-rationalism, it is in reality a new determinism close to theological determinism ("everything is written"), which abandons reason in the sense of the Enlightenment, that is to say, which dethrones transcendental subjectivity (to speak like Immanuel Kant), which is the basis of subjective rights, otherwise known as human rights.

There is a kind of metabolic inability to digest modern liberation, which leads to the neurasthenic nausea that is precisely the subject of Jean-Paul Sartre's novel of the same name.[6] The weight of freedom can become unbearable, because it is a hole that can be envisaged as a bottomless precipice (abyssal to the letter), which makes us definitively (abysmally) responsible for everything that we did not try to prevent, but first of all for our slightest actions and decisions. The only limit of freedom thus discovered is that we cannot choose not to be free:[7] "We are condemned to freedom"[8] because it is a fact that cannot be escaped under any pretext. By this very fact that it is freedom, "it is free neither to not exist nor to not be free."[9] The fact of fabricating (necessarily false) pretexts to get rid of freedom is what Sartre calls bad faith (*mauvaise foi*), which characterizes the figure of the bastard (*salaud*) in his theater and his novels.

The two extreme by-products of the strategy of disempowerment are extreme rationalism (typical of the first industrialist cycle: the repression of the anguish of the void) and extreme neo-traditionalism (typical of the terminal cycle of industrialism: the return of the repressed anguish of the void). The middle, in-between, normalized version of industrialist disempowerment takes the form of schyzohumanist democracy based on security policies (social, health, economic security, etc.), which leads to what Claus Offe calls the Negative State.[10] In this tendency to be neurasthenic, the feeling that ends up being most widely shared is that nothing is really going well without it being clear why. If nothing is going well, it is because of the others, the neighbors, foreigners, corrupt politicians (which may be true), the immigrants. Democracy degenerates from a regime based on the responsibility of all into a regime of individual irresponsibility.

The resentment caused by the inability to assume the modern discovery of one's own freedom is not aimed at a personal social situation but at the condition of being alive in general. It is a resentment of powerlessness without a specific object. The repressed awareness of irreducible uncertainty leads to the (unconscious) desire not to be born, to forget oneself as a living organism. Abolishing existence itself, which is unbearably indeterminable, by returning to the state of a determined thing, in other words making oneself a corpse, is one of the manifestations of the death drive.[11] Like the lizard that self-mutilates itself in the face of danger, according to the example given by Jacques Lacan, man mutilates himself in the face of the danger of losing the moral security of traditional adherence. Nihilism is therefore not an intensification of modernity, but on the contrary its repression, in a first cycle, followed by the regression toward a neo-traditional adherence (yet impossible, and therefore all the more anxiety-provoking). Nihilism fulfilling itself in extreme materialism is, moreover, from the start an anti-tradition as indisputable as a tradition (it is a neo-tradition). It imposes itself as a system of self-evidences designated as facts (this is what constitutes positivism) with a dogmatic background of a unique and perfectly abstract universal law, the absolute determinism of nature (from which all other laws follow, as with divine law).

The obstinate destruction of all traditions is a way of denying that one is in fact in search of the lost childhood, that is, in search of the lost tradition. It is to blame the whole world for not being able to go back to the life before responsibility and to blame oneself secretly for not feeling capable of one's own freedom.

The mortifying preference that leads to the industrialist anti-ontology—which is probably the first anti-ontology in history—is incomprehensible as a conscious decision, that is, as a deliberate choice. It can only be seen clinically as an organic rejection reaction. It is immediately reactive and only then ideologically reactionary (as a system of rational justifications for the immediate irrational reaction). What is rejected is the anguish of the void, more precisely it is the dizzying doubt (without possible resolution) that results from it; the critical instability of modernity, which testifies to individual freedom, is indeed irreversible once it has been experienced. Such a collective historical experience prevents a return to the old traditional morality (reassuring because it is unique and certain); in the case of the West, this unitary certainty functioned from the void (uncertainty) rejected in the distance in Almighty God, himself represented in the figure of all paternities: that of the paterfamilias as well as that of the feudal lord, of the king, and of all authority immediately felt without any doubt. The irreducibility of doubt and criticism of all authorities has given rise to a particular anguish that is omnipresent like a background noise, itself irreducible to the modern situation. It is this anguish that *homo industrialis* seeks to evacuate, to avoid hearing it resonate within him at all costs, by re-creating certainty through the projection of all possible determinisms.

It Is Not Anxiety but Its Repression That Produces the Anxiety Culture

Jacques Lacan asserted that anxiety is the only revealing feeling, whereas all other affections serve to conceal the real, including the reality of anxiety itself (which in fact has not disappeared but is continually felt). The real is the Object a,[12] the point of origin of being, infinite, absolutely singular, and therefore unknowable since all knowledge is established by resemblance allowing the identification of regularities of situations and categories of objects).[13] The collective discovery of the Object a, which is the real, places us ipso facto in front of its anguishing [anxiety building] in definition. So that anguish is no longer anxiety for something in particular: it is not the fear that this or that will happen, but the tension of the real itself within us. The authentic psychoanalytic treatment, which is only of interest in a modern situation, does not aim to overcome anxiety or to annihilate it, but on the contrary to face it in its version unadulterated by avoidance strategies, of which materialist resentment is the most destructive. Science, technology, and money become religious substitutes, fetish objects, because instead of remaining means of knowledge, action, and payment, they take the place of transcendent ends in which man can no longer believe.[14]

The materialist cult is the very language of the repressed anxiety of the void. This is why it is expressed first of all by the obsession with filling the lack of being by (necessarily inadequate) material processes. Such a substitution, like a macabre conjuring trick, deprives us of an authentically modern life and at the same time of an authentically traditional life. It is a double loss. *Homo industrialis* either completes himself in the fragmentation of the self (what Heidegger calls "the oblivion of being," which manifests itself in schyzohumanism: the display of humanistic principles or sentiments in which one does not really believe), or overreacts in the paranoid (desperate and therefore often violent) quest for lost uniqueness (this is identitarianism).

From a Lacanian perspective, paranoia is not in itself pathological since it is the basic situation of the ego, in other words, the basis of what I have called in other works the desire to be:[15] the original feeling of singular unity and at the same time of participation in something greater than oneself. In the opposite direction, schizophrenia is the fragmentation of the ego.[16] The modern worldview, by relativizing (not eliminating) regimes of truths, creates a potentially heartbreaking, if liberating (if faced as one would face the abyss), tension between paranoia (unifying) and schizophrenia (dispersing). I hypothesize that it is this tension which, when not assumed, accomplishes the tear it believes it wants to avoid. Instead of sublimating the anguishing tension between the unifying and the dispersing polarity, which would then allow transcendental subjectivity to emerge (the acceptance of the singular greatness of oneself and of others), it violently represses it until it breaks. But since we cannot live without the desire to be, the only way to survive anyway is to project before us a replacement paranoia, morbid and reactive (which we can also call secondary paranoia to distinguish it from the primary paranoia originally constitutive of the ego). *Homo industrialis*, no longer believing in his own ego (in his unity), creates a false ego that he defends all the more bitterly (and desperately) through externalizations (of which digital social networks have become amplifiers).

The oscillation between a schizoid structure (the disintegrating general fiction) and false paranoia (which one does not really adhere to) constitutes the heart of the industrialist world in which we survive like animals in distress. This oscillation calls itself realism in its middle intensity (gently and cynically schizoid) but can at any moment intensify into a dangerous secondary and frenzied paranoia, which takes the most varied forms: nationalism, republicanism, regionalism, neo-traditionalism (religious or not), in short, the whole range of identitarianism.

It is because we cannot seriously believe in facts alone, in mechanistic reason alone (which is nothing other than reason without reason), but are no longer able to believe in anything else, that our world has become a fiction. That is, it is discreetly false in our own eyes, but we pretend it is not. Materialism needs to constantly pretend that it is not completely materialist, as if it could have an ideal (the typical oxymoron of our time is that of the materialist ideal), which can take the empty form of humanitarian ethics, bioethics, a subsidized but unfelt love of neighbor. Not believing in itself, in the least of its principles, however outrageously exhibited, this world is structurally depressed and therefore in vital need of antidepressants in all possible forms—medicinal, entertaining, monetary, consuming. The list is of course not exhaustive, because in such a world, anything can take the place of an antidepressant. In fact, psychoanalysis would have no use in a traditional world; its only legitimate object being to allow one to face the typically modern anxiety of emptiness without slipping either into schizophrenia (the dispersion that threatens) or into a substitute paranoia. Facing reality and thus remaining modern is its only legitimate aim. In this sense, a certain failure of psychoanalysis is an indicator of the victory of industrialism. A failure that is all the more bitter when psychoanalysis is itself industrialized, that is to say, used as one antidepressant among others, as a way of resolving a conflict (and thus closing the space of doubt) instead of leaving it in suspense. This is the meaning of Gilles Deleuze and Felix Guattari's critique of psychoanalysis when it tries to denomadize, to tame the individual instead of letting it be, that is to say, to let it go as one would ask a nuisance to let go.

Anxiety Culture and Morbid Choice

The modern freeing from the immediate imposition of a unique destiny has simultaneously released a formidable charge of anxiety. This anxiety inherent to the human condition was already there, but it had until then been contained by tradition, as it were, enclosed within it (in its rites, its obvious visions of hell, paradise, good, evil, punishments and beatitudes). Structural anxiety, no longer enclosed by tradition, bursts out in the face of humanity. This is what existentialists call existential anguish. It does not constitute a problem in itself, if it is admitted, lived without diversions, and even embraced, as Lacan has shown. It manifests the supreme degree of realism, that is, the assent to the incompleteness of all reality, that is, of all phenomena (including our own inner reality[17]). The indeterminacy of reality is nestled at the edge of all prehensile realities, as on the crest of a cliff. The deepest wisdom of the moderns consists in making this limit point a place of contemplation, in making vertigo a liberating energy and in making anxiety a virtue, that of the critical mind.[18] Industrialism consists, on the contrary, in throwing oneself into the void by refusing vertigo and by rejecting anxiety, otherwise by the anguish of anguish. The industrialist disfigurement of modernity that takes place in the nineteenth century in this liberating context is equivalent to the choice of death to put an end to existential anxiety instead of assuming it: it is the metaphysical choice of nonbeing (what we call nihilism) and the epistemological choice of determinism (manifested by positivism).

However, and this is the whole problem, one cannot put an end to existential anxiety (just as one cannot put an end to freedom, and to the responsibility inherent in it) unless one puts an end to existence itself. This is why industrialism is divided into two great cycles that lead to nothing less than ending existence. The first cycle is that of the repression of existential anxiety behind productive enthusiasm and the display of humanistic values (in other words, through schyzohumanism); it is the cycle of the maintenance of material, biological, and social determinism that would be simultaneously and paradoxically liberating. But by nature, repression is not a permanent solution. The semblance of compatibility between material determinism and subjective freedom can only be exhausted after having deployed all the entertaining devices of material accumulation, technical acceleration, and massively shared self-images.

When the smiling semblance of success that characterizes the first cycle (proper to the schyzohumanist state in its three positivist-materialist, neoliberal, and correlationist phases) crumbles, the second and final cycle of industrialism begins, that of the return of the repressed (which leads to the degradation of the rule of law and the rise of identarism). The indentitarian anger, the all-out retro-utopian quest, is the return of the repressed caused by schyzohumanism at its maximum intensity, and therefore becomes unbearable (inaudible). It is the moment when larger and larger portions of the population realize that, beyond all the impressive successes that are being marketed in front of their eyes, all reason for being has evaporated. This is the moment when humans feel trapped in a life-size show of which they are the recalcitrant actors, as in the film *The Truman Show*, when the perfect insurance agent Truman Burbank (played by actor Jim Carrey) seriously begins to doubt the reality around him, the sincerity of his best friends, the reality of institutions, and finally the authenticity of his own existence. From that moment on, he tries to escape at all costs, in a desperate search for authenticity. But unlike Truman Burbank, who finally discovers the reality of his puppet existence, entirely devoted since birth to entertaining millions of spectators, the people of the 21st century can find nothing of the sort behind the curtain of appearances. There are no demons or directors pulling the strings. Even if, indeed, people are filmed, classified, entertained, exploited, they are being filmed for nothing. Even more than the insurance agent in *The Truman Show*, these populations resemble a demultiplication of Ulrich, the man without qualities from Robert Musil's novel of the same name. We are in the situation where "ideals and morals (which) are the best means of filling the great hole called the soul"[19] no longer give the impression that they do. Ulrich is searching for an event that cannot be found. The world is hopelessly uneventful, nothing is an event anymore, everything is inconsistent: "we end up floating only on reports, reactions, on the dishwater of reactions and formulas, on something that we wonder if it is an object, a process, a ghost of thought or a God-knows-what!"[20]

Everything seems so normal, so sanitized, so formal, including feelings, so correct (so politically correct) that people no longer feel they are adhering to anything, in the sense of sticking to what surrounds them. It is as if the world in which they live is foreign to them. They want to pinch themselves, but nothing can resolve this impression of floating. A grand gesture is needed, a grand restoration of grandeur, something. This is the impossible and derisory project of *The Man Without Qualities* in the 1,800 pages of this great unfinished novel, which is like a description of the insignificance of the European world in which the totalitarian storm about to erupt is potentiated. The first volume was in fact published in Germany in 1930 and part of the second volume in 1932, just before Hitler came to power. It is more or less the same disillusioned, neurasthenic atmosphere, punctuated by superficial and often confused debates, which presides over the disintegration of European culture, that haunts Stefan Zweig's memories,[21] with the nagging question: How in such a short time did faith in principles that were taken for granted, almost intangible, get swept away? In fact, beyond the factual course of events, the opportunities cynically seized by leaders, the totalitarian slide became inevitable. The Second World War interrupted this totalitarian experiment in 1945, but it was only an interruption, not an overcoming. In the long term, we can even say that we are experiencing a relapse of this atmosphere, albeit at a new cost. A relapse is not the same illness, even if it comes from the same cause. It is not a repetition but a new development of the illness, often redoubled, because its cause is still there: in this case the loss of primary paranoia, that is, the basic feeling of being in the world (of being at the center of my world), and loss of the primary ego around which humans positively relate. This is not the spectacular ego of egoism. It is, moreover, from this primary adherence (simultaneously to oneself and to the world) that one can live as authentically generous, tolerant, ambitious, modest, discreet, and enthusiastic. Modernity, far from destroying this basic (unreflexive) ego, confirms its centrality, which is the meaning of transcendental subjectivity and universalism.[22] The Copernican Revolution of transcendental subjectivity calls into question the univocal and indisputable transmission of a unique sense of being, which is characteristic of traditional societies, but does not call being into question.

It is not modernity but the inability to assume the emancipation from traditional determinisms (offered by modernity) that has engendered industrialism, which consists in its foundation in replacing one determinism by another. Material determinism replaces divine determinism. Industrialism responds to a need for determinism. This operation of substitution destroys the adherence to the world and simultaneously to being (Heidegger could say that it destroys the being of being), because the new determinism (contrary to the traditional determinism which refers to the otherness of the unknowable, to the All Other) is circular: the being is closed on itself, in other words, all the world is circularly conditioned (and all living things, including man, are only a modality of this conditioning, in the sense of a conditioned product, since the whole of reality is ultimately industry), and technique (determined product of matter) is only a new stratum of universal industrial conditioning. Industrialist universality is thus a by-product of the great factory of nature (of nature conceived as a factory).[23]

The destruction of the being of being no longer allows primary paranoia, healthy paranoia if you like, to play its creative role. Thus, in the 19th century, we entered the first nihilistic and ostentatiously deterministic cycle of industrialism (when materialistic determinism replaces traditional determinism). This is the cycle of the repression of the anxiety of the void, and more specifically here the anxiety of the loss of determination (what today we call the loss of meaning); a repression that manifested itself in practice by the double race of filling up (centripetal) and showing off (centrifugal), which is the very dynamic of success. But this centripetal/centrifugal balloting without adherence, at a certain point of intensity, makes industrialist society a borderline society, as we speak of borderline individuals, on the edge of madness. It is at this point that we enter the second cycle of industrialism, with the fabrication of turnkey paranoia, of substitute egos that are designated as identities. These are negative representations of identity, struggling to regain what is seen as lost. In the psychoanalytical sense, identitarianism is a psychic regression that aims to re-fix desires on predetermined products (in this case identities) and thus prevent the epidemic extension of an eventual emancipation (which became possible again at the point of crisis, that is, at the end of the first cycle, at the point of exhaustion of schyzohumanism).

These identities are comparable to prefabricated houses disguised as traditional homes, or ready-made clothes fitted to retro-utopian imaginaries. In this context, the new identity entrepreneurs abound, and no longer present themselves only as politicians, journalists, writers, or even professional communicators. The range of organic intellectuals (according to Gramsci's expression) has exploded with the use of digital media. The major identity entrepreneurs are the YouTube influencers with the most varied styles.

Schyzohumanism (lack of primary adherence) at its peak produces surrogate egos who, to remain credible, attempt to exist in extreme self-expression (either through symbolic violence, or physical violence, or both). The god (or gods) of the neo-traditionalists and the principles of the neo-rationalists are false gods and false principles because nobody really believes in them. It is because nobody really believes in them that one constitutes them in the negativity of resentment. They are nostalgic gods and principles, which can only be experienced in the pain of estrangement, of being torn away from oneself, and which only manage to make themselves heard by naming and violating the culprits of their absence. The cry for authenticity has become the highest degree of kitsch, falsity squared, the most adulterated promise.

The Industrial Making of Retro-Utopias

The circular race to holistic happiness (framed by schizohumanist ethics) is akin to a perpetual motion in constant acceleration.[24] This race, which has been characteristic of the neoliberal era since the middle of the 20th century, has been amplified in the correlationist era via the new digital technologies set up as platforms where profiles are displayed and met. Through Tinder, Grinder, LinkedIn, Facebook, and Instagram, crowds of self-profiled individuals evaluate, inform, select, eliminate, congratulate, judge, insult, meet physically and sometimes make love, spew invective, hire each other, among other things. In short, they adapt themselves to the market.[25] This algorithmic life of general self-tracking incorporates a feverish sense of urgency and causes a feeling of dizziness (which is sought after like a drug shot). Like in a noisy, blinding amusement park, one must go from one attraction to another, faster and faster, from dizziness to dizziness; until there is so little time between two attractions that the dizziness turns into a daze. It is at this point that the individual is entirely available, self-controlled, and dependent.[26] The person becomes fuel. It is not presentism that neoliberalism, which has been overtaken and accomplished by correlationism (general self-profiling), leads to, but the absence of the present, the deprivation of temporality, and, finally, the absence of the self altogether (zombification). In the vocabulary of phenomenology, we would say that retentions (the different strata of memories) and protentions (the different strata of anticipations, of projects) shrink and tighten until the being-present is suffocated. It is in this sense that Bernard Stiegler speaks of our era as the era of the absence of an era.[27]

No longer does any adhesion (to ideas, parties, communities, friends, lovers, nations, even things) rest on a stable adherence. Individuals reduced to profiles (for others and for themselves) slide faster and faster (from one adherence to another), carried along more and more passively by the force of the attractions constantly coproduced in the comanaged amusement park that society has become.[28]

This constant and ecstatic acceleration (due to a growing lack of adhesion) is obviously only in appearance a perpetual motion. The machine necessarily becomes tense in the long run and must be constantly repaired, revised, and reassembled. If the dizziness provoked by the dizzying driving force of the attractions destroys possible psychic resistances with a view to optimizing self-exploitation (there is no longer the material time to question, to wait, to see what is coming, one has to throw oneself forward without thinking), it cannot in fact stem the surges of nausea or even of panic. Nausea and panic are the counterparts of the vertigo of acceleration and of the loss of control that it engenders (and which is nevertheless sought after). As with a roller coaster, the ecstatic fever can turn into panic at any moment: one wants to get off at all costs, to stop the machine, to stop the nausea. These desperate reactions, seeking to land somewhere, to stop the dizziness, the vertigo, and the speed fever, as well as to stop the feeling of unreality, the feeling of the falseness of everything, are inherent to the system while risking at any moment to seize up its functioning. If the fever of speed indeed allows the feeling of unreality to be diluted and thus allows the industrialist semblance to function, when the panic of vertigo sets in it brings to the surface the awareness of the facticity of the setting—like an enchantment that dissipates.

The panicked player is then ready to cling to the most immediate promise of braking or even stopping. Such a promise, to be credible, proposes extreme solutions, which can go as far as a call to murder; the player, no longer able to bear the game, is ready to do anything to get off. The marketing images of success are no longer effective, the personal development practices (based on bungee jumping, relaxation, and mindfulness) no longer support the enchantment of success. The schyzohumanist force of persuasion is exhausted. This is where the last spring of the system comes in: the set of neo-traditionalisms that promise to put the brakes on, to stop, to get out of the infernal circus.

The neo-traditionalist trick is to project or, if you like, to put on display backward-looking, reassuring, slow, hierarchical worlds, where everyone seems to occupy a stable and orderly place: the retro-utopias. The schyzohumanist enchantment that is about to dissipate in the panic is replaced in extremis by these retro-utopias. The individual on the verge of dezombification is thus immediately rezombified. This is why the system itself markets the retro-utopias (ancient worlds that have never existed), which present themselves as emergency exits, to capture the panicking eyes. But these are false emergency exits that actually open onto paths that lead nowhere. These false exits are only there to deceive attention. When I say "the system markets," I don't mean that it is a conspiracy with evil machinists pulling the strings of manipulation. The "system" is the desperate demand that is met by marketers in search of immediate profits; the "system" is the communicators, the market experts, the specialists in the "evolution of values" who, seeing the number of panicked profiles in need of a lost identity in their statistical surveys (a panic that is partly produced by their own actions as marketers, that is to say, as manufacturers of fashions), coproduce (along with political, cultural, economic, and religious experts) reactionary discourse on the tragic loss of "our" identities and the return to a world of the past. The reactionary image, the retro-utopia, is in fact conceived as a falsely anti-fashion fashion, which serves as an outlet. It is the reconstitution of an attraction that presents itself as an anti-attraction, that is, as the very image of authenticity in a world where everything seems adulterated.

At the origin of the success of a politician who relies on retro-utopian tricks, there is almost always an enterprise rationally set up and orchestrated by communicators (i e , by marketers, specialists in statistical profiles) The hyper-retro-utopian inflection of the French far-right party the Front National (agglomerating since 2003 the national left-wing retro-utopias, such as "the ideal French secular republic," with the right-wing retro-utopias already mobilized by the party, such as "France united around Joan of Arc") is almost exclusively attributable to Florian Philippot, whose closest adviser is his brother Damien, a former executive of the IFOP polling institute, a statistical profiling specialist. Former French president Nicolas Sarkozy's political line of defending French identity during the 2012 presidential campaign is also due to the pure communicator Philippe Buisson. Similarly, the US president Donald Trump did not appear out of nowhere in the American political landscape. He did not seize the presidency at the end of 2016 by chance. He is first and foremost a media actor in search of maximum profit, a television host, a sitcom actor, a showman, a specialist in pseudo-scandalous staging of himself, permanently connected to social networks, all this before being a businessman or a politician. Trump is not a priori obsessed with defending the lost American identity, he is an opportunistic dandy who loves luxury and glitter, who has seized a promising niche like an actor who would try his luck in the register that is most suited to his game. His most notable impresario, agent, and scriptwriter in the 2016 election campaign was the communicator Steve Bannon, who provided him with most of his talking points about defending American authenticity against the rest of the world, against the insidious infiltration of evil (corrosive progressive forces, immigrants, traitors from within), against the conspiracy of the Deep State.

The retro-utopias are like artificially aged postcards (just as some goods are artificially worn to give them a patina, the weight of the years) with black-and-white images from the past. The tenderness felt converts the nausea into nostalgia and gives the impression of having stepped off the ride, or at least of having one foot out of the amusement park. When one's eyes are riveted to these idealized images, it seems to the panic-stricken individual that he can finally breathe, calm his nervousness, that his existence has slowed down and finally weighs something. But the lull is superficial, because the retro-utopias are not outside the theme park; they are part of it. The image of a perfect world (in which men would finally have a role to play), by its very nature of fantasy, remains elusive. But the individual is then trapped, because he cannot under any circumstances admit the facticity of this projection, on pain of plunging back into the unbearable vertigo of the Great Eight. All that remains for him to do to stabilize his evil is to crusade against the enemies who deprive him of his mirage and prevent him from enjoying himself, that is, his authentic identity. Since not everyone has the same world as before, identity entrepreneurs compete intensely in a market that today is also the internet. The antagonistic authenticities are fueled by the energy of their imaginary exclusivities and generate a climate of permanent confrontation.

The disoriented *homo industrialis*, afflicted with melancholy,[29] mobilizes for the great return to a lost religious tradition, a lost republic, a lost democracy, a lost secularism, a lost universality, a lost reason, a lost science, a lost morality, a lost God, a lost culture, a lost nature. The most opposite (and contradictory) values, symbols, ideas can then be mobilized in turn or at the same time, it does not matter. We will even have the image of lost progress. Progress is what by definition aims at its own overcoming and therefore cannot be preserved like a relic; progress cannot be a heritage to be defended, since it presupposes its own overflow to fulfill its promise. But the meaning of words, ideas, concepts, customs, principles is blurred and replaced by the obsessive simulacrum of their inexorable loss. It is no longer the meaning of progress to which we refer in reality, nor the meaning of the Republic, nor the meaning of secularism, nor of this or that religion, nor of this or that tradition, but the meaning of loss. It is the image of a heritage that by nature belongs to us and that is unjustly taken away. The feeling of deprivation of this natural heritage as our identity (the feeling of being deprived of oneself) overwhelms all meanings. Identitarianism is the most appropriate generic term for this desperate pursuit of the self through retro-utopian projections, which allow the industrialist system to repair itself.

From Identitarianism to Violence

This is why, in the face of this pace, which continues to accelerate because the authenticity pursued remains an unattainable mirage, the only thing that is left in extremis is the demonstration of explicit violence in the public space, the spectacle of ostentatious killing and sacrifice, in short, terrorism. It must be understood that the new jihadism has become liquid. Its highly flammable fuel, resentment, does not drive any coherent ideological body, as was still the case with the Al Qaeda model in the 1990s. In a frantic search for power, adventure, grandeur, self-existence, the new jihadist wanders between hyperrealistic video games, a desperate quest for exceptional success, social networks, and social humiliation.[30] An organization like the Islamic State (Daech)—which does indeed have an ideological project derived from the former Al Qaed—has been able to adapt to these new wanderings amplified by the internet by offering a turnkey identity, a role of hero/martyr of the lost civilization without trying to transmit a solid ideology (which would require a certain cultural stability, including learning classical Arabic, and several years of internalization of religious practices). The leaders of Daech have adapted wonderfully to the new market of frustration with a simple and unstoppable managerial model entirely centered on the stigma of humiliation. The recipe is straightforward: to promise the reversal of the meaning of discriminatory stigmas, in other words, to turn the feeling of humiliation into a chivalrous coat of arms and thus transmute the mal-à-être into a raison d'être; which amounts to turning the signs of a failed (and frustrating) life into the signs of a heroic destiny (of an accomplishment in total war[31]). It is the old myth of the chosen one: the one who seems to be left on the sidelines, despised at the beginning of the story, turns out to be the real hero at the end of the story. The archetypal narrative of the chosen one was brilliantly updated in Dar al Islam, the online magazine of the Islamic State in particular (mainly in French and

English and very little in classical Arabic, inaccessible to most of the target audience) in a dreamlike grammar mixing Manga and Marvell placed in an Islamic-utopian setting.[32]

This new form of dissemination of violence, which no longer requires a complex logistic structure, rigorous training, and ideological internalization, can be captured and exploited in any direction: by Islamist movements (like most attacks in France), by anti-multiculturalist and/or anti-Islamic nationalist movements (like Anders Breivik's attack on Utoya Island in Norway in 2011, in which he killed 77 people and wounded 151, mostly Social-Democratic teenagers, none of whom were even Muslims, or like the 2019 Christchurch attacks on mosques in New Zealand, which killed 51 people. The terrorist was an Australian immigrant who wanted to defend the West, especially Europe, from Islamic invasion by attacking New Zealand mosques! It is not insignificant that he announced and broadcast his "exploits" online. A few years later in the same country, in September 2021, an individual inspired by ISIS, without benefit of any logistics, murdered six people with a knife in a supermarket). Contrary to appearances, religion is not the cause but rather the packaging for this new violence. The attacks (sometimes mass killings) committed by individuals linked to the Incel (Involuntary Celibate) movement in North America and Western Europe bear witness to this. These young men feel frustrated about their right to enjoy the world, especially to enjoy a sexual life. They murder people (mostly women) in places that symbolize the enjoyment and culture they feel deprived of (their fundamental frustration is the same as that of jihadists): six people were killed on the campus of the University of Santa Barbara in 2014, nine people on the campus of Umpqua Community College in 2015 again in the United States, 10 people in a German chicha bar in 2020, a woman stabbed in a Toronto spa again in 2020. The list goes on.

The Incel movements are characteristic because they push to the extreme the functioning of what is still sketched in jihadism. The murderous gesture is entirely potentiated by the powerlessness complexes of young men who feel humiliated and lost (a much more fundamental variable than belonging to an Islamist or extreme right-wing group; with the Incels this is all that remains, the core of frustration), the internalization of frustration is deployed on the internet, without ideological solidity, but traversed by phantasmic images of extraordinary success by the only mainspring that seems to remain: extreme violence. The 19-year-old man arrested by the police in France on September 28, 2021, typically had this profile, frequenting Incel sites, wanting to be a neo-Nazi, and boasting of being a "white fighter," but not being able to decide whether to attack a mosque or his former high school; he was not sure of his target, the main thing for him being to "do worse than Columbine," in reference to the mass massacre in an American school in 1999 which traumatized North America for several years.[33] The Cornelian hesitation of our white fighter to attack either his old high school or a mosque is paradigmatic; it shows that it is not a question of ideology, that times have changed; it is only a question of what could be the more remarkable feat ("to do worse than Columbine"). It is the spectacular effect of the act itself, its visibility, and the number of likes (and) or anti-likes (which amounts to the same thing in this case) of horrified expressions (especially on the internet) that counts. In the end it is an accounting issue. You have to make the biggest number, kill as many people as possible to leave a deeper mark, to distinguish yourself more durably, in other words, to feel the significant weight of your action (and that, at the same time, the rest of the world cannot help but feel it either). It is a jihad against the unbearable lightness of being. Clearly, this dissemination of empty violence has nothing to do with a possible war of civilizations or ideologies. It is in the continuity of neoliberal logic, in which the ideological label is no more than a brand chosen for the optimization of visibility. By reaching an impressive number of brutally massacred individuals, one can become somebody, in other words, one can become successful. In short, it is a matter of acquiring an indisputable quality through an impressive quantity of victims.[34]

The Internet as an Amplifier of the Anxiety Culture

The new element in the 21st century is the existence of global identities fueled by de-territorialized spaces of desire through the internet.[35] Digital spaces are indeed spaces in which individuals meet (envy each other, admire each other, imitate each other, hate each other, share knowledge, even practice religious rituals, to name a few[36]), but they do not meet in a physically located territory. These spaces of interaction do not have circumscribed territories. They are spaces of existence that abolish physical distances. So much so that an individual living in New York who is used to a social network where he or she meets people located in Japan, France, or Argentina on a daily basis may feel closer to them than to his or her next-door neighbor, because they share a practice, a hobby, opinions, or an obsession. The classic logics of solidarity, imitation, belonging, and local rivalries are thus short-circuited (without disappearing, they can even be amplified; for example, a feeling of exclusion due to living in an unhealthy urban periphery can be exacerbated by frequenting de-territorialized spaces of desire, in other words through digital existence).

Moreover, everyone can make an event by filming a murder or a suicide, which is immediately relayed from one end of the planet to the other. Everyone can control and be controlled. Everyone can inform and misinform, monitor themselves and be monitored by those they monitor (or by others). There can no longer be any monopolistic or even oligopolistic producers of information in a given territory. Each person becomes a producer of information that can be disseminated on a large scale, beyond their region, nation, or continent. All feelings (love, hate, jealousy, compassion, anger, etc.) and representations (of wealth, poverty, success, failure, greatness, baseness, etc.) are massively co-constructed without a determined local perimeter.

Globalization has amplified industrialism because it has produced a system of culture that is inter-reactive, subject to constant manipulation, imitation, marketing, and to constant outbursts of hatred, frustration, and violent reactions. To put it another way, if no centralized censorship is entirely possible, no limit to violence can be effectively set a priori either. The real risk in this context is, on the one hand, a surge of violence, without any responsible administration or government, but with operators of opinions who play on feelings and representations for their own benefit and on an unprecedented scale, and, on the other hand, the slide toward authoritarian regimes that lock down feelings and representations.

NOTES

1. This text of this chapter has been elaborated from unpublished passages (remodeled and summarized) of a study that has kept me intensely busy for the last three years and which has been published in full as a book in August 2023: *Khaos. La promesse trahie de la modernité* (Paris: Les Liens qui Libèrent).

2. The notion of *correlationism*, has been elaborated in *Khaos*, is not identical to correlationism in the philosophy of knowledge, although there are correspondences between the two meanings.

3. The concept of *schyzohumanism*, elaborated in my previous research, has been considerably deepened in *Khaos*.

4. The repression never completely represses the anguish of the void, and the repressed anguish of the void never completely rises to the surface of the collective consciousness.

5. Sartre compares freedom to a hole; Jean-Paul Sartre, *L'être et le néant* (Paris: Gallimard, 1943), 551.

6. I am of course referring to the novel *La nausée*; Jean-Paul Sartre, *La nausée* (Paris: Gallimard, 1938).

7. This is what Sartre calls "the facticity of freedom," to which he devotes more or less the last part of *Being and Nothingness*, but above all the first chapter of this fourth part, and more particularly title 2 of this first chapter titled "Freedom and Facticity: The Situation'"; Sartre, *L'être et le néant*, 527–598.

8. Sartre, *L'être et le néant*, 530.

9. Sartre, *L'être et le néant*, 531.

10. Claus Offe, *Zur Klassentheorie und Herrschaftsstruktur im staatlich regulierten Kapitalismus* (quoted from Jürgen Habermas, *La technique et la science comme "idéologie"*) (Paris: Gallimard, 1978), 41.

11. The death drive can be a general safeguarding principle, such as cellular suicide, as well as the quasi-sacrificial suicide of the hero who offers his life. The death drive corresponds here to a desire for self-annihilation without organic benefit. See Sigmund Freud, *Beyond the Pleasure Principle* (first published in 1920).

12. In the two convergent senses of Object a, the incomparable singularity of the ego (which can be said to be transcendental subjectivity, the soul, etc.), and Object A, as the incomparable greatness of the real (which can be said to be God).

13. Jacques Lacan, *L'angoisse, Séminaire 10*, 1962–1963, accessed May 20, 2024, http://staferla.free.fr/S10/S10.htm.

14. See Slavoj Žižek, *The Sublime Object of Ideology* (London: Verso, 2009).

15. I distinguish three layers of desire in humans: the desire to survive (to continue to exist), the desire to live (objective improvement of the conditions of existence), and the desire to be (to tell oneself what I am through the doubling of the inner language and the external staging of oneself).

16. See Frédéric Baitinger, "Jacques-Alain Miller, Paranoia: A Primary Relation to the Other," *The Lacanian Review*, no. 10 (2020): 52–91.

17. The incompleteness of psychic interiority is the metaphysical meaning of the unconscious, of which a certain industrialist psychoanalysis has made, on the contrary, a reservoir of unconscious causes but entirely already there and therefore absolutely determining.

18. Søren Kierkegaard, *The Concept of Anxiety: A Simple Psychologically Orienting Deliberation on the Dogmatic Issue of Hereditary Sin*, ed. and trans. Reidar Thomte. (Princeton, NJ: Princeton University Press 1980). Original work June 17, 1844, pseud. Vigilius Haufniensis.

19. Robert Musil, *The Man Without Qualities*, original German editions 1930 and 1932; for the French edition, (Paris: Seuil, 1954), 233.

20. Musil, *The Man Without Qualities*, 84.

21. Stefan Zweig, *Le Monde d'hier: Souvenirs d'un Européen* (Paris: Belfond, 1982).

22. *Transcendental subjectivity* for adherence to the self, and *Universality* for adherence to the world.

23. This is what Heidegger means when he assimilates technique to metaphysics. Metaphysics would be an ontology without being, therefore an ontology without reason to be, therefore a nonontology.

24. For a complete analysis of the concept of retro-utopia, see *The horror of the void*.

25. See Roland Gori, *La fabrique des imposteurs* (Paris: Les Liens qui Libèrent, 2013).

26. Barbara Stiegler, « *Il faut s'adapter* ». *Sur un nouvel impératif politique* (Paris: Gallimard, 2019).

27. Bernard Stiegler, *Dans la disruption: Comment ne pas devenir fou?* (Paris: Les Liens qui Libèrent, 2016).

28. This is the cause of the social acceleration observed by Edmund Rosa.

29. Cioran has wonderfully identified this illness without an object that is melancholy. It is the lack of everything, and above all of oneself, and therefore the obsessive focus on oneself, that produces melancholy: "Melancholy is the dream state of egoism . . . Feeding on what corrupts it, it hides, under its melodious name, the Pride of Defeat and Self-pity"; Emil Cioran, *Précis de décomposition* (Paris: Gallimard, 1949).

30. See Raphaël Liogier, *La guerre des civilisations n'aura pas lieu. Coexistence et violence au XXIème siècle* (Paris: CNRS Éditions, 2016, new revised edition, 2018).

31. Liogier, *La guerre des civilisations n'aura pas lieu*. I would like to take this opportunity to mention the fact that a number of journalists questioned me about this latest book at the time

of its release, asking me in substance, "Wouldn't you be a little too optimistic in claiming that the war of civilizations will not take place?" Apart from the fact that such a remark showed that they had either not understood or simply not read the book, I invariably replied to them, in substance, "Certainly the war of civilizations will not take place, but it would be less serious if it did take place than what we are really in danger of experiencing: an internal war, with no civilizational exteriority, no stable ideological structure. In short, I am not optimistic, because what we are risking is much more destructive."

32. The psychoanalyst Fethi Benslama has shown to what extent this image of the superhero is present among the new jihadists, in contradiction with Islamic traditions; Fethi Benslama, *Un furieux désir de sacrifice: Le surmusulman* (Paris: Seuil, 2016). For example, the famous exclamation *Allah 'akbar* (Allah is great), which traditionally expresses modesty, the feeling of smallness in the face of God's immeasurable greatness, will become, in the opposite direction, a war cry expressing the exorbitant power of the superhero-terrorist.

33. Pierre Plottu and Maxime Macé, "Bulles de haine. Projet d'attentats en Seine-Maritime: suprémaciste, fan de tueurs de masse, "incel" . . . le profil du suspect se precise," *Libération*, October 5, 2021, https://www.liberation.fr/societe/police-justice/projet-dattentat-contre-un-lycee
-et-une-mosquee-radicalise-sur-internet-le-suspect-admirait-les-tueurs-de-masse-20211005
_J4YEK7HSVVG47JR7JWBFOPXFTI/.

34. In *Khaos, La promesse trahie de la modernité,* I call this process *qualitatization.*

35. Global identities as I have tried to define them in my work are not equivalent to de-territorialized identities specific to internet social networks (taking the notion of social networks in a broad sense, including, for example, massively multiplayer online games). Classical territorialized identities (e.g., regional) and inter-territorial identities (e.g., diasporas) do not disappear but form a system with the de-territorialized identities that characterize digital spaces. It is this system of connected identity strata that constitutes global identities; See Liogier, *La guerre des civilisations n'aura pas lieu.*

36. See Olivier Servais, *Dans la peau des gamers (Continent digital)* (Paris: Karthala, 2020).

CHAPTER SEVENTEEN

Fear and Technology in Modern Europe

A Call for Researching Fears as Drivers of Technology Development

KARENA KALMBACH

When we think of fear in relation to technology, we usually have a very specific kind of relationship in mind—namely, fear that is produced by technology: the fear of nuclear fallout, the fear of traffic accidents, the fear of computer hacking. But what if we turn this relationship upside down, add a time perspective, and ask: Which technologies have been produced by fears?

The fear of terrorism, the fear of mass migration and the fear of global warming—to name but a few of the current most prominently expressed fears in Europe—are important references in public debates and political decision-making. What is more, these fears strongly impact research agendas and lead to the development of new technologies.[1] Surveillance technologies in city centers, identification technologies at state borders, and carbon capture facilities are all offshoots of these fears. Did similar dynamics of fear drive technological development in the past?

Despite that fears are deeply inscribed in many technologies that shape our daily lives, social sciences and humanities research has mainly focused on people's fears of technologies. Enormous resources have been dedicated to developing strategies that analyze and diminish these fears and thus increase the acceptance of technologies.

So far, hardly any attention has been paid to how fears have driven technological innovation and implementation—neither in history, nor in science and technology studies.[2] In fact, no theoretical framework exists that reflects on the interrelationship and coproduction of technology and fear. This is remarkable, considering the prominent role that both fear and technology play in the current public discourse, as well as in academic endeavors to conceptualize modernity.

This essay's starting point is the principle that technologies not only nurture and perpetuate fears, but fears also act as driving forces for technological development. The invention and implementation of new technologies sustain existing fears and cause new fears, which again trigger technology development. This means that fear and technology coproduce each other in a dialectic manner: fear is both the source and the result of technology—and vice versa.

If we consider large-scale implementations of technology and fast spinning innovation circles as the cornerstones of "modernity"—and at the same time take seriously the claim that since the dawn of the 20th century, we are living in an "age of fear"—we need to investigate and conceptualize the entanglement of fear and technology. Such an investigation has three significant benefits. First, it broadens our understanding of why certain technologies actually came into being. Second, it allows further exploration of the narratives and worldviews interwoven in these technologies and thus a broader perspective on "technology resistance." Third, it enables a reconceptualization of modernity that pays due credit to the role of fear and technology in shaping the era. To be able to make the connection with modernization theory, I argue that the historical time and space that offers itself most for such a research endeavor is Western Europe in the 19th and 20th centuries: the center stage of what has been labeled "modernity."

The Coproduction of Fear and Technology

The following theoretical reflections on the reciprocal relationship between fear and technology are based on the research I have conducted in the framework of the interdisciplinary working group "Fearful Technologies," which I established at Eindhoven University of Technology in 2017.[3] I have presented this conceptualization at numerous conferences and received valuable feedback from colleagues in both the fields of History of Technology and History of Emotions.[4] My theoretical reflections on this interrelationship have led me to the conclusion that we can differentiate five basic forms of causal relations between fear and technology.

1.　*Fear of Technology*

Fear of Technology can act out in several different dimensions. The first dimension is the fear of a technological artifact. This refers to the actual use of a technological artifact; thus, the fears implied are mostly linked to the integrity of one's own body. Sometimes these fears are strongest when a new technology is introduced, as was the case for gas ovens in the late 19th century. However, these fears can also be detached from the time of the technological implementation, as demonstrated by the fear of flying, which has always existed in the history of aviation.

The second dimension is the fear of the societal and cultural effects of a technological artifact. Here, not so much one's own body is the object of concern, but rather the societal norms and customs that will probably change through the mass use of a technology. The fears expressed in relation to the development of the film and photography industry around 1900 are as much examples of this dimension as today's fears about artificial intelligence. These fears are closely linked to what has become known under the term *cultural pessimism* and imply a negative outlook on the further development of society.[5]

The third dimension of Fear of Technology is the fear relating to the politics inscribed in a technological artifact. The strong opposition to mass implementation of nuclear power plants in the 1970s and 1980s is a telling example. Particularly in German-speaking countries, anti-nuclear activists mobilized the narrative of the "atomic state."[6] In their reading, nuclear power plants required an authoritarian police state and the state's backing for the nuclear bomb—if not, the technology would be unfeasible, both politically and economically. These activists looked on pro-nuclear politics as a form of reimplementing a political mindset in society very much akin to Nazi ideology.

2.　*Fear by Technology*

This is closely related to the category Fear of Technology. Whereas Fear of Technology does not specify the purpose of the technology, this purpose is at the very heart of the category Fear by Technology. Here, we are dealing with fears created deliberately and induced by the technology. For instance, we could not be afraid of becoming the victim of a nuclear bomb attack if nuclear bombs did not exist. But technologies can also provoke fears in a positive sense, like a roller-coaster ride. A crucial differentiation lies in the carrier of the fear: is it the users of the technology themselves who become afraid, or is the technology applied to provoke fear in someone else?

3.   *Fear for Technology*

Technological artifacts can become objects of high value for the owner or user—to a point where the person becomes afraid of losing the pleasure or service the technology provides or the aesthetics or social value of the technological object itself. This can happen to an individual, but it also can occur on a wider societal level. The fear that a beloved new car (be it the Volkswagen Beetle in the 1950s or Tesla Model S in the 2010s) might become the victim of vandalism is an example of this fear for technology on an individual level. The fear that a critical infrastructure might break down is an example of this fear playing out on a wider societal level. Group or individual identities can be inscribed in a technology. If this is the case, the fear for technology becomes directly linked with existential questions. The French Minitel system is a typical example: the decline in the technology was strongly linked with France's fear of losing its reputation of national technological grandeur; it thus became a struggle against "surrendering" to the United States internet.

The three dimensions of Fear of Technology, Fear by Technology, and Fear for Technology all take the technological artifact as starting point for the causal relationship between fear and technology. This perspective is what we usually find in the literature and public discourse. However, this causal relationship can also be turned around to highlight fear as the main agent in this interconnection.

4.   *Technology against Fear*

The dimension Technology against Fear is almost the opposite of Fear by Technology. Instead of triggering fears deliberately, Technology against Fear aims to reduce existing fears. Examples are technologies that calm a person before or during medical treatment. Technologies against fear do not only work on an individual's body. If we consider the example of flood protection infrastructures, we see that their purpose is highly discursive: removing the fear that a serious flood could hit any time. The Dutch Delta Works considerably reduced public fears of extreme North Sea floods after the major flood in 1953. Acting on people's fears, technology against fear embodies both: technologies of prevention and technologies of resilience. Highlighting the aspect of fear in these technologies, preventing an event from happening or preparing to better cope with the event's aftermath (thus making the event appear less scary) are both forms of fear management—of course with very different (bio)political implications.[7]

5.   *Technology by Fear*

As with the categories Fear by Technology and Fear of Technology, Technology against Fear and Technology by Fear are closely related and can overlap. To account for the major differences in the forms of fears and objects on which these fears play out, I consider it crucial to differentiate Technology against Fear and Technology by Fear. This differentiation becomes clearer when we apply Kierkegaard's distinction of *fear* and *anxiety*.[8] He conceptualized fear as the unease directed at a specific object or phenomenon (which can peak in phobias, like arachnophobia), whereas anxiety is not directed at a precise target. Applying this distinction to the causal link between fear and technology, I consider Technology against Fear to be driven by a concrete fear directed at a specific object or phenomenon (like medical treatment or a flood). Technology by Fear, on the other hand, relates to wider, more abstract fears, and we cannot directly act on the object of these fears. This implies that the technology invented or implemented by this fear has to take a kind of "detour" to fight the object that causes the fear. Because this does not concern general anxieties about being in the world, I refrain from using the term *anxiety* but stick to the term *fear*. To clarify my argument, consider the fear of the global population explosion, a fear that became widespread in the 1970s and 1980s, mostly thanks to the success of the study "The Limits to Growth."[9] The fear of the world's population growing too large is a concrete fear, yet one that is located somewhere between a general anxiety about being in the world and the fear of an individual person or group of persons. This fear did not lead (fortunately, in most cases) to directly killing other people, but rather it led to the invention and implementation of mechanisms geared to reducing the growth of the world population (like the one-child policy in China) or accommodating more people on planet earth. A key mechanism was developing new technologies; for example, genetically modified crops, labeled as a means to "feed the growing population of the world," can thus be considered a Technology by Fear.

State of the Art in Research

Of the five dimensions of fear–technology interrelationships, Fear of Technology is the dimension academic researchers have mainly investigated. A seminal example is Spencer Weart's work on Nuclear Fear.[10] Often, historical investigations into fear of technology stress the irrationality of past fears from a contemporary point of view. Wolfgang Schivelbusch's work on train passengers' fears of traveling at high speed is an often-quoted anecdote.[11] Another common phenomenon, particularly in social sciences research, is a focus on strategies or instruments to overcome Fear of Technology and thus increase technology acceptance. The research fields of Public Understanding of Science and Public Risk Perception strongly emphasize increasing technology acceptance. These studies often start their argument by clearly distinguishing "unjustified public fears" and "rational expert knowledge," particularly in relation to nuclear technology.[12]

In recent years, it has become popular to link the Luddite movement to the contemporary debate on the political implications of judging Fear of Technology as legitimate or not. While historians have discussed the Luddites in the context of the British working class,[13] contemporary (non-historian) authors completely disconnected the term *Luddite* from this context, using it as a synonym for technology resistance.[14] They interpreted the Luddites' destruction of machines as an act of rebellion against the societal and cultural effects of a technological artifact. So, while there are some broad claims circulating in the public and academic discourse about the interrelationship between fear and technology, historians of technology have remained silent on this issue.

This silence likely stems from the fact that the history of technology has not yet paid much attention to emotions. The German Society for the History of Technology (GTG) recently addressed this lacuna and dedicated its annual conference in April 2018 to *Technikemotionen*. It was Martina Heßler who had pushed for this topic. In the framework of her reflections on the technological futures of work,[15] she is one of the few historians of technology who has started to investigate fears of the societal and cultural effects of technological artifacts.

Not only has the history of technology shown little interest in emotions; likewise, the flourishing field of history of emotions[16] has not paid much attention to technology. The recent conference held at George Mason University in June 2018—promoted as the first big history of emotions conference in North America—did not include a single presentation on technology.[17]

This missing connection between the history of technology and the history of emotions is also apparent when we look at our particular emotion of interest: fear.[18] Although cultural historians (some of whom are historians of emotions) have a long-established interest in fears,[19] they have not investigated the impact of these fears on technology development. This is also true for historians' involvement in interdisciplinary endeavors.[20] It is a telling example that the recent interdisciplinary *Handbook on Fear*[21] only considers one single technology and the corresponding fear of technology: nuclear power.[22]

Thus, academic research has indeed addressed the dimension of Fear of Technology by touching on its three dimensions: fear of a technological artifact, of the societal and cultural effects of a technological artifact, or of the politics inscribed in a technological artifact. The dimension Technology by Fear—which I consider the opposite side of this relationship—is a topic entirely overlooked so far. It is thus precisely this dimension that I think needs to be addressed much more profoundly. Investigating technology by fear implies approaching from the perspective of fear.

I will refrain from discussing the state-of-the-art research on the dimensions Fear by Technology and Fear for Technology. Both dimensions stress technology as the driving force of fear–technology interrelationships. As this essay is a call for putting the focus on fear as a driving force for these interrelationships, I turn my attention to historical research on fear.

In the area of social history, a strong interest has recently developed in the topics of resilience and prevention. Both research areas strongly rely on the notions of *risk* and *uncertainty* and thus deal with fears about what is to come. German historians have published on this topic in particular, coining the term *Versicherheitlichung* (securitization).[23] However, in these social history works on *Zukunftsängste* (fears about the future and fears projected onto the future), the link with technology is once again distinctly lacking. These works mainly investigate the social regimes of coping with risk and uncertainty[24] and pay particular attention to insurances.[25] Yet these works do not ask: How did *Zukunftsängste* drive technological innovation?

The aspect of *Zukunftsängste* and the mechanisms implemented to prevent negative possible futures bring us to the core focus of the research endeavor I call for and thus require elaboration. After all, it is this very aspect of *Zukunftsängste* where the theorization of fear–technology interrelationships and modernization theory interconnect. As Reinhart Koselleck prominently pointed out, the historic era which we have come to know as modernity began at the moment when people started to conceptualize the future as a time and space which they can proactively shape and re-shape.[26] At the dawn of modernity, people conquered the future as an open space of possibilities by expanding their expectations or *Erwartungshorizont*. Despite repeatedly mentioning the accelerated development of technologies as a key feature of modern times, Koselleck did not unpack the black box of technology. He reflected neither on the nature and variety of technologies that we came to know as "modern," nor on the potential interconnections between these modern technologies and the uncertainties implied in the open and contingent (and thus uncertain) futures he described.[27] Lucian Hölscher, another prominent figure in academic research on the history of the future, likewise did not engage with technology.[28] The paragraphs he dedicates to this subject contain anecdotes about promising new technologies for the 20th and 21st centuries. Although his entire book focuses on political utopias and thus the political shaping of future times, he does not even politicize the technologies he mentions. What is interesting about his findings, however, is his claim that future scenarios have become less and less positive. If this is true, it means that there are probably growing fears about negative future scenarios becoming reality. How do these increased fears impact technology development? And are these fears actually produced by technologies?

Also, recent works on the history of future thinking have not engaged more structurally with technology development;[29] research on forecast regimes and technologies are an exception to the rule.[30] However, the importance of future visions for technology development has recently become a central field of research in science and technology studies (STS). The concept of sociotechnical imaginaries developed by Sheila Jasanoff and Sang-Hyun Kim has become a buzzword and features in numerous publications and research projects. [31] The focus of future imaginaries so far has been much more on positive, utopian scenarios than on negative, dystopian ones. Researchers using this concept are asking: What futures do societies want to make come true by developing and implementing certain technologies? The focus on positive narratives and scenarios that drive technology innovation is also central in innovation studies[32] and has recently entered economic theory. Jens Beckert points out: "utopian visions of a pretended future reality—imagined futures—are an impetus for innovative activity."[33] But what about dystopian visions? What future technologies do they stimulate? We could argue that these positive narratives already incorporate the flip side of the coin: constructing a positive future scenario means simultaneously constructing a counterstrategy for a negative future scenario. But does this justify sweeping under the carpet these negative future scenarios and the fears they trigger? I do not think so. Focusing on these negative future scenarios and their impact on technological innovation and implementation not only widens our understanding of why certain technologies have come into being, but it also allows for an investigation of the narratives and worldviews interwoven in these technologies.[34] And last but not least, it enables a reconceptualization of modernity, which pays due credit to the role of fear and technology in shaping this era.

More and more scholars claim that fear is "the most pervasive emotion of modern society."[35] We read in numerous publications that in the context of the Cold War and 9/11, fear has become a central driving force in politics,[36] and that fear has colonized every single aspect of our lives, so that today we are living in an "age of fear."[37] Various culprits are blamed for this development. Secularization is a prominent candidate: with the loss of belief in divine forces came the fear of facing the unknown, or even worse, the fear of facing nothingness. Yuval Harari is currently spreading this argument across the globe in his popular book *Homo Deus*.[38] We also find the secularization thesis in more sophisticated work, like Lars Koch's introduction to his interdisciplinary *Handbook on Fear*.[39] Another candidate is mass media, enabling large-scale "fear communication," along with consumer society, which relies on fear for creating demand. Relating to the role of fear in modern capitalism, Schumpeter conceptualized the role of fear in entrepreneurial action already more than a century ago.[40] Considering the prominent role of fear in the theorization of modernity, it is remarkable that recent historiographic works on fear are criticized for lacking theoretical engagement,[41] and that historians researching fear have to lobby for more comparative works.[42] Even more remarkable is the fact that in theoretical contemplations on modernity, technology and fear are not brought together in a structural way. A historical investigation into the interrelationship of fear and technology within the time span labeled "modernity" is thus a crucial lacuna of modernization theory. Filling this gap might challenge basic assumptions about this era. For Koselleck—a major reference for historians when it comes to localizing the *Sattelzeit*, thus the passage from premodern society to modern society—apocalyptic thinking is a key characteristic of premodern times. But what if we find, while investigating fears as drivers of technology development in 19th and 20th century Western Europe, that modern technologies are coagulated fears of apocalyptic thinking? According to Koselleck, modernity is fueled by the "expectation that scientific inventions and discoveries will bring about a new world. Science and technology have stabilized progress as the time difference between experience and expectation."[43] What if this "new world" was mainly imagined and narrated as a negative future, a future that needed to be prevented by science and technology? What if these "modern" future expectations were not mainly positive (as the concept of "sociotechnical imaginaries" and mainstream innovation studies literature suggest), but fearful?

Conclusion: What Would We Gain from Researching Technology by Fear?

So far, research into fear and technology has been driven by efforts to overcome challenges in technology implementation, not by the desire to understand where the urge to implement certain technologies originated. This needs to change. Without a deeper historical understanding of the processes that stir technology developments, we run the risk of leaving the popular concept of "technological fixes" unchallenged. In recent decades, resorting to technological fixes has become commonplace in international policymaking in the area of grand societal challenges. We expect technology to come up with solutions for the problems humanity and its environment are facing. Politics has to settle for second row. At least that is what believers in the concept of technological fixes claim—and their voices dominate the current research and development (R&D) discourse. For certain industries, technology acceptance is no longer just a matter of economic interest. The issue has quickly escalated. Today, not accepting a certain technology is quickly construed as putting the very existence of humankind at risk: How can we feed the world without genetically modified crops? How can we guarantee safety for our society without surveillance cameras? A person who refuses to embrace new technology is therefore no longer only considered in marketing terms as a late adopter, but is associated with a certain political conviction. Meanwhile, technology R&D has become depoliticized on a broader societal level through the master narrative of technological fixes. To appreciate these changing dynamics of politicization and depoliticization of, on the one hand, technology R&D and implementation and, on the other hand, technology adaptation, acceptance, nonacceptance, and resistance, we need to better understand why certain technologies emerged. This approach also allows us to critically question the very concept of technological fixes and brings the politics of technology R&D back into play.

NOTES

At the time of writing, Dr. Kalmbach was an assistant professor at Eindhoven University of Technology, Netherlands.

1. Karena Kalmbach et al., "Crises and Technological Futures: Experiences, Emotion, and Action," *Technology and Culture* 61, no. 1, (January 2020): 272–281.

2. Karena Kalmbach et al., "Crises and Technological Futures," 276.

3. The working group consisted of Karena Kalmbach (history), Andreas Spahn (philosophy), and Ginevra Sanvitale (cultural anthropology). The working group investigated how promot-

ing new technologies has appealed to fears, thus focusing on the role of fear in pro-technology discourses.

4. I presented this conceptualization at the following forums: Interdisziplinäres Zentrum für Wissenschafts- und Technikforschung, Bergische Universität Wuppertal, November 2016 (invited speaker); Conference: Angst! Zeithistorische Konjunkturen eines gesellschaftlichen Phänomens, Zentrum für Zeithistorische Forschung Potsdam, February 2017 (keynote); Society for the History of Technology, Annual Meeting October 2017 (panel convener); Gesellschaft für Technikgeschichte, Annual Conference May 2018 (panel convener); and Conference: The Multifaceted Relationship of Fear and Technology, Max-Planck-Institute for Human Development, October 2018 (conference co-convener). For individual discussions on specific dimensions of fear–technology interconnections, I am grateful to Christian Götter (Fear *for* Technology), Bettina Hitzer (Technology *against* Fear) and Mikael Hård (Fear *by* Technology).

5. For a discussion on the ethical responsibilities of individual scientists, see Raphael Sassower, *Technoscientific Angst: Ethics and responsibility* (Minneapolis: University of Minnesota Press, 1997).

6. Robert Jungk, *Der Atomstaat: Vom Fortschritt in die Unmenschlichkeit* (Reinbek: Kindler, 1977).

7. On the biopolitics of resilience, see Eva Horn, "Die Enden des Menschen: Globale Katastrophen als biopolitische Phantasie," in *Apokalypse und Utopie in der Moderne*, eds. Reto Sorg and Stefan Bodo Würffel (Paderborn: Wilhelm Fink, 2010), 101–118; Ulrich Bröckling, *Gute Hirten führen sanft: Über Menschenregierungskünste* (Berlin: Suhrkamp, 2017); and Orit Halpern, "Hopeful Resilience," *E-flux Accumulation*, April 2017, https://www.e-flux.com/architecture/accumulation/96421/hopeful-resilience/.

8. Søren Kierkegaard, *Der Begriff Angst* (Hamburg: Europäische Verlagsanstalt, 1844, 2002).

9. For earlier debates on global population growth, see Marc Frey, "Experten, Stiftungen und Politik: Zur Genese des globalen Diskurses über Bevölkerung seit 1945," *Zeithistorische Forschungen* 4, no. 3 (September 2007): 137–159.

10. Spencer Weart, *Nuclear Fear: A History of Images* (Cambridge: Harvard University Press, 1988).

11. Wolfgang Schievelbusch, *Geschichte der Eisenbahnreise: Zur Industrialisierung von Raum und Zeit im 19. Jahrhundert* (München: Carl Hanser, 1977).

12. Karena Kalmbach, *Meanings of a Disaster: Chernobyl and Its Afterlives in Britain and France* (New York/Oxford: Berghahn, 2020); and Karena Kalmbach, "Revisiting the Nuclear Age: State of the Art Research in Nuclear History," *Neue Politische Literatur* 62, no. 1 (May 2017): 49–69.

13. Edward Palmer Thompson, *The Making of the English Working Class* (London: Victor Gollancz, 1963); and Eric Hobsbawm, *Labouring Men: Studies in the History of Labour* (London: Weidenfeld & Nicolson, 1964).

14. Kirkpatrick Sale, *Rebels Against the Future. The Luddites and Their War on the Industrial Revolution: Lessons for the Computer Age* (New York: Perseus, 1995); Steven Jones, *Against Technology: From the Luddites to Neo-Luddism* (Oxfordshire: Taylor & Francis, 2006); and Richard Conniff, "What the Luddites Really Fought Against," *Smithsonian Magazine*, March 2011, https://www.smithsonianmag.com/history/what-the-luddites-really-fought-against-264412/?no-ist=&page=2.

15. Martina Heßler, "Angst vor Technik und das Kontingentwerden 'des Menschen'," in *Ermöglichen und Verhindern: Vom Umgang mit Kontingenz*, eds. Markus Bernhardt, Stefan Brakensiek, Benjamin Scheller (Frankfurt: Campus, 2016).

16. The major research groups are based at the Max Planck Institute for Human Development, Berlin ("History of Emotions," Max Planck Institute for Human Development, https://www.mpib-berlin.mpg.de/en/research/history-of-emotions), Queen Mary University of London

("Welcome," Centre for the History of the Emotions, https://projects.history.qmul.ac.uk /emotions/), and the Australian Research Council Centre of Excellence for the History of Emotions. For an overview of the field, see Birgit Aschmann, "Heterogene Gefühle: Beiträge zur Geschichte der Emotionen," *Neue Politische Literatur* 61, no. 2 (July 2016): 225–249; Jan Plamper, *The History of Emotions* (Oxford: University Press, 2015); Ute Frevert, *Emotions in History— Lost and Found* (Budapest: Central European University Press, 2011); Ute Frevert, et al., *Emotional Lexicons: Continuity and Change in the Vocabulary of Feeling 1700–2000* (Oxford: University Press, 2014); and Bettina Hitzer, "Emotionsgeschichte—ein Anfang mit Folgen," *H/Soz/Kult*, November 23, 2011, www.hsozkult.de/literaturereview/id/forschungsberichte-1221. *Emotionology* (Peter Stearns and Carol Stearns, "Emotionology: Clarifying the History of Emotions and Emotional Standards," *The American Historical Review* 90, no. 4 [October 1985]: 813–836), *Emotional Community* (Barbara Rosenwein, *Emotional Communities in the Early Middle Ages* [Ithaca: Cornell University Press, 2006], and *Emotional Regime* (William Reddy, *The Navigation of Feeling: A Framework for the History of Emotions* [Cambridge: University Press, 2001]) have become the key analytic concepts in History of Emotions. History is, however, not the only discipline to develop a strong interest in emotions. The "emotional turn" also occurred in philosophy (Martha Nussbaum, *Upheavals of Thought: The Intelligence of Emotions* [Cambridge: University Press, 2003], Sabine Roeser, *Moral Emotions and Intuitions* [London: Palgrave Macmillan, 2011], Sabine Roeser and Cain Todd, eds., *Emotion and Value* [Oxford: University Press, 2014]), as well as in the Social Sciences, which coined the term "affect" (Melissa Gregg and Gregory Seigworth, *The Affect Theory Reader* [Durham: Duke University Press, 2010]).

17. See the conference program: "Program," History of Emotion: 2018 Conference at George Mason University, https://emotionshistory.wordpress.com/about/.

18. Karena Kalmbach et al., "Crises and Technological Futures," 277.

19. Michael Laffan and Max Weiss, eds., *Facing Fear: The History of an Emotion in Global Perspective* (Princeton: University Press, 2012); Susanne Michl and Jan Plamper, "Soldatische Angst im Ersten Weltkrieg: Die Karriere eines Gefühls in der Kriegspsychatrie Deutschlands, Frankreichs und Russlands," *Geschichte und Gesellschaft* 35, no. 2 (November 2009): 209–248; Peter Stearns, *American Fear: The Causes and Consequences of High Anxiety* (Oxfordshire: Routledge, 2006); and Johanna Bourke, *Fear: A Cultural History* (London: Virago Press, 2005); Jean Delumeau, *La Peur en Occident (XIVᵉ au XVIIIᵉ siècle)* (Paris: Fayard, 1978).

20. Jan Plamper and Benjamin Lazier, eds., *Fear: Across the Disciplines* (Pittsburgh: University of Pittsburgh Press, 2012).

21. Lars Koch, ed., *Angst: Ein interdisziplinäres Handbuch* (Heidelberg: J. B. Metzler, 2013).

22. Bernd Rusinek, "Atomkraft," in *Angst: Ein interdisziplinäres Handbuch*, ed. Lars Koch (Heidelberg: J. B. Metzler, 2013), 331–341.

23. It is no coincidence that historical research on risk and uncertainty is particularly strong in the German-speaking research community. First, some of the most prominent social scientists conceptualizing risk and uncertainty originate from this context: Ulrich Beck, Niklas Luhmann, Wolfgang Bonß, and Helga Nowotny (Ulrich Beck, *Risikogesellschaft: Auf dem Weg in eine andere Moderne* [Berlin: Suhrkamp, 1986], Ulrich Beck, *Weltrisikogesellschaft: Auf der Suche nach der verlorenen Sicherheit* [Berlin: Suhrkamp, 2008], Niklas Luhmann, *Soziologie des Risikos* [Berlin: De Gruyter, 1991], Wolfgang Bonß, *Vom Risiko: Unsicherheit und Ungewissheit in der Moderne* [Hamburg: Hamburger Edition, 1995], Adalbert Evers and Helga Nowotny, *Über den Umgang mit Unsicherheit: Die Entdeckung der Gestaltbarkeit von Gesellschaft* [Berlin: Suhrkamp, 1987]); and historians have just started to historicize their main assumptions (Rüdiger Graf and Kim Christian Priemel, "Zeitgeschichte in der Welt der Sozialwissenschaften: Legitimität und Originalität einer Disziplin," *Vierteljahreshefte für Zeitgeschichte* 59, no. 4 [October 2011]: 479–508, and Soraya Boudia and Nathalie Jas, "Risk and 'Risk Society' in Historical Perspective," *History and Technology* 23, no. 4 [December 2007]). Second, Lutz Raphael's and Anselm

Doering-Manteuffel's highly influential research program, "After the Boom" (Anselm Doering-Manteuffel, "Nach dem Boom: Brüche und Kontinuitäten der Industriemoderne seit 1970," *Vierteljahreshefte für Zeitgeschichte* 55, no. 4 [October 2007]: 559–581, Anselm Doering-Manteuffel and Lutz Raphael, *Nach dem Boom: Perspektiven auf die Zeitgeschichte seit 1970* [Göttingen: Vandenhoeck & Ruprecht, 2009])—which conceptualized the 1970s and 1980 as the era when (post–World War II) hopes for future prosperity were replaced by disenchantment with the promises of modern progress—inspired many German historians to place the topics of risk, prevention, uncertainty, and contingency in a *longue durée* perspective.

24. Nicolai Hanning, *Kalkulierte Gefahren: Naturkatastrophen und Vorsorge seit 1800* (Göttingen: Wallstein, 2019); and Peter Itzen and Simone Müller, eds., "Risk as an Analytical Category: Selected Studies in the Social History of the Twentieth Century," *Historical Social Research* 41, no. 1 (2016).

25. Christoph Wehner, *Die Versicherung der Atomgefahr: Risikopolitik, Sicherheitsproduktion und Expertise in der Bundesrepublik Deutschland und den USA 1945–1986* (Göttingen: Wallstein, 2017); and Cornel Zwierlein, "Sicherheit und Epochengrenzen," *Geschichte und Gesellschaft* 38, no. 3 (September 2012).

26. Reinhart Koselleck, *Vergangene Zukunft: Zur Semantik geschichtlicher Zeiten* (Berlin: Suhrkamp, 1979).

27. Karena Kalmbach et al., "Crises and Technological Futures," 273.

28. Lucian Hölscher, *Die Entdeckung der Zukunft* (Frankfurt am Main: Fischer, 1999).

29. Lucian Hölscher, ed., *Die Zukunft des 20. Jahrhunderts: Dimensionen einer historischen Zukunftsforschung* (Frankfurt/New York: Campus, 2017); Joachim Radkau, *Geschichte der Zukunft: Prognosen, Visionen, Irrungen in Deutschland von 1945 bis heute* (München: Carl Hanser, 2017).

30. Elke Seefried, *Zukünfte: Aufstieg und Krise der Zukunftsforschung 1945–1980* (München: De Gruyter Oldenbourg, 2015).

31. Sheila Jasanoff and Sang-Hyun Kim, "Containing the Atom: Sociotechnical Imaginaries and Nuclear Power in the United States and South Korea," *Minerva* 47, no. 2 (June 2009): 119–146; and Sheila Jasanoff and Sang-Hyun Kim, eds. *Dreamscapes of Modernity: Sociotechnical Imaginaries and the Fabrication of Power* (Chicago: University of Chicago Press, 2015).

32. Ingo Schulz-Schaeffer, "Scenarios as Patterns of Orientation in Technology Development and Technology Assessment," *Science, Technology & Innovation Studies* 9, no. 1 (September 2013): 23–44; Harro van Lente, "Promising Technology: The Dynamics of Expectations in Technological Development" (PhD diss., University of Twente, 1993); and Harro van Lente and Arie Rip, "The Rise of Membrane Technology: From Rhetorics to Social Reality," *Social Studies of Science* 28, no. 2 (April 1998): 221–254.

33. Jens Beckert, *Imagined Futures: Fictional Expectations and Capitalist Dynamics* (Cambridge: Harvard University Press, 2016), 169.

34. Karena Kalmbach et al., "Crises and Technological Futures," 274.

35. Johanna Bourke, *Fear: A Cultural History* (London: Virago Press, 2005), 1.

36. Douglas Walton, *Scare Tactics* (Berlin: Springer-Science, 2010); Bernd Greiner, Christian Müller, Dierk Walter, eds., *Angst im Kalten Krieg* (Hamburg: Hamburger Edition, 2009); Patrick Bormann, Thomas Freiberger, Judith Michel, eds., *Angst in den internationalen Beziehungen* (Göttingen: Vandenhoeck & Ruprecht, 2010); Veith Selk, "Neue Beiträge zur Politik der Angst im Zeitalter des War on Terror," *Neue Politische Literatur* 57, no. 2 (January 2012): 267–291; Veith Selk, *Das Regieren der Angst: Eine politische Ideengeschichte von der Tyrannis bis zum Leviathan* (Hannover: Wehrhahn, 2016); and Corey Robin, *Fear: The History of a Political Idea* (Oxford: University Press, 2004).

37. Heinz Bude, *Gesellschaft der Angst* (Hamburg: Hamburger Edition, 2014); Zygmunt Bauman, *Liquid Fear* (Cambridge: Polity, 2006); Frank Furedi, *Culture of Fear Revisited:*

Risk-Taking and the Morality of Low Expectation (London: Continuum, 2006); Peter Stearns, *American Fear: The Causes and Consequences of High Anxiety* (Oxfordshire: Routledge, 2006); Christophe Lambert, *La société de la peur* (Paris: Plon, 2005); Renata Salecl, *On Anxiety* (Oxfordshire: Routledge, 2004); and Brian Massumi, ed., *The Politics of Everyday Fear* (Minneapolis: University of Minnesota Press, 1993).

38. Yuval Harari, *Homo Deus: A Brief History of Tomorrow* (London: Harvill Secker, 2016).

39. Lars Koch, ed., *Angst: Ein interdisziplinäres Handbuch* (Heidelberg: J. B. Metzler, 2013); for a strong critique of this argument, see Birgit Aschmann, "Heterogene Gefühle: Beiträge zur Geschichte der Emotionen," *Neue Politische Literatur* 61, no. 2 (July 2016): 225–249.

40. Joseph Schumpeter, *Theorie der wirtschaftlichen Entwicklung* (Berlin: Duncker & Humblot, 1912).

41. Lars Koch, "Sammelrezension Angst—globale und interdisziplinäre Perspektiven," review of *Facing Fear: The History of an Emotion in Global Perspective*, by Michael Laffan and Max Weiss, *H/Soz/Kult,* April 7, 2014, http://hsozkult.geschichte.hu-berlin.de/index.asp?id=20135&view=pdf&pn=rezensionen&type=rezbuecher.

42. Peter Stearns, "Fear and History," *Historein* 8 (May 2009): 17–28.

43. Reinhart Koselleck, *Vergangene Zukunft: Zur Semantik geschichtlicher Zeiten* (Berlin: Suhrkamp, 1979), 374, translation by the author.

CHAPTER EIGHTEEN

Fear and Freedom in Technology

On Prometheus as an Ambiguous Figure of Technology in Philosophy

CHRISTINE BLAETTLER

Since the modern age, and increasingly since the late 18th century, countless reformulations of the myth of Prometheus have again and again served for imagining the hopes and fears, desires and anxieties toward a historical dynamic objectified in technology.

Cultural history still likes to refer to Prometheus. The character of Prometheus is used to illustrate processes of humans trying to shape the world, to appropriate it and to make their stand in it; that is, they create culture while they themselves are being shaped by it. In the forefront of these cultural achievements is human creativity, unfolding both through the arts and through technology. Referring positively to Prometheus as a cultural hero provides him with an emancipatory moment and a time vector pointing at a future that is to be created and is considered better. On the other hand, negative references to Prometheus have been dominating the modern critique of technology up to the present and renders Prometheus into a paradigm of fear in imagining modern technology. This critique starts out from the observation that although modern technology is man-made, it has become independent and now is turning against humans.

The figure of the Titan Prometheus from ancient Greek mythology has been associated with the idea of an ambivalent founder of culture. The story goes that Prometheus, whose name means the forward-thinking one, stole fire from the gods and brought it to the weakly endowed humans, thus enabling them to handle fire and teaching them cultural techniques. Decisive for the history of impact is, on the one hand, that already in European antiquity there are several strikingly different versions of the Prometheus myth, with especially influential ones by Hesiod, Aeschylus, and Plato. Equally relevant, on the other hand, is that all versions express an inner problematic that links human culture and civilization to Prometheus's sacrilege against the gods. In addition to the type of the tragic hero, which finds its continuation in the formula of a "tragedy of culture," a contrasting evaluation of the figure is particularly striking. Whereas Prometheus is still seen as the epitome of a hero creating himself, his works, and his environment in the versions that grasp him as a creator and liberator of humans, he is also stigmatized as a great sinner against the existing (divine) order. He serves his just punishment, in which he is forged to the Caucasus for thirty-thousand years and an eagle daily eats his liver, which grows back each night. In all versions, the field of technology occupies a prominent place and allows us to realize a change in the understanding of technology in the respective Prometheus figuration. The different versions as well as their inherent problems are opposed to any self-evident and unambiguous acceptance of this myth and make it a task to examine it in its historically specific context and regarding its respective function. Thus, the investigation starts from (1) today's appearance of the Prometheus figure in visualizing technology; (2) analyzing two specific strands of tradition in imagining the ambiguous power of technology; and (3) undertaking a rereading of Hans Blumenberg's philosophical enterprise of a "work on myth," which is focused on the Prometheus mythologem with regard to its relevance in thinking about technology today.

Technology and Prometheus Today
Promethean Culture

With this book title, a recent volume of cultural studies on the Prometheus myth explores the question of energy. On the one hand, the contributions deal with stages in the history of the impact of the Prometheus figure on the arts. On the other, they refer to Promethean culture as a metaphor for a human culture based on production in the broadest sense.[1] The introductory contribution by Hartmut Böhme looks at the ancient foundations of the myth of Prometheus, which are also briefly recalled here, and it lays out tracks of the history of its impact. Through this myth, Böhme examines the question of the emergence of culture and touches on anthropological, cognitive, technical, and socio-ethical "foundations."[2] If *physis* in

Greek stands for nature, something that is there by itself and maintains itself, culture marks something that only comes into being through intervention. The area of culture is marked in Greek with the word *techne*,
which in turn is translated with artistry, practical ability, and professional
knowledge. Culture is to be understood here as contingent in the sense
that the dynamics it denotes do not necessarily proceed like laws of nature
but are equally not impossible. Even if cultural practices and products are
improbable, they are still possible and can be examined for their conditions and effects.

In Hesiod, the titanic Prometheus tries to outwit the Olympian father-god
Zeus in the service of sacrifice for the benefit of humankind and proves to be
philanthropos, philanthropist, also here, not only in the creation of man and
his animation by fire. Zeus does not punish the Titan with the sacrifice fraud
but the human race, which is henceforth compelled to work for its survival,
or as Böhme writes: "Humans do not live in an energetic equilibrium with a
nourishing nature, but they must raise energy"[3] and invest in (agriculture) work.
Thereby they were deprived of the "energetically most vital element fire,"[4] so
they could not cook and had to eat raw food. Until Prometheus's (second) fire
theft (for which he himself was punished with chains and torture, and the
people were punished with the evils of Pandora's box), fire belonged to the gods.
If one follows the distinction of Claude Lévi-Strauss, according to which the
cooked marks the transition to culture, the human race is at this time still in
the "state of nature." The appropriation of fire thus offers itself as a distinguishing feature between man and animal. Böhme speaks in this respect ten-
tatively of "anthropological distinction,"[5] without which there would have been
no cultural development "at least for 500,000 years." He clearly emphasizes the
problem that in this narrative the emergence of culture is linked to transgres-
sion and the breaking of taboos and is staged in a "break with nature,"[6] as can
still be seen in Freud's concept of culture as a sublimation achievement. This
problematic makes culture appear as hopeless toil and punishment compared
to a paradisiacal prehistory. In all its versions, the narrative of the emergence
of culture made via the Prometheus mythologem is technical in several respects: On the one hand, it connects technology with the breaking of taboos
and, to a certain extent, "alienation"; on the other, it connects just as much
with self-assertion and self-empowerment. Both aspects can be found in the
history of its effects up to the present day, and they are specifically virulent in
the current debate about a modern Prometheanism. This will be shown by
two examples.

Cosmotechnics

In his book *The Question of Technology in China*, Yuk Hui starts from the following hypothesis: It is true that technology is an anthropological and world-wide phenomenon; however, the concept of technology that accompanies practices and products is exclusively European and does not exist in this way in other cultures, at least in the Chinese tradition of thought. For Hui, technology is an "ontological category" that must, therefore, be considered within the larger cosmological context of a given culture.[7] Before he sets out to find a specifically Chinese concept of technology, that is, technology as a philosophical object, he turns to the European concept of technology. He considers this to be instrumental, characterized by dual categories such as subject-object and human-world-god-world, as well as decisively determined by Greek philosophy. He turns to the myth of Prometheus via Plato's version,[8] and one chapter of Hui's book is titled "The Becoming of Prometheus." Against a universal understanding of becoming man and technology based on this Greek myth, he cites Chinese mythology. This mythology presents a different "origin" for technology, which is not based on the separation of divine and human world, because the divine is presented naturalistically.[9] By "cosmotechnics," Hui aims to unify cosmic and moral order through technical activities, referencing ritual practices in the case of the Chinese tradition of thought. In this way, Hui wants to develop a specifically Chinese understanding of technology that is in harmony with nature and morality and can serve to "overcome modernity."[10] For Hui, this modernity is determined by a direct and extensive reference to Heidegger, on the one hand, and characterized by the global domination of a European understanding of technology on the other. For Hui, Prometheus and a Prometheanism based on it with a universal claim stand for this. With his Chinese cosmotechnology, Hui wants to counter this with a postcolonial, more social and ecological alternative.

Acceleration

In the recent theoretical strand of accelerationism, the figure of Prometheus is programmatically taken up in a "*Promethean* approach." This wants to bring rationality into connection with "concrete historical, economic and biological developments." At the same time, it turns "against various cardinal virtues of a cozy and self-satisfied left,"—namely, "the fetishization of grassroots democratic processes and the associated nostalgia for authenticity."[11] Here, the figure of Prometheus is brought into conversation anew by Alberto Toscano and Ray Brassier. Against the widespread blanket identification of human self-idolatry and hubris with "Promethean activism,"[12] Toscano recalls Marx's Prometheus: this figure was the "most distinguished saint and martyr in the philosophical calendar," whose "confession"[13] for "human self-consciousness" against "all heavenly and earthly gods" Marx made a philosophical creed in the preface to his dissertation. Toscano, with Marx, reads the Promethean act first and foremost as an "emblem" of revolt against the infinite supremacy of an authority that considers the unconditional claim to human emancipation to be sin.[14] While those who despise Prometheus follow this authority, Toscano points out that "Prometheus is the bearer of the open question of how we, creatures that draw their breath in gasps, can manage not to be subject to the violent prerogatives of sovereignty."[15] This thrust, also with recourse to Marx, is also pursued by Ray Brassier, who, against what he calls the "right-wing Prometheanism" of neoliberal optimization projects in capitalist competition, pleads for a kind of left-wing Prometheanism: "Prometheanism is the attempt to participate in the creation of the world without having to defer to a divine blueprint."[16] Brassier as well as Toscano take up the figure of Prometheus in order to intervene in a current field of discourse, which in turn is grounded in a certain tradition of the mythologem of Prometheus.

The Ambiguous Power of Technology

German-language philosophy of the 20th century, concerned with the figure of Prometheus in several vogues, articulates a connection of technology and myth in different directions,[17] which can be regarded as decisive for today's discussion of technology in relation to anxiety culture. Then as now, the question of a power of technology is up for debate. Is there an instrumental understanding insofar as humans invent technology, make use of it, and thereby increase their effective powers? This view is part of a European philosophical tradition dating back to antiquity, which makes technology a topic primarily through a relationship of means and purpose and is reinforced by the romantic pathos of a creative subject in the arts and in industry. Since around 1800, the power of technology also has been attributed to technology itself. Thus, technology is imagined as something that is created by humans but has become independent and now exercises power over humans. Two historical examples that visualize the two sides via the figure of Prometheus are given by Goethe's poem *Prometheus* on the one hand and Mary Shelley's novel *Frankenstein, Or the Modern Prometheus*, on the other. The German phrase "*Macht der Technik*" is ambiguous depending on whether one reads it with *genitivus subjectivus* or *objectivus*.[18] If one considers the inherent dynamics of emergence and effect in technology, this linguistic ambiguity does make sense. The formulation alone, however, leaves open whether power is to be understood in the sense of new possibilities or violence, which can only be inferred from the respective context.

In postwar West Germany, philosophical criticism of technology was sparked by the invention and use of the atomic bomb as well as by the increasing mechanization of industrialized society. On the one hand, this criticism of technology was directed against a technocratic paradigm of feasibility, which did not realize how it was technology that determined people. On the other, this criticism goes hand in hand with a negative evaluation that declares human self-empowerment in modernity to be presumptuous and sees the punishment of the modern subject as a logical consequence. The figure of Prometheus lent itself to both approaches. This becomes most apparent in the works of Günther Anders, whose writings critical of technology are once again finding a lively reception today. For him, Prometheus serves to illustrate the tragic character of the human–technology relationship. First of all, in contrast to the tool as a means, he now states a separation of man and his products and names this with "Promethean gradient."[19] Although the Promethean human being sees its pride in "owing everything, even itself, exclusively to itself," in fact it has not only lost control over the objects it has produced, but it can no longer keep up with their own dynamics in any way.[20] Here, technology is no longer understood as a means for free human objectives, but as a system or "*macro-device*,"[21] which makes "*the* preliminary decision." This is a decision that is made "*before*" people "get to act." This decision makes technology an "*epochal*"[22] "destiny" that encompasses all continents, political systems, and ideologies. Anders focuses his critique on the "peculiar destiny of Prometheanism."[23] In 1956, he writes that "in the last 175 years (from Goethe to Shelley to Ibsen to Sartre's 'Mouches')" everyone, "our fathers and even we ourselves," have imagined themselves with Prometheus "allegorically"; this concerns both the mockery and the "presumptuous claims" and the "mangling."[24] Via Prometheus, human creative power could be imagined as a defiant as well as a proud attitude toward the world, as Anders notes not only with regard to the *self-made man*.[25] But the "Prometheus of today," according to Anders, has become a "court dwarf of his own machinery"[26] who is "no longer equal to his products"[27] and feels inferior to them and is ashamed. From the high and effective quality of self-made things, Anders diagnoses a "Promethean shame" of the human being, who had once started out with Promethean defiance and pride.[28] Anders refers to the fate and tragedy of the ancient myth. At the same time, he reflects on the literary representation of the problem with technology and correlates the transmission of the myth with his rhetoric of exaggeration. Nevertheless, this understanding of technology remains heroic and tragic and is oriented toward the possible extinction of the human species through *human engineering* and the atomic bomb. Here, technology remains a means to an end, even in its turn against those who produced it.

While Anders identifies a tragic trait of technology with the help of Prometheus, Friedrich Georg Jünger identifies technology on the one hand as the epitome of human hubris, and on the other as a fateful doom, as hostile to human beings as it is to life. Technical intervention in an existing fixed order is denounced, and the "striking back" of a technology that has taken on a life of its own is taken as a signal to turn back and return, or even considered as a punishment. In the last chapter, *The Perfection of Technology* illustrates F. G. Jünger's conception of technology through a particular turn of the Prometheus myth.[29] The author identifies the fall of Prometheus not in the theft of fire, but in the sacrificial fraud. It is this sacrilege against the old divine order that marks the beginning of the history of the decay of the human being, now called Promethean. The human being has enthroned itself as Lord instead of God and is made a "victim" by the perfect Promethean technology of modernity. Here, no reflection on a contemporary problematic situation takes place via the myth. Instead, the myth is reduced and evoked as existential, Prometheus is stylized as an archaic proto-technician, and hostility to technology is paired with closeness to nature.[30] Together with Martin Heidegger's 1949 Bremen Lectures devoted to the question of technology, F. G. Jünger's book had a lasting effect in post–World War II West Germany. Both are still positively received today, especially in academic ecological discourse, further reinforced by anthropogenic climate change and the concept of the Anthropocene. Heidegger and F. G. Jünger were in continuous exchange and agreed on the conception of modern technology as an autonomous agency, which was bottomless, nihilistic, and totalitarian in its predatory exploitation of human beings and nature. They also agreed in correlating such a demonized technology with the industrial and bureaucratic killing in the Holocaust and in conducting a discourse of apology about technology; this kind of critique of technology thus proves to be "exculpative."[31] Technology, demonized into an abstract power and a large subject, thus becomes the systematic point of application of a fundamental critique of modernity, which laments the "disenchantment of the world" through rationalization, economization, and mechanization as a one-sided decline. In addition to science, technology, which is materially more manifest, becomes the prominent subject area to which the suspicion of the illegitimacy of modern times is attached. In this suspicion, Prometheus is also assigned his place.[32]

This critique of technology appeared at the same time as cybernetics. Computer-based automatic control technology was developed during World War II, and it is not surprising that the aforementioned critique of technology is of great interest today. Technology is addressed in its autonomy and its inherent power, and the question is raised as to whether technology determines human beings. In the age of digital technologies, people are confronted with a technological eigen momentum that configures their experiences of power and powerlessness in a specifically historical way. Neither a liberalist concept nor the complete suspension of subjective agency can adequately account for these experiences on a theoretical level. Theoretical deployments that decenter the position of the human being attempt to reflect critically on the changed conditions, for example, via genealogical and archaeological procedures following Nietzsche and Foucault. Others, conversely, try to take this decentering as evidence for a technological a priori. Provided with normative weight, this decentering is also defended in large parts in the debate on the Anthropocene as a counterstrategy to human hubris.[33] In this way, humanism becomes a negatively valued cipher of human domination, culminating in technically assumed godlikeness and the new religion of "*dataism.*"[34] However, this decentering of the human being is also referred to with utopian intentions to suggest human-technical ensembles;[35] indeed, an antecedent technology is welcomed within the framework of a critique of anthropocentrism.

The figure of Prometheus recurs even in times of computer simulation and serves to mark a categorical difference to the age of creative design, exemplified by Goethe's ode on Prometheus. "Even conceivably simple algorithms" deliver, in contrast to the linguistic codes of modern art, "results beyond all conceivability," and it is precisely in this that Friedrich Kittler sees the "concept of a Promethean or poetic creative power itself disappearing."[36] So-called randomly generated data create new images, which are unprecedented and unpredictable, and create a new order in the sense of an order from noise, and precisely in this way attempt to make the "unpredictable predictable."[37] In the "pure syntax of commands or algorithms" new things are indeed generated that were never there before. But Kittler aptly remarks that "master discourses and chains of command" would by no means, and certainly not for all time, have been abolished by Prometheus rebelling against Zeus.[38] They would only have changed sides, because now they originate from technology itself. The medial, even war-technological a priori, does not only concede technology a status prior to humans but drives it on and before itself, turns it into agents of technology, and thus unhinges a concept of autonomously acting individuals. In this sense, this techno-subject is still to be understood as a shadow of God, as Kittler suggests by now calling humans "subjects of a dead God."[39] Kittler describes the resounding power of validity of digital technology and thus rejects a strong notion of action of human subjects that operates via freedom. In contrast, the sayings of *dataism* or "technological totalitarianism"[40] address this power of technology as a danger and, unlike Kittler, lament the loss of human agency.

Work on Myth

For some, the Prometheus figure serves to mythically underpin and titanically exaggerate a doom of the modern human being manifested in technology. Blumenberg, on the other hand, turns it into a depotentiated "guiding fossil"[41] through which he theoretically reflects, historically traces, and himself carries out a "work on myth." In this bringing together of myth and technology, he practices an enlightenment enterprise that is neither self-evident, nor conclusive, nor immune to mythicizing reversals.

Blumenberg traces the mythologem of the origin of human culture in its various forms and evaluations through the various versions, their receptions and mediations, rewritings, and adaptations up to the present day. In doing so, he makes clear how conditional and inauthentic every access to this myth already is at the time of its creation: "To speak of beginnings is always suspicious of the mania for originality. To the beginning, to which converges what is spoken of here, nothing wants to return. Rather, everything measures itself at a distance from it."[42] Because for Blumenberg myth is neither supratemporal nor universal, it is also not the "material of the myth"[43] that is decisive, but "the distance of the listener and spectator granted to it." Thus, the Prometheus myth is by no means to be understood as archetypal, prescribing something once and for all, but as a mythologem that becomes visible through its formations.[44]

For Blumenberg, myth is a cultural form that people create through "artifices."[45] Especially in the case of the figures of the gods and the stories associated with them, it becomes apparent how attempts were made to name the nameless and to explain the incomprehensible. Blumenberg first points to the function of rationalizing anxiety into fear.[46] In this respect, myth is able to visualize fear. As soon as "the stories of the gods no longer frighten and no longer bind,"[47] Blumenberg discovers an "approach to the freedom of stories."[48] This opens up a poetic playing field that finds new sensibilities in *poiesis*, human making and creating, not only in poetry.[49] Its "lightness, its non-commitment and plasticity, its disposition for playability in the broadest sense"[50] virtually disposes the myth for "aesthetic reception" and further shaping. In contrast to a "sense content of ancient sagas"[51] asserted as timeless, Blumenberg is interested in "the interlocking of the formally opposing tendencies of constancy and variation, of binding and digression, of tradition and innovatory boldness." Significantly, he compares myth to the "theme of musical variations,"[52] which, even when "modified to the limit of unrecognizability," remains recognizable and thereby proves its specific "validity." Instead of asserting a real and true origin and wanting to restore it mythically, Blumenberg tries to read off the "respective state of history and concept of reality" from the individual forms.[53]

Why does Blumenberg focus on Prometheus as the guiding fossil in his work on myth? After all, it could have been another mythological figure, such as Odysseus in Max Horkheimer and Theodor W. Adorno's *Dialectic of Enlightenment*. In postwar Germany, however, as Christian Voller notes, it was Prometheus who became "the yardstick of the Enlightenment and thus of distance from both 'pure being' and the Third Reich."[54] In the German postwar period, Prometheus, "the hero of the Enlightenment and of the self-empowerment of the human species," "fell out of favor."[55] If a return to the mythical order in combination with immediate subordination is desired, all that remains of Prometheus is the sacrilegious "proto-technician" whose titanic power could only be broken by a god of Zeus's stature.[56] In contrast to such a depotentiation of Prometheus, Voller points to Blumenberg's depotentiation of a completely different kind, which downplays the Titan: "The Prometheus of comedy is 'only the little crook who steals the sacrificial flesh from the gods.'"[57] Blumenberg equally depotentiates the myth in formal terms: instead of asserting an archetypal grand narrative, Blumenberg's "sprawling studies" approach "the myth only by means of a never-ending chain of quotations (often enough quotations of quotations), allusions, and ironic refractions" "to remain fragments at last."[58] His "ironic pathos of inauthenticity"[59] virtually deconstructs the prevailing conception of myth, even though his approach, in contrast to dogmatic "fixedness,"[60] relies on the "variable scriptural unbundling"[61] of myth.

In contrast to the demonization of Prometheus on the part of conservative critics of modernity, who thereby demonize modern technology and want to conceptualize it directly from an original ancient myth, Blumenberg de-demonizes both Prometheus and modern technology. Against the suspicion of illegitimacy of modern science and technology, a genuine cultural–philosophical reflection on technology is formed in Blumenberg's work via various paths and detours. It is not about a specific justification of concrete technological phenomena and effects or a philosophical support of technocracy. Instead, an uneasiness in technology is registered and technology is considered in a broader and historical context of human culture. Blumenberg countered the fixation on Prometheus coming from the critique of technology in postwar Germany, with which he was very familiar, with his work on myth. Yet, he responded to it, so to speak, with his earlier project of an "intellectual history of technology," which he had pursued for decades. In this project, the figure of Prometheus plays no role, and this blank space is revealing in several respects. For example, Blumenberg almost ostentatiously does not refer to the proto-technician and the contemporary mythicization of a fateful power associated with it, and takes a different path instead. In contrast to the well-known anthropological topic of explaining technology from the human deficiency structure, he starts with the aspect that understands technology as a historical phenomenon. This aspect includes the anthropological aspect of a deficient being, but exceeds it insofar "as technology, from this point of view, does not consist in being an instrument of securing existence and elementary satisfaction of needs."[62] Blumenberg is concerned here with the fact that the human species "perceives its technicality and grasps it as the subject and signature not only of self-assertion, but also of its self-interpretation and self-realization."[63] Thereby no apology of modern technology is represented, but an objection against the suspicion of its illegitimacy is raised. This objection also concerns Heidegger's "Gestell" and his *Question About Technology*, which is widely and across many disciplines regarded as the first authority for philosophically addressing technology until today. Although Blumenberg's early project of an "intellectual history of technology" did not lead to a monograph and the later works do not fall under philosophy of technology in the narrow sense, technology manifests itself as a "life theme,"[64] which continued to shape his thought. A striking example of this is given by *Work on Myth* with Blumenberg's approach of a theory of myth and the history of the Prometheus mythologem full of windings and variants. This work deals with the discomfort and anxieties in the face of a power of technology. Technology is not demonized as something alien, but it is reflected upon in its medial formation and always considered in terms of possible margins and degrees of freedom.

NOTES

1. See Claus Leggewie, Ursula Renner, and Peter Risthaus, eds., *Prometheische Kultur. Wo kommen unsere Energien her?* (München: Wilhelm Fink, 2013); Peter Sloterdjik, *Die Reue des Prometheus. Von der Gabe des Feuers zur globalen Brandstiftung* (Berlin: Suhrkamp 2023); and Wolfgang Storch and Burghard Damerau, eds., *Mythos Prometheus. Texte von Hesiod bis René Char* (Leipzig: Reclam, 1995).

2. Hartmut Böhme, "Was ist und zu welchem Ende studieren wir die prometheische Kultur?," in *Prometheische Kultur. Wo kommen unsere Energien her?*, eds. Claus Leggewie, Ursula Renner, Peter Risthaus (München: Wilhelm Fink, 2013), 23.

3. Böhme, "Was ist und zu welchem Ende studieren wir die prometheische Kultur?," 26.

4. Böhme, "Was ist und zu welchem Ende studieren wir die prometheische Kultur?," 26.

5. Böhme, "Was ist und zu welchem Ende studieren wir die prometheische Kultur?," 26.

6. Böhme, "Was ist und zu welchem Ende studieren wir die prometheische Kultur?," 28.

7. Yuk Hui, *The Question Concerning Technology in China. An Essay in Cosmotechnics* (Falmouth: Urbanomic, 2016, 2018), 10.

8. See Hui, *Question Concerning Technology in China*, 12–13.

9. Hui, *Question Concerning Technology in China*, 17.

10. The formula "overcoming modernity" runs like a leitmotif through Hui's entire book. It comes from an essay published in 1942 by Keiji Nishitani, a major representative of the Kyôto School who studied with Heidegger in the 1930s and who, as a Japanese fascist, called for total war during World War II; see Hui, *Question Concerning Technology in China*, § 24, who distances himself from the fascist consequences of this enterprise to overcome modernity.

11. Armen Avanessian, "Einleitung," in *#Akzeleration*, ed. Armen Avanessian (Berlin: Merve, 2013), 9.

12. See also John S. Dryzek, *The Politics of the Earth. Environmental Discourses* (Oxford: University Press, 1997, 2012).

13. Karl Marx, "*Differenz der demokritischen und epikureischen Naturphilosophie*" (PhD diss., University of Jena, 1841), in Marx Engels Werke MEW, vol. 40 (Berlin: Dietz, 1968), 262–263.

14. Alberto Toscano, "A Plea for Prometheus," *Critical Horizons. A Journal of Philosophy and Social Theory* 10, no. 2 (August 2009): 254.

15. Toscano, "A Plea for Prometheus," 255.

16. Ray Brassier, "Prometheanism and its Critics," in *#Accelerate#. The Accelerationist Reader*, eds. Robin Mackay and Armen Avanessian (Falmouth/Berlin: Urbanomic, 2014), 485.

17. See primarily Christian Voller, "Wider die 'Mode heutiger Archaik:' Konzeptionen von Präsenz und Repräsentation im Mythosdiskurs der Nachkriegszeit," in *Zwischen Präsenz und Repräsentation. Formen und Funktionen des Mythos in theoretischen und literarischen Diskursen*, eds. Bent Gebert und Uwe Mayer (Berlin: De Gruyter, 2014).

18. See also Christoph Hubig, *Die Kunst des Möglichen III. Macht der Technik* (Bielefeld: Transcript, 2015), 7–11.

19. See Günther Anders, *Die Antiquiertheit des Menschen 1. Über die Seele im Zeitalter der zweiten industriellen Revolution* (München: C. H. Beck, 1956, 1994), 16–18.

20. Anders, *Die Antiquiertheit des Menschen 1*, 24.

21. Anders, *Die Antiquiertheit des Menschen 1*, 2.

22. Anders, *Die Antiquiertheit des Menschen 1,* 7.

23. Anders, *Die Antiquiertheit des Menschen 1,* 24.

24. Anders, *Die Antiquiertheit des Menschen 1,* 49.

25. See Anders, *Die Antiquiertheit des Menschen 1,* 24.

26. Anders, *Die Antiquiertheit des Menschen 1,* 25.

27. Anders, *Die Antiquiertheit des Menschen 1,* 45.

28. See Anders, *Die Antiquiertheit des Menschen 1,* 21–95.

29. See also F. G. Jünger, *Griechische Mythen,* ed. Ernst A. Schmidt (Frankfurt am Main: Klostermann, 1947, 2015), 78–101.

30. See Voller, "Wider die 'Mode heutiger Archaik.'"

31. See Daniel Morat, *Von der Tat zur Gelassenheit. Konservatives Denken bei Martin Heidegger, Ernst Jünger und Friedrich Georg Jünger 1920–1960* (Göttingen: Wallstein, 2007), 455–497.

32. Concerning Heidegger, see Christine Blättler, "Heideggers Technikbegriff und der verstellte Blick auf die Ökonomie," *Navigationen—Zeitschrift für Medien- und Kulturwissenschaften* 16, no. 2 (2016): 65–81. Bernard Stiegler builds substantially on Heidegger and for this, in addition to Prometheus, above all brings the figure of Epimetheus into play; see Bernard Stiegler, *La Technique et le Temps 1. La faute d'Épiméthée* (Paris: Galilée, 1994).

33. See Bernd Scherer and Jürgen Renn, eds., *Das Anthropozän. Zum Stand der Dinge* (Berlin: Matthes & Seitz, 2017).

34. See Yuval Harari, "On Big Data, Google, and the End of Free Will," *Financial Times,* August 26, 2016, https://www.ft.com/content/50bb4830-6a4c-11e6-ae5b-a7cc5dd5a28c.

35. See Bruno Latour, *Nous n'avons jamais été modernes. Essai d'anthropologie symétrique* (Paris: La Découverte, 1991); and Heidrun Allert, Michael Asmussen, and Christoph Richter, eds., *Digitalität und Selbst. Interdisziplinäre Perspektiven auf Subjektivierungs- und Bildungsprozesse* (Bielefeld: Transcript, 2017).

36. Friedrich Kittler, "Fiktion und Simulation," in *Aisthesis. Wahrnehmung heute oder Perspektiven einer anderen Ästhetik,* eds. Karlheinz Barck et al. (Leipzig: Reclam, 1992), 202–203.

37. Kittler, "Fiktion und Simulation," 206.

38. Kittler, "Fiktion und Simulation," 201, 199.

39. Kittler, "Fiktion und Simulation," 212.

40. See Frank Schirrmacher, ed., *Technologischer Totalitarismus. Eine Debatte* (Berlin: Suhrkamp, 2015).

41. Hans Blumenberg, "Wirklichkeitsbegriff und Wirkungspotential des Mythos," in *Ästhetische und metaphorologische Schriften,* ed. Anselm Haverkamp (Berlin: Suhrkamp, 1971, 2001), 348.

42. Hans Blumenberg, *Arbeit am Mythos* (Berlin: Suhrkamp, 1979, 2006), 28.

43. Blumenberg, "Wirklichkeitsbegriff und Wirkungspotential des Mythos," 335.

44. See Blumenberg, *Arbeit am Mythos,* 192.

45. Blumenberg, *Arbeit am Mythos,* 11.

46. Blumenberg, *Arbeit am Mythos,* 11.

47. Blumenberg, "Wirklichkeitsbegriff und Wirkungspotential des Mythos," 335.

48. Blumenberg, "Wirklichkeitsbegriff und Wirkungspotential des Mythos," 344.

49. See Blumenberg, *Arbeit am Mythos,* 68.

50. Blumenberg, "Wirklichkeitsbegriff und Wirkungspotential des Mythos," 335.

51. Blumenberg, "Wirklichkeitsbegriff und Wirkungspotential des Mythos," 348.

52. Blumenberg, "Wirklichkeitsbegriff und Wirkungspotential des Mythos," 341.

53. Voller, "Wider die 'Mode heutiger Archaik,'" 245.

54. Voller, "Wider die 'Mode heutiger Archaik,'" 251.

55. Voller, "Wider die 'Mode heutiger Archaik,'" 251.

56. Voller, "Wider die 'Mode heutiger Archaik,'" 240, 252.

57. Blumenberg, "Wirklichkeitsbegriff und Wirkungspotential des Mythos," 349.

58. Voller, "Wider die 'Mode heutiger Archaik,'" 255.

59. Voller, "Wider die 'Mode heutiger Archaik,'" 240.

60. Blumenberg, *Arbeit am Mythos*, 242.

61. Blumenberg, *Arbeit am Mythos*, 241.

62. Hans Blumenberg, "Ordnungsschwund und Selbstbehauptung. Über Weltverstehen und Weltverhalten im Werden der technischen Epoche," in *Schriften zur Technik*, eds. Alexander Schmitz and Bernd Stiegler (Berlin: Suhrkamp, 1960, 2015), 138.

63. Blumenberg, "Ordnungsschwund und Selbstbehauptung," 138.

64. Rüdiger Zill, "Von der Atommoral zum Zeitgewinn: Transformationen eines Lebensthemas. Hans Blumenbergs Projekt einer Geistesgeschichte der Technik," *Jahrbuch Technikphilosophie* (2017), 291.

CHAPTER NINETEEN

Technology Policy in Society 5.0

A Comparison of the Technological Innovation Strategies of Germany and Japan

MARKUS LEMMENS AND
IRIS WIECZOREK

Japan and Germany are as different as they are comparable. An insular industrial power on the one hand, a country in the heart of the European Union with nine borders to neighboring states on the other. Taking a comparative look at the strategic efforts of technology and innovation policies of Germany and Japan with regard to the "Anxiety Culture," both countries offer a frame for an exemplary discourse. Such a comparison shows how the dynamics of technological options and the feelings of uncertainty and fear among citizens might interact in modern societies and reveals how the two systems deal with it. The traditional approval of technology by Japanese society suffered a huge setback by the nuclear disaster of Fukushima in March 2011. And the shifting pro and con attitude toward technological progress in Germany, well known for the "German Angst," invites a closer look. The aim of this chapter is hence a reflection on the conceptual and strategic developments in the technology and innovation policies of Germany and Japan. We believe our analysis could help inform policy decisions about how to confront and get along with societal uncertainties.

The guiding question is: How important is a strategic sociocultural dialogue on research and technology to balance the opportunities of technologies with the uncertainties citizens might feel viewing changes through the innovations in their individual future? How do citizens think about the current innovative topics like artificial intelligence; fusion or hydrogen energy supply;

digital health or smart materials; and livable city concepts, public transportation, and mobility (just to name a few discoveries and developments)? Citizens might feel uncertain and could express fear and anxiety while facing the
rapid pace of technological change in this new world.

The starting point for the German–Japanese comparison is the following:
Japan and Germany have fumbled their way forward in their research, innovation, and technology policies with multiyear strategies since the mid-1970s
(Japan) and the mid-1990s (Germany) of the last century. Now, in the 2020
decade, a connectable concept could find followers. Japan, for example, has
brought up the new paradigm of a "Society 5.0." The idea behind it was first
put forward in 2016 along with the Japanese government's Fifth Basic Plan for
Science, Technology and Innovation (STI) and it could be understood as a
progression of the concept of "Industry 4.0," which has been intensively discussed and deepened in Germany.

The Society 5.0 paradigm requires (first) that technological improvements
should provide real and measurable benefits for individuals. And (second), the
science behind these innovations should be communicated as transparently
as possible to the public. Within the discourse of anxiety culture as a "New
Global State of Human Affairs," this understanding of an open societal dialogue offers some promises and potential pathways.

By comparing the planning scenarios at the beginning of the Japanese 1970s
and the German 1990s until today, everything began with the relevant Delphi
Studies that Tokyo had designed at that time. These surveys among experts
asked about future challenges, trends, and topics in technology and innovation. In the late 1980s, Germany was still rather reluctant for planning the
future of research according to the Delphi approach. But changes came along:
From the mid-1990s onward, the Minister for Research and Technology at that
time—Heinz Riesenhuber (a Christian Democrat) and his department—
began to understand the benefit of strategic scenarios and the chance to listen to the citizens' feelings about technology and innovation. This position
garnered growing support over the decades, until today.

Japan was ahead then and wanted to understand the technosocial future
through expert consultation in an evidence-based manner. This knowledge
was used to underpin Japan's technology policy. Germany, however, needed
until the mid-1990s to apply this method as well. One reason for this restraint
could be found in the country's constitution. The Basic Law (Germany's
Grundgesetz) guaranteed the freedom of research and teaching for individual
scientists and still does (Article 5 of the Constitution). Accordingly, scientists

can determine research questions, topics, and methods themselves. Along with the understanding at the time, this was not compatible with a research and technology policy that relied on forecasting and planning. (Incidentally, this is still an argument when German scientists critically question the strategy in research and science management.)

Insights from the German Debate

Three main formats were developed in the 1990s, influenced to some extent by the Japanese Delphi surveys. Their effect on overcoming technological reservations cannot be rated highly enough. These instruments are now considered to be strategic instruments of Germany's research, technology, and innovation policy. Embedded in an open social dialogue, which also includes a centrally funded concept of Citizen Science cooperation, this is an attempt to promote a positive understanding for new developments and innovations in the civil society. It is assumed that an open and critical dialogue with citizens within the civil society might raise the chance for an acceptance of technology and innovation in the long run. Along with the growing knowledge and better understanding of the pro and con of new developments, uncertainty, fear, and anxiety could decrease. Citizen Science is understood as an instrument to foster the public-private dialogue on science and innovation. So far, German policymakers have made efforts to bring about a societal dialogue on future decisions in science and technology. This is the background to understanding the dialogue instruments.

The German Instruments

Since its launch in 2006, the (first) "High-Tech Strategy" has been a so-called learning strategy. This means that it is continuously developed and adapted to technological and societal changes, as the recent Federal Report on Research and Innovation 2020 outlines. This mechanism is also reflected in the associated consultation process of the High-Tech Forum, in which stakeholders from science, business, and civil society get together. The Forum continuously publishes results in the form of fundamental papers and can also propose new consultation topics.

The (second) "Innovation and Technology Analysis" examines and evaluates interdisciplinary social and technological future topics with a time horizon of a good five years with regard to their opportunities and risks. Its well-founded data contribute to a better understanding of new developments and a transparent dialogue process. Citizens are specifically involved in the impact assessment. The analysis of topics in the area of tension between technological possibilities, societal values and developments, and economic requirements supports the design of future innovation policy.

Finally (and third) in the course of "Foresight Processes," technological trends and societal changes with a long time horizon are described with the help of experts to discuss them with representatives from politics and society. Foresight is a strategic anticipation. It analyzes possible and desirable developments with a time horizon of up to 15 years. The "Bundesministerium für Bildung und Forschung" (BMBF), the German Federal Ministry of Education and Research, has been conducting Foresight Processes with different focuses since the 1990s. In 2019, the Third Foresight Process started and takes a look at the (expected) values of German society up to 2030.[1]

Current Innovation Policy Thematic Framework in Germany

Today, in the decade of the 2020s, German civil society faces the identical major challenges that apply to all nation-states of the world, and these circumstances are drivers for uncertainty and anxiety. To address and solve the megatopics of energy, health, climate and environment, future work and artificial intelligence, to name just a few, four pivotal questions need to be addressed during the present decade to 2030. First, how can an acceptance of new technologies be achieved socially to help reduce uncertainty, fear, and anxiety about innovations? Second, how can the transfer of knowledge and technology to society be improved? Third, how can the digital transformation of society as a whole be accomplished? And fourth, how can the transparency and ethics of scientifically based findings and their global compliance be guaranteed?

In all these surveyed subareas, the new tasks are to be measured, values are to be negotiated, and logics of action are to be understood. Not all of them correspond primarily to a classical understanding of the task of science (generating new knowledge and the transfer of knowledge in exchange for funding).

Is the German Angst Still at Stake?

The German Academy of Technology (Acatech) publishes with partners the *Technology Radar* (*Technik Radar*) on a regular basis. The recent issue points out the health system, which has been stressed by the COVID-19 pandemic:

> Contrary to what is often assumed, the media analysis of the Technology Radar 2021 does not show any sceptical reporting. Similar findings in the Technol-

ogy Radar 2020 have been focused on the bioeconomy. In terms of numbers more opportunities than risk-related arguments and the sceptical arguments and the skeptical statements refer to only a few direct challenges. Scepticism relates to a few direct challenges—for example data protection—but hardly any indirect side-effects such as the economisation of health care.[2]

Regarding the BMBF's most recent Foresight Process (2020), it says:

The task of strategic foresight is to anticipate technological, economic, legal or geopolitical developments at an early stage, to relate them to each other and to identify possible fault lines. Consequently, it is not only necessary to record and analyze scientific and technological trends, but also to identify social developments and corresponding transformation processes and to consider them in terms of their impact. Science, research and technology development are explicitly understood as processes that interact with political, economic, social and cultural phenomena.[3]

And for the anticipated "landscape of value" in the Germany of the future, the Foresight Process states:

In the 2030s, Germany is on the move towards a society in which not only social participation and economic equality have increased, but also the concept of prosperity has been redefined. Noneconomic forms of prosperity are at the center: quality of life, sustainability, temporal prosperity and social cohesion. However, the new scope for development is also accompanied by new fears and lines of conflict.[4]

Expanded Knowledge and Technology Transfer

An expanded KTT model, designed with the scientifically motivated entrepreneur, must be embedded in the recognizable innovation policy cornerstones in Germany of this current decade. This inward view leads first to Rafael Laguna de la Vera. He is the director of Sprin-D, the first federally owned agency for the big leap and disruptive innovations, based in Leipzig. He and his team are working for the really big technological breakthroughs, as they call it. Driven by the idea of a next big thing, which German politicians sometimes associate with the hope of a German Google or a similarly groundbreaking innovation plus a scalable business model, the successful entrepreneur Laguna ideally promotes a completely new approach to the transfer and innovation market in Germany. The agency's approach writes the politics of

Germany for decades to come: a broad and socially stable middle class has always been the guarantor of the democratic system since World War II. As in many other countries, this middle class is increasingly coming under economic pressure. Likewise, many industrial and overall commercial sectors in Germany are feeling the effects of global competition. That is why Germany must turn scientific knowledge into resilient and successful business models more quickly.

Laguna states unequivocally in the *Frankfurter Allgemeine*, one of the leading German daily quality papers in his (still remarkably frank) interview: "Between basic research and the finished product lies a valley of death. To bridge that in innovations that involve new, complex technologies, you need a lot of money for a long time. In Germany, there is a lack of that."[5] This position is heated and still fuels fiery discussions on innovation policy in Germany. The outcome of technology and innovation policy for the discourse of anxiety culture will be nurtured by the following question: Is technology a benefit to solve problems or does technological change create insecurity and fear in the population?

From Entrepreneurial State to Mission Economy

For some years now, Mariana Mazzucato has been framing the debate on technology, innovation, and science policy in Germany. In her view the state—with the capacity to act—takes on the complex issues of research, transfer, and innovation by creating supportive framework conditions and with a committed coordinating role. Mazzucato works, teaches, and conducts research at University College London, where she heads the Institute for Innovation and Public Purpose. In Germany, her ideas are also being received by the current federal government.[6]

With the idea of the "Entrepreneurial State," Mazzucato has comparatively elaborated the strong position of the administration in the United States for the European innovation discourse. [7] In doing so, she has also put the myth of Silicon Valley into perspective. After all, she is sure, not everything was created there, in the United States, out of purely private impetus and money. Both military research and the US Defense Advanced Research Projects Agency (DARPA), as well as the Advanced Research Projects Agency–Energy (ARPA-E), which focuses on energy research, are proof of the impulse role the United States has always had and continues to play in the country's science-business-society transfer triangle.

European Trends in Technology Policy:
Understanding the German Strategy

The European Union (EU) is trending in a similar direction and it followed suit in the summer of 2021. The European External Action Service has presented a non-paper, which, according to an exclusive report by the *Handelsblatt*, the leading economic daily in Germany, was discussed by the EU foreign ministers.[8]

Germany's central EU partner, France, views the topic from a different perspective, following in the tradition of the United States and Israel. The French President Emmanuel Macron has high expectations for the Agence de l'innovation de défence (AID), founded in 2018. It is intended to link civil and military research. The big role model is again DARPA. With state funds from the United States defense budget, groundbreaking innovations were made possible. (A lot of money went into Silicon Valley or America's private world dream missions.) This is now to be organized from Paris to Europe as well.[9]

France, as a high-tech country, is also aware of the importance of deep technology and sees new opportunities in the close cooperation between civilian and military research. The discussion will also arise in Germany until the end of the decade around 2030.

Finally, Germany is continuing the High-Tech Strategy and will transform it into a new research and innovation strategy by 2025. One of the hallmarks will be the inclusion of traditional French elements with a strong emphasis on research but that will have an industrial policy weighting, too.

Insights From the Development in Japan

The starting point for Japan looking into the field of STI policy nurtures and rests with one pivotal question: Does a focus on the needs and concerns of society help to reduce feelings of uncertainty, fear, and anxiety among citizens? One step ahead might be found in the STI-Strategy. In March 2021, the Japanese government published its Sixth Science, Technology and Innovation Basic Plan for the next five years, stating in the introduction that the central message is as follows:

> Looking back, science and technology served as the basis for Japan's recovery from the devastation of the postwar period. If that is the case, then in an era facing a global crisis, also called the Anthropocene epoch, we will put Society 5.0 to the forefront as a universal and global image of our future society in order to

achieve what the Constitution of Japan declares, "we desire to occupy an honored place in an international society."[10]

The concept of Society 5.0 has been formulated in the previous Fifth STI Basic Plan (2016–2020), which strongly stipulates that STI policy has to secure the understanding, trust, and support from the society in order to meet social expectations. Society 5.0 is described as "an initiative merging the physical space (i.e., the real world) and cyber space by leveraging ICT to its fullest, where we are proposing an ideal form of our future society" with "a series of initiatives geared toward realizing this."[11] The core notion of Japan's STI and growth strategy is that a "super smart society" shall enhance the quality of life of all citizens.[12] Behind the eye-catching expression Society 5.0 lies a fundamental shift in how economies and societies may be structured in the future to achieve a digital transformation of the society itself, thus going beyond the notion of Industry 4.0, which was Germany's response to digital transformation in manufacturing since the 1990s.

Early Shifts in Policymaking: Toward the "Needs" of Society and "Innovation"

By the 1980s, Japan had moved from catching-up to that of a global leader. Yet, when the global economy entered into a new phase, and even faster technological progress enhanced the crucial link to science, the Japanese system of innovation came under criticism. The political leadership started to debate how to design a "post-catch-up innovation system."[13] The enactment of the S&T Basic Law in 1995 marked a visible and significant turning point in this respect, acknowledging that Japan—as a small, resource-poor nation facing a rapidly aging population—had no choice but to restore the competitiveness in science and technology to remain a global leader in the 21st century. S&T Basic Plans for consecutive five-year periods became the main tool of policy planning, forcing the S&T community to periodically review and reflect on the national innovation system. The First S&T Basic Plan (1996–2000) largely emphasized the "seeds" of science and technologies and aimed at systemic changes of Japan's Research & Development (R&D). With the Second S&T Basic Plan (2001–2005), we see already a shift toward the "needs" of society in policymaking: A vision was formulated to apprehend technological and societal changes and to promote R&D activities which are in line with policy priorities to solve national and social issues. The Council for Science and Technology Policy (CSTP) was established in 2001 and was placed directly under the jurisdiction of the Prime Minister to function as a control tower for policy implementation. The country's foresight activities, which started in the 1970s, became strongly interlinked with the S&T policymaking and the formulation of the S&T Basic Plans. With the Third S&T Basic Plan (2006–2010) an explicit shift to "innovation" became apparent.[14] At the outset, the plan stated that "Japan intends to be a leading country in innovation" and that S&T has "to be supported by the public and to benefit society."[15] The urgent need to develop human capital was newly emphasized.

Citizen Science and Co-Creative STI Policy

The 3/11 Fukushima disaster had a dramatic impact on Japan, and the effects linger today. The catastrophe caused severe human distress, wide-scale devastation, and highlighted the lack of interface between science, policy, and society backed by mutual trust in times of emergency in Japan. Public opposition to nuclear power generation quickly strengthened, and in response to a growing distrust in the political elites and bureaucracy, interest in citizen science has grown in Japan as elsewhere. The term *citizen science* entered governmental policy documents under the auspices of a co-creative STI policy, but it becomes obvious that the Japanese government has a top-down understanding of participation in which citizens contribute data or local knowledge to science.[16] The Fourth STI Basic Plan (2011–2015) underlined the importance of the "roles of human resources and their supporting organizations" and the "implementation of STI policy created together with society."

After the 3/11 Fukushima disaster, the urgency to bring about Japan's "rebirth" became immense.[17] The CSTP became henceforth responsible for formulating the STI policy and ensuring its sound implementation, and it was renamed the Council for Science, Technology and Innovation (CSTI) in 2014. This change in vocabulary indicates that the role of government has also changed from pursuing "industrial policy" to "innovation policy."[18]

Society 5.0 and a Vision of a Desirable Society

From the Fifth STI Basic Plan (2016–2020), back-casting policy-making processes were introduced to discuss policy implications based on the vision of a desirable society, the Society 5.0. The Basic Plan stipulates that STI has to obtain the understanding, trust, and support from the society to meet social expectations; thus the Japanese government is addressing themselves to communicate and collaborate with various stakeholders in the society. To spread new STI into the society, it is necessary to get public comprehension and acceptance.[19]

Despite these buzzwords, however, the plan's main thrust remains largely unchanged. It places strong focus on fostering open innovation and diversity, the promotion of R&D-type startups, and emphasizes the cultivation of an entrepreneurial mentality. Moreover, the plan puts high priority on unleashing the full potential of universities as engines of economic growth. Narratives of crisis now strongly include Japan's isolation from the global (scientific) community. Increasingly, newspapers, scientific articles,[20] and various governmental documents point out that Japan's innovative output is rapidly declining in international comparison, and that there is a great danger that Japan will be left behind.

These crisis narratives again suggest an urgent need for increasing government R&D spending. Since the Third STI Basic Plan, a government R&D investment target of 1% of the gross domestic product (GDP) had been set but still not achieved. Hence, the powerful Japan Business Federation urged the government to increase spending to bring about the "rebirth of Japan,"[21] and it became a strong advocate of the Society 5.0 concept as a way to resolve Japan's economic crisis.[22]

What is remarkable is that the preparation of the Fifth STI Basic Plan was initiated with a new methodological approach, which consisted of brainstorming discussions among CSTI's executive members and external stakeholders, all with a view to identify shared guiding principles for the Fifth STI Basic Plan. This was run in parallel to a formal assessment of 20 years' worth of experiences of Basic Plans and benchmarking exercises of STI policies around the world. Industry 4.0 was intensively discussed as an appropriate concept also for Japan. Nevertheless, the executive members identified the preparedness of the entire society for an unpredictable and unforeseeable near future of rapid digital transformation as the most fundamental challenge to be addressed. "The capacity to design future industry and society will be instrumental, and to this end, investing in people and providing the space to test their ideas will be the key. What we observe here is the shift from the traditional technology-driven to a more society-centred and challenge-driven innovation policy."[23]

Japan's Eleventh Foresight Survey, published in November 2019 and looking ahead to the year 2050, was conducted by combining four methods: First, understanding trends in science, technology, and society (scanning method); second, examining the future images of society (visioning method); third, examining the future images of science and technology (Delphi method); and fourth, examining the future images of society brought about by the development of science and technology (scenario planning).[24]

To further pave the way to realize Society 5.0, in March 2020, the Japanese government renamed the Science and Technology Basic Law to the "Science, Technology and Innovation Basic Law," making substantial amendments for the first time in 25 years.[25] "Humanities and Social Sciences," which had been excluded from the provisions of national STI policies, were added to the Law.[26] This marked a fundamental policy change,[27] especially when one recalls that the humanities and social science departments at Japanese Universities had been under attack by the Ministry of Education, Culture, Sports, Science, and Technology Japan in 2015.[28]

Moreover, innovation "is now seen as an activity by a wide range of actors that creates major changes in the economy and society, and is evolving into the concept of transformative innovation which focuses on the creation of new value and the transformation of society itself."[29]

The Sixth STI Basic Plan (2021–2025), which was published directly after these amendments, is focusing on the implementation of Society 5.0, calling for "a society that is sustainable and resilient against threats and unpredictable and uncertain situations, that ensures the safety and security of the people, and that individual to realize diverse well-being. . . . This is also in line with the SDGs [Sustainable Development Goals of the UN]."[30] STI policies are being accelerated under road maps focusing on carbon neutrality, digital transformation, countermeasures against infectious diseases, and human resource development.

Outlook: Germany's High-Tech Confession, Japan's Unique and Long Journey Toward Society 5.0

Politics in Germany is fanning out. A change of course can be seen for the current decade: The topic complex of "research-transfer-technology-innovation" will no longer be negotiated and pursued in universities, academies, institutes, and non-university institutions alone. Technology policy has become the geopolitics of the industrial nations and alliances of states. Berlin, Brussels, Washington, Beijing, Tokyo, and many other capitals of the world have declared the subject area a matter for government. Whether it is research on 6G, quantum computers, artificial intelligence, smart materials, brain research, and energy, to name just a few, they have all become benchmarks for economic prosperity and democratic freedoms of the future. This has consequences for the knowledge and technology transfer practiced in Germany thus far; this area of activity must expand and integrate the requirements of deep technology in the future.

Thematically, the deep technology fields of Industry 4.0, quantum computing, automotive, life sciences, energy, chemicals, and smart materials represent Germany's specialty of combining specialists' deep expertise with industrial scalability and thus still being able to maintain almost 24% (2019) industrial manufacturing as a contribution to gross national product. The development of deep-technology solutions extends far beyond the usual transfer periods (greater than 15-year horizons).

With its flagship program of Society 5.0, Japan started a societywide experiment, putting the transformative power of STI policy to the test. The outcomes are yet open. Japan's government always used many foreign STI policies for inspiration without properly evaluating them before their implementation, which often resulted in the impression of frenetic change for change's sake. With the concept Society 5.0, the Japanese government tried a new way, along with and through new mechanisms of STI policymaking. The concept of Society 5.0 is also born out of necessity, to justify increased public funding in R&D at an unprecedented—yet in international comparison, still low—scale. The question is whether the concept of Society 5.0 will gather enough traction to gain acceptance and commitment from all key stakeholders, whether the portrayed threats and anxieties are able to mobilize the society to transform. Innovative disruption is needed everywhere, which is a real challenge in the Japanese innovation system that is still dominated by a centralized culture where big companies and ministries have a central position in the decision-making process. Nevertheless, we see new actors, new mechanisms, a new diversification, and disruption in the innovation system in Japan and in other countries, also caused in part by the COVID-19 pandemic, for better or for worse.

Like in many other countries, the COVID-19 pandemic exposed Japan's digital backwardness—despite its rollout of 5G technology in 2020. Thus, it is not technological capacity but structural problems of the Japanese innovation system that have caused the delay of digital reforms, which are the cornerstone of realizing Society 5.0. Japan's traditional mindset and unadventurous bureaucracy has, for years, resisted digital changes within the system. Moreover, the system of rotating posts in ministries every two years has created hurdles in attaining specialization; many bureaucrats that are able to acquire digital knowledge are transferred to other sections after two years. Apart from bureaucracy, many interest groups and unions have historically resisted digitalization policies in Japan.

In May 2021, as a response to the exposure of Japan's digital backwardness, the Japanese government passed a law to establish a new government agency, called the Digital Agency, to ramp up its ambitions in digitalization. The Digital Agency started its operation in September 2021 and consists of 600 officials, one-third of whom are from the private sector (for comparison, Singapore's Government Technology Agency had 1,800 officials at its inception in 2016).[31] The Digital Agency thus can be a seen as a test bed for the aspirations of Society 5.0.

Conclusion

Based on the preceding discussion, we draw the following conclusions from the German–Japanese comparison for our reflection on its implications for anxiety within a political-decision context. First, maximizing democratic participation of the society seems to be the key to reducing uncertainty, fear, and even anxiety about new technologies and innovations. Second, the strategic Foresight Process (plus the other instruments) in Germany, as well as the Society 5.0 approach that has been used in Japan, show how understanding and (possible) acceptance can be achieved by communicating the benefits of technological progress to citizens in a transparent way. Finally, the fact that scientists are daring to engage in more open knowledge and technology transfer will nurture a contemporary discourse around anxiety culture.

NOTES

1. Bundesministerium für Bildung und Forschung (BMBF), ed., *Bundesbericht Forschung und Innovation 2020: Forschungs- und innovationspolitische Ziele und Maßnahmen* (Frankfurt: Zarbock, 2020), https://www.bmbf.de/SharedDocs/Publikationen/de/bmbf/1/31611_1_BUFI _2020_Hauptband.pdf?__blob=publicationFile&v=7.

2. Acatech, Körber-Stiftung, Universität Stuttgart, eds., *Technik Radar 2021: Stakeholderperspektiven* (2019), https://www.acatech.de/wp-content/uploads/2021/06/Langfassung-Technik Radar-2021-Einzelseiten-final.cleaned.pdf.

3. Prognos AG and Z_punkt GmbH The Foresight Company, eds., *Zukunft von Wertvorstellungen der Menschen in unserem Land: Die wichtigsten Ergebnisse und die Szenarien im Überblick* (2020), https://www.vorausschau.de/SharedDocs/Downloads/vorausschau/de/BMBF _Foresight_Wertestudie_Kurzfassung.pdf;jsessionid=E60FBA07450FE717B955DAD1248613 CD.live471?__blob=publicationFile&v=1.

4. Foresight Company, eds., *Zukunft von Wertvorstellungen der Menschen in unserem Land*.

5. Rafael Laguna de la Vera, "Deutschland scheitert in kleinen Schritten," *Frankfurter Allgemeine*, May 30, 2021, https://zeitung.faz.net/fas/wirtschaft/2021-05-30/deutschland-scheitert -in-kleinen-schritten/616039.html.

6. Mariana Mazzucato, *Mission Economy: A Moonshot Guide to Changing Capitalism* (Dublin: Allen Lane/Penguin Books, 2021).

7. Mariana Mazzucato, *The Entrepreneurial State: Debunking Public vs. Private Sector Myths* (Cambridge: Anthem Press, 2013).

8. Moritz Koch, "Digitale Diplomatie. Europas Technologieplan," *Handelsblatt*, July 23–25, 2021, 12.

9. Thomas Hanke and Larissa Holzki, "Wie bei Star Wars: Mit Magnetwellenkanonen gegen Drohnen. Das französische Militär soll Innovationstreiber werden—auch für den zivilen Sektor," *Handelsblatt*, July 24, 2021, 24–25.

10. Council for Science, Technology and Innovation (CSTI), ed., *Science, Technology and Innovation Basic Plan* (2021), https://www8.cao.go.jp/cstp/english/sti_basic_plan.pdf.

11. Council for Science, Technology and Innovation (CSTI), ed., *Kagaku gijutsu kihon keikaku* [Basic plan for science and technology] (2016), https://www8.cao.go.jp/cstp/kihonkeikaku/5honbun.pdf.

12. CSTI, *Kagaku gijutsu kihon keikaku* [Basic plan for science and technology] (2016).

13. Kazuyuki Motohashi, "Innovation Policy Challenges for Japan: An Open and Global Strategy," *Asie.Visions* 45, November 2011, http://www.mo.t.u-tokyo.ac.jp/seika/IFRI_asievisions45kmotohashi.pdf.

14. Kerstin Cuhls and Iris Wieczorek, "Changes in the Japanese Innovation System and Innovation Policies," in *Competing for Global Innovation Leadership: Innovation Systems and Policies in the USA, Europe and Asia*, ed. Rainer Frietsch and Margot Schüller (Stuttgart: Fraunhofer Verlag, 2010), 143–168.

15. Council for Science and Technology Policy (CSTP), *Science and Technology Basic Plan*, March 28, 2006, https://www8.cao.go.jp/cstp/english/basic/3rd-BasicPlan_06-10.pdf.

16. J. Kenens et al., "Science by, with and for Citizens: Rethinking 'Citizen Science' after the 2011 Fukushima Disaster," *Palgrave Commu* 6, 58 (2020).

17. Cabinet Office, ed., *Comprehensive Strategy for the Rebirth of Japan: Exploring the Frontiers and Building a "Country of Co-Creation"* (2012), https://www.cas.go.jp/jp/seisaku/npu/pdf/20120731/20120731_en.pdf.

18. Sébastien Lechevalier, *The Great Transformation of Japanese Capitalism* (Abingdon: Routledge, 2014).

19. CSTI, *Kagaku gijutsu kihon keikaku* [Basic plan for science and technology] (2016).

20. Nicky Phillips, "Japanese Research Leaders Warn About National Science Decline," *Nature*, October 17, 2017, https://www.nature.com/articles/550310a.

21. Keidanren (Japan Business Federation), ed., *Toward the Establishment of a "Venture Eco-system" in Japan* (2015), https://www.keidanren.or.jp/en/policy/2015/118_outline.pdf.

22. Keidanren, *Toward the Establishment of a "Venture Eco-system" in Japan*.

23. CSTI, *Kagaku gijutsu kihon keikaku* [Basic plan for science and technology] (2016).

24. National Institute for Science and Technology Policy (NISTEP), Science and Technology Foresight Center, *The 11th Science and Technology Foresight: S&T Foresight 2019, Summary Report*, https://www.nistep.go.jp/en/?page_id=56.

25. CSTI, *Kagaku gijutsu kihon keikaku* [Basic plan for science and technology] (2016).

26. CSTI, *Kagaku gijutsu kihon keikaku* [Basic plan for science and technology] (2016).

27. Shuzo Yui, "Gov't to Promote Humanities, Social Sciences Amid Advances, AI, Life Sciences," *The Mainichi*, January 8, 2019, https://mainichi.jp/english/articles/20190108/p2a/00m/ona/007000c.

28. On June 8, 2015, Ministry of Education, Culture, Sports, Science and Technology Japan (MEXT) sent a 10-page directive to all 86 national universities in Japan, calling on them to abolish or reorganize their humanities and social sciences departments. National and international heated discussions and fears about funding and the role of humanities and social sciences

followed. See Ministry of Education, Culture, Sports, Science and Technology Japan (MEXT), ed., *Kagaku gijutsu hakusho* [White Paper of science and technology] (2015), https://warp.ndl .go.jp/info:ndljp/pid/11293659/www.mext.go.jp/b_menu/hakusho/html/hpaa201501/detail /1358751.html.

29. MEXT, *Kagaku gijutsu hakusho.*

30. MEXT, *Kagaku gijutsu hakusho.*

31. Leo Lewis, "Japan's Innovators Seek Their Lost Mojo," *Financial Times*, March 7, 2021, https://www.ft.com/content/bd51a6b8-e084-42fe-8b9a-4dd9361ac33b.

PART SIX

CODA

Introduction

JOHN P. ALLEGRANTE

This final part contains selections that we hope will provoke the reader to consider some of the broader consequences of anxiety culture in relation to the issues and interpretations raised by the essays in this volume. The chapters that compose part VI constitute three discrete but nevertheless related essays that raise provocative questions about the contours of anxiety culture and its impact on our lives. How does the coarsening of public political discourse and the flirtation with illiberal democracy contribute to anxiety culture? What can we learn from how climate anxieties are represented in discourse and how do these shape the possibilities for human action? Is the conventional Western therapeutic culture that has evolved in the treatment of individual anxiety, with its emphasis on positive psychology and achieving happiness, relevant to coping with anxiety on cultural and social levels? The essays in this part provide insights into these and other questions that this book raises.

First, Dirk Nabers and Frank Stengel's chapter, "Discourse, Fantasy, and Anxiety in Trump's America," takes up the question of how growing political polarization and the fascination with autocrats is contributing to anxiety culture, not only in the United States where elections have become fraught with fears and suspicion but across much of Europe and other places around the globe. Nabers and Stengel focus their analysis on the impact of former president Donald Trump in the United States and the ongoing threat that he and the extremist far right he has succeeded in mobilizing is widely thought to pose for democracy—and the governing principles that liberal democracies can offer in addressing the challenges of climate change, population health, migration, and technology. From the perspective of illiberal democracy, their chapter could just as easily have been written about the rise of Viktor Orbán of Hungary, Xi Jinping of China or, of course, Vladimir Putin of Russia. Thus, their perspicacity calls on us to think about the consequences of the broader movement toward the autocratic political right in fostering an anxiety culture from the unique domestic American perspective.

Next, Konrad Ott and Maren Urner analyze how feelings and passions can be addressed in discourse in their chapter, "Climate Anxieties in Discourse: From Mental States to Arguments." First, they outline a terminology that integrates both ethics and psychology. Next, they analyze anxieties as special feelings from a biopsychological perspective. Finally, they clarify the modes by which anxieties can be represented in validity claims and argumentation. Thus, they take climate change as a paradigm case and conclude with a commentary on the dialectics of anxieties in troublesome times. Although their chapter could readily have been placed in part II, we chose to include it here because of the existential threat that climate change presents as perhaps the most pressing planetary challenge we face. For if we cannot resolve a global path forward to wean the planet from fossil fuels, develop and scale new sources of clean energy, and bring down the rising temperature of the planet, then all else is potentially lost.

Finally, this section concludes with a trenchant analysis by Julie Reshe, a philosopher and psychoanalyst, of the limits of conventional, post-Freudian therapeutic culture—with what is perhaps its misplaced emphasis on positive psychology and the mirage of happiness—and the implications this poses for living and coping in an age of anxiety culture. In her essay, "No Longer Waiting for Messiah: The Antidote for the Tyranny of Happiness in Therapeutic Culture," Reshe deconstructs the popular myth that the goal of society is to achieve happiness and argues that such happiness is elusive, concluding that living in an anxiety culture requires rethinking purpose and the "universally shared collective aspect of our lives."

CHAPTER TWENTY

Discourse, Fantasy, and Anxiety in Trump's America

DIRK NABERS AND
FRANK A. STENGEL

What role did anxiety play in the rise and persistence of Trumpism, a unique ideological blend of white supremacy, misogyny, and patriarchy as well as populism that informed much of former President Donald J. Trump's election campaign and term in office? Trumpism represents a particularly interesting case for anyone interested in the nexus between discourse, fantasy, and in particular anxiety, commonly understood as "a sense of uncertainty or unease over something that cannot quite be identified."[1] In politics, constructing anxiety also serves the crucial function of maintaining quiescence and delegitimizing dissent.[2] This argument seems to be at least partly responsible for the (1) almost complete immunity of Trumpism's followers to opposing evidence, and (2) their stubborn refusal to hold Trump and other advocates of Trumpism to any moral or legal standards.[3] Thus, many Trumpists not only refused to accept a vaccine that is widely considered very effective against COVID-19,[4] some of them preferring a horse dewormer that the US Food and Drug Administration has explicitly warned against,[5] but many also believed, barring any evidence, that the 2020 US presidential election was fraudulent.[6] Neither did Trump's pursuit of liberal economic policies appear to have had any meaningful effect on his support among poor white voters whose class interests these policies directly contradict. Similarly, the breaking of moral and even legal norms by Trump and members of his administration seem not to have had any meaningful implications for either his base or his supporters in

Congress. Even his followers' attempt, incited by Trump's claims that his election victory had been "stolen by emboldened radical-left Democrats" and the "fake news media,"[7] to violently stop the certification of Joe Biden's election victory in Congress on January 6, 2021, a de facto armed insurrection, did not lead to his removal from office.[8] Also, his election loss appears to have done zero damage to Trumpism's appeal. Indeed, if anything, the Republican Party (GOP) continued its movement toward embracing Trumpism even more than before. In sum, truth and morality appear to be suspended when it comes to Trump—a fact that has led commentators to refer to him as "Teflon Don."[9]

How should we understand this phenomenon? Theoretically, this chapter draws on poststructuralist discourse theory (PDT) and Lacanian psychoanalysis[10] (in particular, its reformulation by Slavoj Žižek[11]) to make sense of the appeal of certain discourses and in particular the role that anxiety plays in this context. In a nutshell, we argue that the appeal of Trumpism can be explained by the discourse's fantasmatic dimension or category of enjoyment—*jouissance* in Lacanian terms[12]—which promises essential identities and social stability in times of crisis. That is, what made, and continues to make, Trumpism so appealing is its (ultimately empty) promise of a fully constituted, "essential" American identity. Ultimately, what makes "make America great again" (MAGA) successful is its unapologetic quest to restore "real"—that is, white, male, Christian, heterosexual, cis-gendered—Americans to the privileged position in society that they not only think they deserve but whose absence they perceive as oppression. This appeal, we argue, is further multiplied by anxiety among Trumpists produced by political practices that openly challenge white supremacy, patriarchy, and neoliberal capitalism as naturalized political practices shaping US society. Understood this way, Trumpism's appeal is not in spite of its obvious racist and misogynist references and its open contempt for moral and legal norms but (in part at least) because of it.

A focus on fantasy and affect can add new dimensions to research on so-called populism, which has briefly pointed to anxiety as a factor[13] but has—aside from a few notable exceptions[14]—not systematically explored this important concept. We thus build on existing studies and complement them in two respects: (1) by drawing on the notions of fantasy and jouissance, we foreground the role of anxiety as well as white supremacy and patriarchy as structural conditions of possibility; and (2) we empirically include the period beyond Trump's time in office. While the next section introduces central concepts from PDT and Lacanian theory, the subsequent section provides a tentative illustration of the theoretical arguments made here, drawing mainly on statements made by Trump, members of his administration and accompanying media coverage. Using the example of Trumpism, we show how the very concept of the political is based on the identification of the enemy and the creation of anxiety, which is best understood through an exploration of the fantasmatic logic at play in this discourse. The conclusion sums up the main findings and outlines avenues for further research.

Anxiety, Fantasy, and Discourse

How can we make sense of phenomena like Trumpism and the grip it has on subjects, even in the face of overwhelming contrary evidence, as the Big Lie shows?[15] Before we jump into the theoretical argument itself, we first need to locate Trumpism in ontological terms. What kind of a thing is Trumpism? Understood in discourse theoretical terms, Trumpism is a specific discourse. Discourses from a poststructuralist perspective are understood as "relational systems of signification," that is, networks of related discursive elements (words, nonverbal practices, and so on) that acquire their specific contextual meaning as a result of how they are arranged vis-à-vis each other.[16] Put simply, what the term *apple* refers to in the context of a supermarket is different from what it means in an IT discourse because the discursive elements it is linked to differ between the two contexts (bananas, raspberries, and pineapples in one; IBM, Microsoft, and Google in the other).[17] The connection of previously unconnected elements transforms these elements into moments of a specific discourse. We call this transformation *articulation*. Articulation signifies, both in a linguistic and in a very practical sense, because subjects acquire meaning only through their positioning in a structure, be it linguistic or social. In this perspective, discourse becomes coterminous with the social; in fact, it can be highly material when it becomes institutionalized.[18] Discourses are relevant for political and sociological analysis because meaning—the way we come to understand the world around us—is not naturally given but instead the result of discursive struggles between different competing articulatory practices. Two aspects are worth accentuating here. First, although meaning is not unproblematic, people do take it for granted most of the time,[19] and as a result, what comes to be accepted as the truth has a potentially significant impact on how we engage with the world. For how we understand reality—which phenomena we see as policy problems to be solved, whom we consider a friend or an enemy, whether human beings are matter or walking wave functions—unavoidably influences how we behave toward others. For instance, if I think the coronavirus pandemic is a hoax cooked up by Bill Gates to implant microchips in people's bodies,[20] it is very likely I will not get the vaccine and as a result, risk my and other people's health as well as contribute to the pandemic turning into a very unpleasant version of *The NeverEnding Story*.[21] Second, contrary to common sense, reality itself does not function as a neutral arbiter here, rejecting "false" discourses and making truthful ones more effective (otherwise, no one would believe Trump's Big Lie). Instead, which representation manages to assert itself as the only valid truth depends on factors other than an allegedly objective reality, which brings us to the role of fantasy.

Lacanian theory, which has been widely used to amend PDT,[22] delivers a model that explains, at least in part, how some discourses manage to assert themselves in struggles between different competing depictions of reality. Fantasy, and its connection with anxiety, is crucial in this respect. From a Lacanian perspective, anxiety is a chronic condition of human life, constitutive of the futile drive toward identity.[23]

If we want to understand this, we need to turn our attention to the Lacanian conception of the subject. For Lacan, the subject is constituted by the symbolic. The symbolic order refers to what from a discourse theoretical perspective would be called discourse or the social; it is the entirety of social structures, roles, subject positions, practices, institutions, and so forth, "into which individual human beings are thrown at birth."[24] The symbolic order however fails to capture reality in its entirety. It is marked by a "constitutive incompleteness"[25] or what Laclau refers to as "dislocation."[26] As Nabers shows, dislocation has two crucial dimensions:[27] First, it implies translocation, referring to a situation in which a signifier that is seen as foreign to a particular discourse enters and destabilizes the internal structure of that discourse, an example being the allegedly "Chinese virus" that has entered the Western world. Subjects, practices, and institutions are continuously called into question by such translocatory discourses. Second, dislocation denotes inarticulation and is often related to trauma, that is, a situation that is hard to describe and yet desperately demands to be communicated. As an omnipresent feature of the social, dislocation thus creates unstable subjects, as well as ambiguous and incomplete symbolic structures. The "stuff" that is left out of the symbolic by translocation and trauma, which exceeds the limits of discourse and cannot be represented, is what Lacan calls the real. Most notably with respect to the subject, the real includes the subject's affective side, or enjoyment.[28] Affect here refers to the "unconscious bodily intensity" that, once articulated in discourse, becomes a specific emotion, such as anger or joy.[29] Comparable to dislocation, the real disrupts the symbolic, constantly transcending its limits.

As a result of the constitutive role of dislocation and the disruptive character of the real, the subject is necessarily "split"[30] or "traumatized."[31] This is where anxiety comes into play, as the gap between the subject's strive for completeness and the affective subject's dislocated character constitutes it as fragile, insecure and open to apprehension.[32] In other words, anxiety stems from the subject being confronted with an inaccessible desire, or, more precisely, it is "the very experience of this inaccessibility."[33] Lacanian psychoanalysis presumes that precisely because the subject cannot ever attain a full identity (because the lack is constitutive), it has a never-ending desire for a stable identity. The question turns from "Who am I?" into "Who do I want to be?" However, desire in Lacanian terminology should not be confused with demand or need, for example, hunger. Desire is, in Glynos's words, "what emerges in the dissatisfaction felt when the demand is actually met,"[34] for instance in Post-Tenure Depression Syndrome. Indeed, a core feature of desire is that it cannot ever be fulfilled.[35] Desire works because it remains "forever *dis-satisfied*."[36] In Johnston's words, "[n]o object" the subject "gets its hands on is ever quite 'IT.' "[37] As a result, the subject is in constant pursuit of the unreachable (nonexistent) object of its desire.

In that sense, desire and enjoyment are closely related to the concept of fantasy. Broadly speaking, fantasy refers to specific discourses that blame the lack of "our" identity on another (immigrants, terrorists, billionaires, capitalism, the deep state, etc.) and propose a certain course of action that will not only overcome the Other but in doing so will restore the lost fullness of the subject's identity. As Moran Mandelbaum argues in his work on Brexit, fantasy does at least two things: (1) it "produces a sense of loss" in that it gives an ontic form to a lack that is actually ontological (for example, by blaming detached or corrupt elites for the loss of an allegedly better past); and (2) it promises a way forward to regain that lost fullness (for instance, by claiming that a return to that mythical past can be realized by taking certain actions).[38] Fantasy is ideological in Laclau's sense in that it covers over "the radical contingency of social relations."[39] It pretends that if only action XYZ were taken, the (constitutive) lack could be overcome and a fully constituted identity could be realized, giving the subject an object to desire. We can distinguish here between a "beatific" and a "horrific side of fantasy," where the former refers to the promise of wholeness and the latter to potentially catastrophic consequences if a certain course of action is not taken.[40] As Eberle points out, "[t]he structure of a fantasmatic narrative . . . pictures our very identity as threatened and offers a particular policy as the way of making identity whole again, or at least averting some irreparable damage to it."[41] In doing so, a fantasmatic discourse structures and directs the subject's enjoyment and sustains its desire.[42]

Because fantasy gives a form to desire, it is not supposed to be realized either. In Žižek's words, "fantasy, at its most elementary, is inaccessible to the subject, and it is this inaccessibility which makes the subject 'empty.' "[43] In fact, as Glynos explains, if the subject were to get too close to the realization of its fantasy, this would not have a satisfying effect on the subject but, quite to the contrary, the subject would "experience an unbearable anxiety as a result of suddenly being confronted not with lack (since it is upon this very lack that desire is founded), but with the *lack of a lack*."[44] In Lacan's words, "that what is feared is success."[45] Anxiety is linked to the need to stabilize the subject as a subject of desire.[46]

Fantasy has another function with respect to anxiety—namely, to manage it. For instance, Ali and Whitham claim that fantasies about Muslims allow British society to "avoid confrontation with contradictory and upsetting aspects of our social 'Real.' "[47] Similarly, drawing on an ontological-security framework, Steele and Homolar have argued that in times of anxiety, people tend to stick to routines, which can manifest itself as resistance to expertise. In such a case, ignorance can function as a "coping mechanism," lending support to populist anti-intellectual projects.[48] On the flip side, one could argue that the dislocation of and political practices that challenge fantasmatic discourses should contribute to anxiety among the subjects that have identified with a specific fantasmatic discourse.

Fantasy highlights the moment of the subject; it links affect and discourse together. Subjects affectively invest in certain fantasies, and it is this investment that explains different discourses' longevity. In Eberle's words, "it is the affective investment that holds discursive orders together."[49] Understood this way, it is not their rationality or purportedly objective truthfulness that makes certain representations credible for certain audiences but primarily their ability to channel enjoyment by providing the illusion of a fully constituted identity. In that sense, fantasy adds an important aspect by pointing to the affective side of persuasion.[50]

Trumpism as a Fantasmatic Discourse

Lacanian theory's strong suit is to add to our understanding of cases in which people stick to certain ideologies even in the face of overwhelming contrary evidence. What makes Trumpism particularly interesting as a case is that it defies expectations on many fronts. Trump's norm-breaking behavior already during his presidential campaign alone led many observers to expect that he would likely be forced out of the race even before the GOP nomination. Thus, his racist, misogynistic, and anti-democratic remarks (about Mexican "rapists" and grabbing women "by the pussy" as well as his refusal to accept an election loss) were expected to end his campaign.[51] Nevertheless, and against all odds, he not only won the nomination but also the presidency. Equally, his base stuck with him despite that many claims he made during his term in office were in blatant conflict with scientific evidence, such as his claim that climate change was a hoax or that COVID-19 would simply vanish or could be treated by injecting disinfectant.[52] The most infamous example is the Big Lie about the 2020 election having been stolen. In spite of a complete lack of evidence—as pointed out by Trump's own Attorney General William Barr—on January 6, 2021, Trump's supporters stormed the US Capitol to stop the certification of Joe Biden's election victory.[53] Like Brexit[54]—and indeed many other examples of so-called populism—Trumpism's lasting influence even after Trump left office is a phenomenon that is hard to explain with recourse purely to allegedly rational motives. This is why a turn to fantasy and enjoyment can be very fruitful.

So how can we make sense of this remarkably powerful grip that Trumpism seems to exert over people? From a Lacanian perspective, Trumpism's grip is best explained by focusing on its fantasmatic character. And indeed, in many respects, Trumpism appears like an ideal typical example for a fantasmatic discourse. To begin with, Trumpism offers a simple and clear explanation for the lack that the subject experiences as anxiety. According to Trumpism, America has lost its greatness and is currently facing a severe crisis. As Trump claimed in his presidential announcement speech, "Our country is in serious trouble. We don't have victories anymore. We used to have victories, but we don't have them. . . . We got nothing but problems. . . . Sadly, the American dream is dead. But if I get elected president I will bring it back bigger and better and stronger than ever before, and we will make America great again."[55]

Crisis and lack are co-constitutive in this picture, which can be well explained through the theoretical vocabulary presented above. Two dimensions are particularly pertinent in this context: First, what Lacan, Laclau, and others have called an "ontology of lack" directly relates to the absent ground of society, giving identity "the name of what we *desire* but can never *fully* attain."[56] Crisis, as dislocation, becomes a permanent underlying feature of the social to be exploited by political forces. Second, the articulation of crisis is necessarily based on an identification of the enemy. Thus, the reason for America's lost greatness was, according to Trump, the fact that the United States was ruled by incompetent and/or corrupt elites: "We have losers. We have losers. We have people that don't have it. We have people that are morally corrupt. We have people that are selling this country down the drain."[57] This is the point where the fantasmatic is linked with the populist dimension of Trumpist discourse, evident in the claim that ruling elites have become detached from the will of the people and that fixing things will require a restoration of popular sovereignty. As Laclau has maintained, popular identities are articulated on the basis of antagonistic frontiers.[58] In a similar vein, Žižek has aptly shown that, "a nation *exists* only as long as its specific enjoyment continues to be materialized in a set of social practices and transmitted through national myths that structure these practices."[59] National unity, that is, identity, can only be achieved through two interlinked moves: First, the (alleged) complete elimination of all dislocatory tendencies, in which the literal contents of particular social demands recede into the background and a mythical identity is translated into an imaginary horizon which provides the surface for the inscription of various political demands. Second, the articulation of antagonism. As Laclau summarizes: "[T]he only possibility of having a true outside would be that the outside is not simply one more, neutral element but an *excluded* one, something that the totality expels from itself in order to constitute itself."[60]

Especially during Trump's reelection campaign and after President Joe Biden had assumed office, Trumpist discourse took on a conspicuously sinister tone. Trump mainly derided liberal elites as "stupid" during his first campaign,[61] but now there was a dark conspiracy at work. This is the horrific aspect of Trumpism as a fantasmatic discourse, which fell on the fertile ground of a deeply dislocated society. Thus, the GOP claimed that Biden was pursuing "far-left socialist policies."[62] Trump himself maintained that "Biden is a puppet of Bernie Sanders, AOC [Alexandria Ocasio-Cortez], the militant left, the people that wanna rip down statues and monuments to George Washington, Thomas Jefferson, Benjamin Franklin, Jesus, okay, Jesus. They wanna rip down statues to Jesus."[63] Here, Biden, Sanders, Alexandria Ocasio-Cortez, and the "militant left" are articulated as an antagonistic Other threatening not just capitalism but also the Founding Fathers of the American republic and even Christianity itself. Similarly, the right-wing media painted a dark picture of the United States being overrun by, as Fox News host Tomi Lahren put it in October 2021, "illegal immigrants looking to bust in and invade our country," while Biden was functioning as a "puppet" for the left to "ramrod through their radical socialist agenda."[64] Indeed, according to then Fox News host Tucker Carlson, the Democrats were planning nothing less than to open US borders to illegal immigrants with the aim to replace "legacy Americans with more obedient people from far away countries," that is, replacing white Americans with people of color.[65] An ideological, fantasmatic discourse creating widespread anxiety becomes eye-catching in this context, which Žižek summarizes as follows:

> What is at stake in ethnic tensions is always the possession of the national Thing: the "other" wants to steal our enjoyment (by ruining our "way of life") and/or it has access to some secret, perverse enjoyment. In short, what gets on our nerves, what really bothers us about the "other", is the peculiar way he organizes his enjoyment (the smell of his food, his "noisy" songs and dances, his strange manners, his attitude to work—in the racist perspective, the "other" is either a workaholic stealing our jobs or an idler living on our labor). The basic paradox is that our Thing is conceived as something inaccessible to the other and at the same time threatened by him.[66]

Identity building and the creation of anxiety go hand in hand in the process of constructing the American people in Trumpist discourse. We can also see that Trumpism, in particular in its radicalized form, articulates a very specific version of the American society—one that is primarily white. For in Trumpist discourse the category of the people does not refer to the entirety of the American populace. Rather, Trumpist discourse clearly distinguishes between real Americans and others. Real Americans according to this discourse are what Carlson calls "legacy Americans," a code for white people.[67] The national crisis that Trumpist discourse produced seemed ideal for the fruition of a binary discourse relying on a black-and-white picture of the world, based on relations of equivalence, difference, and the articulation of antagonistic frontiers. The notion of "real" Americans—aberrant as it may still be for the many critical minds inside and outside of American society—has thereby been thoroughly normalized in Trumpist circles.

What is more, this kind of division continues along party lines. For the goal to gain and hold on to power, Trumpists claim, the Democratic Party will stop at nothing. Thus, Trump and his supporters continue to assert that the 2020 election was stolen from them. Already during the election night on November 3, 2020, Trump claimed that "we did win this election" and demanded that the counting of absentee ballots be stopped while he was in the lead: "We want all voting to stop."[68] During the following weeks and months, Trump maintained that he and his supporters were fighting for "honesty of our elections and the integrity of our glorious republic" and continued to push the Big Lie.[69] Thus, on January 6, 2021, the day of the certification of Biden's victory, Trump claimed that "our election victory [is being] stolen by emboldened radical-left Democrats, which is what they're doing. And stolen by the fake news media. That's what they've done and what they're doing. We will never give up, we will never concede. It doesn't happen. You don't concede when there's theft involved."[70]

What was at stake was not only the election but the future of the country as such. Thus, Trump demanded that his supporters "[fight] like hell. And if you don't fight like hell, you're not going to have a country anymore."[71] Again, we can identify three of the most important tenets of the logic of fantasy at play in this discourse. First, identity-building requires some kind of enjoyment; while enjoyment cannot be equated with pleasure, it often implies the construction of anxiety. The affective power of Trumpism does not stem from it being able to offer pleasure but "closure."[72] Second, anxiety is based on the articulation of antagonistic frontiers. Accordingly, Trumpist discourse delivers an unambiguous explanation for who is standing in the way of a return to American greatness and thus the continued presence of a lack and, by extension, the subject's continued trauma. Hence, Trumpist discourse can be characterized "as structured around a certain traumatic impossibility, around a certain fissure which *cannot* be symbolized."[73] Third, dislocation is constitutive of the social, making identity necessarily futile, while at the same time triggering a sense of collective identity, on which politics can be conducted. In this sense, inaction would, according to the Trumpists, lead to the complete loss of the country.

Implicit in this articulation is the promise that MAGA success and the overcoming of the leftist obstacle will restore America to greatness and realize a fully constituted identity for the subject. As Trump put it in his announcement speech, "We need somebody that can take the brand of the United States and make it great again. It's not great again. We need—we need somebody—we need somebody that literally will take this country and make it great again."[74] On January 6, Trump claimed that "Our exciting adventures and boldest endeavors have not yet begun."[75] MAGA is turned into a mythical imperative at this stage. Myths essentially depict an absence, but that absence is necessary for social transformation to become an ongoing possibility. It can only be constructed around emptiness, as any precise details or a concrete scheme for the future development path would move the myth into the realm of everyday politics, and it would lose its quality as a myth. Myths are no more than a foil that represents the missing fullness of a nation. The desire for fullness, in turn, is constitutive for the nation's development path toward future greatness. Deborah Madsen rightly points to American exceptionalism as the central myth around which nationalism is constructed in the US context: "American exceptionalism permeates every period of American history and is the single most powerful agent in a series of arguments that have been fought down the centuries concerning the identity of America and Americans."[76]

Here, myths establish a relation to the pure but lost origin, which in Trumpist discourse is articulated through the MAGA slogan. This is the beatific side of fantasy, in which MAGA functions as a master signifier, an empty signifier that its adherents can affectively identify with. What exactly it means to make America great again remains obscure. Trump does not explain what exactly the slogan would entail. But rather than a disadvantage, the emptiness of MAGA as a demand is a big part of its appeal because it allows a broad range of subjects to project their specific demands onto it. That is, the reason why a broad range of subjects can affectively identify with MAGA is precisely because it is whatever they want it to be. Following the January 6 speech, Trump supporters stormed the Capitol. Not only did this armed insurrection not lead to his removal from office, but even after Trump left office the GOP did not return to a more moderate course but instead continued to further radicalize. Subsequently, the GOP embraced the Big Lie and began to reinterpret January 6 as either a false flag operation by the leftist Antifa or instigated by the FBI, or as a patriotic service to democracy, hailing Ashli Babbitt, the woman who was shot and killed by a Capitol police officer during the riot, as a hero and martyr. Later on, the GOP even officially censured Republican Representatives Liz Cheney and Adam Kinzinger for their participation in the House Select Committee to Investigate the January 6 Attack on the United States Capitol.[77] To be sure, aside from a few true believers, GOP leaders' adherence to Trumpism appears to be primarily opportunistic, not ideological,[78] but that does not explain why the Republican base appears to be fully invested in even the most outrageous aspects of Trumpism. Instead, the fantasmatic logic behind the Trumpist discourse seems to have gained hegemonic status with the GOP, implying a position that portrays Trump not just as *one* option among many, but as *the* only alternative to absolute chaos and insecurity.

Conclusion

In this chapter we analyzed Trumpist discourse from the perspective of Lacanian theory, putting the notions of fantasy, enjoyment, and dislocation at center stage to elucidate the nexus between anxiety, identity, and affect. We attempted to illustrate three arguments: First, the articulation of national identity remains an ongoing and ultimately futile endeavor. It rests on lack and can never reach ultimate closure. In effect, the notion of an intrinsically constituted, real American identity loses all its meaning, since it can only be conceived as an identity vis-à-vis the difference that puts it in opposition to something else. This means, second, that antagonism plays a crucial role in this process. Constructing an outside as an antagonist aims at securing the nation's identity by building it on anxiety and fear. Especially in a moment of crisis or discursive dislocation, previously taken-for-granted practices are innovatively articulated and new political communities constructed. Third, the articulation of anxiety is related to what Lacan has conceptualized as enjoyment, implying that every effort to resolve the lack that rests within identity will necessarily fail. Eventually, Trumpist discourse shows its problematic ethical dimension at this point: It can only survive by creating the fantasmatic illusion of a stable identity, that is, by concealing the contingent and highly heterogeneous character of the American society and reducing it to an underlying sameness. However, as the analysis has shown, this comes down to a dangerous and extremely divisive endeavor.

NOTES

An earlier version of this was presented as a paper at the conference "Varieties of Anxiety—A Global Perspective," December 10–11, 2019, New York University. The authors would like to thank the participants as well as members of the Anxiety Culture project for helpful comments.

1. Brent J. Steele and Alexandra Homolar, "Ontological Insecurities and the Politics of Contemporary Populism," *Cambridge Review of International Affairs* 32, no. 3 (2019): 215.

2. Dirk Nabers, *A Poststructuralist Discourse Theory of Global Politics* (New York: Palgrave Macmillan, 2015).

3. Although Trumpism predates Trump's presidential bid, Trump himself personifies this discursive amalgam like few others, although later on, former Fox News host Tucker Carlson as well as Representatives Matt Gaetz, Marjorie Taylor Greene, and a few others appear to have out-Trumped Trump.

4. Ariel Fridman, Rachel Gershon, and Ayelet Gneezy, "COVID-19 and Vaccine Hesitancy: A Longitudinal Study," *PLoS One* 16, no. 4 (2021): e0250123. This has gone so far that Trump himself has faced backlash due to his muted advocacy for the vaccine.

5. See US Food and Drug Administration, "Ivermectin and COVID-19," FDA.gov, May 4, 2024, https://www.fda.gov/consumers/consumer-updates/ivermectin-and-covid-19.

6. Andrew C. Eggers, Haritz Garro, and Justin Grimmer "No Evidence for Systematic Voter Fraud: A Guide to Statistical Claims About the 2020 Election," *Proceedings of the National Academy of Sciences* 118, no. 45 (2021): e2103619118.

7. See Brian Naylor, "Read Trump's Jan. 6 Speech, A Key Part of Impeachment Trial," NPR .org, February 10, 2021, accessed on April 23, 2024, https://www.npr.org/2021/02/10/966396848 /read-trumps-jan-6-speech-a-key-part-of-impeachment-trial?t=1644327730710.

8. Paul Musgrave, "This Is a Coup. Why Were Experts So Reluctant to See It Coming?" *Foreign Policy*, January 6, 2021, https://foreignpolicy.com/2021/01/06/this-is-a-coup-live/. See also David C. Rapoport, "The Capitol Attack and the 5th Terrorism Wave," *Terrorism and Political Violence* 33, no. 5 (2021): 912–916.

9. See Edward-Isaac Dovere, "Teflon Don Confounds Democrats," *Politico*, September 13, 2017, https://www.politico.com/story/2017/09/13/teflon-trump-democrats-messaging-242607.

10. Jacques Lacan, *Anxiety: The Seminar of Jacques Lacan, Book X* (Cambridge: Polity, 2011).

11. Slavoj Žižek, *Tarrying with the Negative* (Durham, NC: Duke University Press, 2008).

12. Jason Glynos and David Howarth, *Logics of Critical Explanation in Social and Political Theory* (London: Routledge, 2007).

13. Pippa Norris and Ronald F. Inglehart, *Cultural Backlash: Trump, Brexit, and Authoritarian Populism* (Cambridge: Cambridge University Press, 2019).

14. See Florentina C. Andreescu, "Donald Trump's Appeal: A Socio-Psychoanalytic Analysis," *Journal for Cultural Research* 23, no. 4 (2019): 348–364; Moran Mandelbaum, " 'Making Our Country Great Again': The Politics of Subjectivity in an Age of National-Populism," *International Journal for the Semiotics of Law—Revue internationale de Sémiotique juridique* 33, no. 2 (2020): 451–476; Chris McMillan, "MakeAmericaGreatAgain: Ideological Fantasy, American Exceptionalism and Donald Trump," *Subjectivity* 10, no. 2 (2017): 204–222; and Emmy Eklundh, "Populism and Emotions," in *Research Handbook on Populism*, ed. Yannis Stavrakakis and Giorgos Katsambekis (Cheltenham: Edward Elgar, forthcoming 2024).

15. The Big Lie refers to Trump's false claim that his 2020 presidential election victory was "stolen by emboldened radical-left Democrats." Jason Glynos, "The Grip of Ideology: A Lacanian Approach to the Theory of Ideology," *Journal of Political Ideologies* 6, no. 2 (2001): 191–214.

16. Jacob Torfing, "Discourse Theory: Achievements, Arguments, and Challenges," in *Discourse Theory in European Politics*, ed. David Howarth and Jacob Torfing (Basingstoke: Palgrave Macmillan, 2005), 14.

17. Frank A. Stengel, *The Politics of Military Force: Antimilitarism, Ideational Change and Post-Cold War German Security Discourse* (Ann Arbor, MI: University of Michigan Press, 2020), 20. Discourse then loosely corresponds to what from a more conventional perspective would be referred to as an ideology, i.e., "configurations of political concepts"; see Michael Freeden, *Ideologies and Political Theory: A Conceptual Approach* (Oxford: Oxford University Press, 1996), 48. The difference is that discourse encompasses any meaningful subjects, objects and practices, not just political concepts; see Ernesto Laclau and Chantal Mouffe, *Hegemony and Socialist Strategy: Towards a Radical Democratic Politics*, 2nd ed. (London: Verso, 2001), 107.

18. Dirk Nabers, "Crisis and Dislocation in Global Politics," *Politics* 37, no. 4 (2017): 418–431.

19. This is for practical reasons as much as anything else, for if we were to question each and every aspect of what we think we know about reality we would very likely not even make it out of the house each morning.

20. See European Union, "DISINFO: Bill Gates and Other Globalists Use the Corona Pandemic to Implant Microchips in the Whole of Humanity," *EUvsDisinfo*, May 3, 2020, https://euvsdisinfo.eu/report/bill-gates-and-other-globalists-use-the-corona-pandemic-to-implant-microchips-in-the-whole-of-humanity/.

21. *The NeverEnding Story*, directed by Wolfgang Petersen, Warner Bros., 1984.

22. For example, see Yannis Stavrakakis, *Lacan & the Political* (London: Routledge, 1999).

23. Lacan, *Anxiety: The Seminar of Jacques Lacan, Book X*.

24. Adrian Johnston, "Jacques Lacan," in *The Stanford Encyclopedia of Philosophy* (Spring 2023 edition), ed. Edward N. Zalta and Uri Nodelman (Stanford, CA: Stanford University, 2022), https://plato.stanford.edu/entries/lacan/.

25. Jason Glynos, "Critical Fantasy Studies," *Journal of Language and Politics* 20, no. 1 (2021): 99.

26. Ernesto Laclau, *New Reflections on the Revolution of Our Time* (London: Verso, 1990), 39.

27. Dirk Nabers, *A Poststructuralist Discourse Theory of Global Politics*; and Dirk Nabers, "Discursive Dislocation: Toward a Poststructuralist Theory of Crisis in Global Politics," *New Political Science* 41, no. 2 (2019): 263–278.

28. Jakub Eberle, *Discourse and Affect in Foreign Policy: Germany and the Iraq War* (New York: Routledge, 2019), 14.

29. Eberle, *Discourse and Affect in Foreign Policy*, 14.

30. Laclau, *Anxiety*.

31. Torfing, "Discourse Theory: Achievements, Arguments, and Challenges," 17.

32. Nadya Ali and Ben Whitham, "The Unbearable Anxiety of Being: Ideological Fantasies of British Muslims Beyond the Politics of Security," *Security Dialogue* 49, no. 5 (2018): 404; Nabers, "Crisis and Dislocation in Global Politics."

33. J. Peter Burgess, "For Want of Not: Lacan's Conception of Anxiety," in *Politics of Anxiety*, Emmy Eklundh, Andreja Zevnik, and Emmanuel-Pierre Guittet, eds. (Lanham, MD: Rowman & Littlefield, 2017), 29.

34. Glynos, "Critical Fantasy Studies," 200.

35. Burgess, "For Want of Not."

36. Glynos, "The Grip of Ideology," 201.

37. Johnston, "Jacques Lacan."

38. Mandelbaum, "'Making Our Country Great Again,'" 457.

39. Jason Glynos and David Howarth, *Logics of Critical Explanation in Social and Political Theory* (London: Routledge, 2007), 15.

40. Jason Glynos, "Ideological Fantasy at Work," *Journal of Political Ideologies* 13, no. 3 (2008): 283.

41. Eberle, *Discourse and Affect in Foreign Policy*, 106.

42. See Glynos, "The Grip of Ideology," 200; and Glynos and Howarth, *Logics of Critical Explanation*, 107.

43. Žižek, *Tarrying with the Negative*, 159.

44. Glynos, "The Grip of Ideology," 201.

45. Lacan, *Anxiety*, 54.

46. Burgess, "For Want of Not."

47. Ali and Whitham, "The Unbearable Anxiety of Being," 401.

48. Steele and Homolar, "Ontological Insecurities and the Politics of Contemporary Populism."

49. Eberle, *Discourse and Affect in Foreign Policy*, 15.

50. Glynos, "Critical Fantasy Studies," 100.

51. Ben Jacobs and Sabrina Siddiqui, "Donald Trump Forced to Apologise as Sex Boast Tape Horrifies Republicans," *The Guardian*, October 8, 2016, https://www.theguardian.com/us-news/2016/oct/08/donald-trump-forced-into-apology-as-sex-boast-tape-horrifies-republicans.

52. Carol Leonnig and Philip Rucker, *I Alone Can Fix It: Donald J. Trump's Catastrophic Final Year* (London: Bloomsbury, 2021).

53. Musgrave, "This Is a Coup"; see also Rapoport, "The Capitol Attack."

54. Christopher S. Browning, "Brexit Populism and Fantasies of Fulfilment," *Cambridge Review of International Affairs* 32, no. 3 (2019): 222–244; and Mandelbaum, "'Making Our Country Great Again,'"

55. See "Here's Donald Trump's Presidential Announcement Speech," *Time*, June 16, 2015, https://time.com/3923128/donald-trump-announcement-speech/.

56. Yannis Stavrakakis, "Passions of Identification: Discourse, Enjoyment, and European Identity," in *Discourse Theory in European Politics: Identity, Policy and Governance*, eds. David Howarth and Jacob Torfing (Basingstoke: Palgrave Macmillan, 2005), 68–92.

57. "Here's Donald Trump's Presidential Announcement Speech."

58. Ernesto Laclau, *On Populist Reason* (London: Verso, 2005).

59. Slavoj Žižek, *Looking Awry: An Introduction to Jacques Lacan through Popular Culture* (Cambridge, MA: MIT Press, 1991), 202.

60. Laclau, *On Populist Reason*, 70.

61. "Here's Donald Trump's Presidential Announcement Speech."

62. See House GOP, "Biden's Far-Left Socialist Policies Have Created Crisis After Crisis," GOP.gov, January 19, 2022, https://www.gop.gov/bidens-far-left-socialist-policies-have-created-crisis-after-crisis/.

63. See "Trump Calls Joe Biden 'Puppet' of the Far Left," ABC News, July 10, 2020, https://abcnews.go.com/US/video/trump-calls-joe-biden-puppet-left-71723819.

64. See FOX News, "Tomi: President Biden Is a Puppet for the Radical Left," YouTube.com, October 26, 2021, https://www.youtube.com/watch?v=1xjHCD4hybs.

65. See FOX News, "Tucker: Why Would Biden Do This to His Own Country?" Youtube.com, September 23, 2021, https://m.youtube.com/watch?v=Z_oiFBJPWoY. Note that Carlson is echoing the white supremacist "Great Replacement" conspiracy narrative. See Milan Obaidi, Jonas Kunst, Simon Ozer, and Sasha Y. Kimel, "The "Great Replacement" Conspiracy: How the Perceived Ousting of Whites Can Evoke Violent Extremism and Islamophobia," *Group Processes & Intergroup Relations* 25, no. 7 (2021): 1675–1695.

66. Slavoj Žižek, *Looking Awry*, 165.

67. See Tom Mockaitis, "'Legacy American' Is the Latest Catchphrase in the Racist Lexicon," *The Hill*, November 11, 2021, https://thehill.com/opinion/civil-rights/580980-legacy-american-is-the-latest-catchphrase-in-the-racist-lexicon.

68. "Donald Trump 2020 Election Night Speech Transcript," Rev.com, November 4, 2020, https://www.rev.com/blog/transcripts/donald-trump-2020-election-night-speech-transcript.

69. Naylor, "Read Trump's Jan. 6 Speech, A Key Part of Impeachment Trial."

70. Naylor, "Read Trump's Jan. 6 Speech, A Key Part of Impeachment Trial."

71. Naylor, "Read Trump's Jan. 6 Speech, A Key Part of Impeachment Trial."

72. Mandelbaum, "'Making Our Country Great Again,'" 457.

73. Slavoj Žižek, "Class Struggle or Postmodernism? Yes Please!,'" in *Contingency, Hegemony, Universality: Contemporary Dialogues on the Left*, eds. Judith Butler, Ernesto Laclau, and Slavoj Žižek (London: Verso, 1990), 249.

74. "Here's Donald Trump's Presidential Announcement Speech."

75. Naylor, "Read Trump's Jan. 6 Speech, A Key Part of Impeachment Trial."

76. Deborah Madsen, *American Exceptionalism* (Edinburgh: Edinburgh University Press, 1998), 1.

77. Philip Elliott, "Why the RNC's Embrace of Trump and the January Sixers Will Backfire," *Time,* February 7, 2022, https://time.com/6145764/rnc-censures-liz-cheney-adam-kinzinger-january-6-donald-trump/.

78. A telling example is Senator Ted Cruz who first repeatedly referred to January 6 as a "violent terrorist attack," just to then backpedal on Tucker Carlson's Fox News show and apologize for his own "sloppy phrasing." In a similar vein, Cruz even claimed that Senate minority leader Mitch McConnell's characterization of January 6 as a "violent insurrection" was "political propaganda;" see Jade Bremner, "Ted Cruz Reverses on Jan. 6 Opposition and Says It Wasn't an Insurrection After All," *The Independent,* February 10, 2022, https://www.independent.co.uk/news/world/americas/us-politics/ted-cruz-mitch-mconnell-insurrection-b2012525.html.

CHAPTER TWENTY-ONE

Climate Anxieties in Discourse

From Mental States to Arguments

KONRAD OTT AND
MAREN URNER

Environmental anxieties are nothing new: The first waves documented for Western societies can be traced back to the 18th and 19th century. There were anxieties about overutilization of natural resources such as timber, anxieties about overpopulation and famines, anxieties about declining fertility of soils, and anxieties of losing pristine nature and even the countryside. In 1962, anxieties about polluted and toxic environments were expressed by Rachel Carson in her "Silent Spring," which advanced the global environmental movement including political and institutional reactions.[1] In 1970, the US Environmental Protection Agency (EPA) was founded largely in response to the publication.[2] Two years later the famous report, "The Limits to Growth," by the Club of Rome predicted scarcity of natural resources, increasing pollution, a decline of food production, and a decline in human population after the year 2000.[3]

Facing anxieties about forest dieback, a shrinking ozone layer, and risks of nuclear energy, including disposal of radioactive waste, the future of the environment looked rather bleak 30 years ago. There was much literature demanding radical change. Hans Jonas proposed a "heuristic of fear" that urged us to face worst case scenarios.[4] Silicon Valley, MIT, and other tech hubs remained headquarters of technological optimism.

Fast forward into the year 2024, the climate crisis and associated ecological anxieties such as biodiversity loss are paradigmatic but not unique for widespread societal fears. The experience of the COVID-19 pandemic taught people to fear infectious diseases but also vaccines and pandemic rules on top of a fear of migrants, criminals, right-wing radicals, terrorism, unemployment, poverty, and more. In the recent past, Western societies have gained a high level of social security for (almost) all members compared to all previous periods in history.[5] Despite all these efforts, feelings of insecurity and unsafety prevail, and a "global risk society" is being built.[6]

Besides parallels to former environmental anxieties, the current situation and the triggered ecological anxieties seem to be unique in their magnitude. At least three aspects are worth mentioning here. First, even though not formerly approved yet, the Anthropocene has been proposed as a new geological epoch[7] acknowledging the profound human impacts on essential planetary processes, including but not restricted to anthropogenic climate change.[8] Second and closely related, an international group of scientists have defined nine planetary boundaries based on the idea that "crossing certain biophysical thresholds could have disastrous consequences for humanity."[9] Six out of nine boundaries have been officially crossed.[10] Third, psychologists and therapists seem to confirm a new level of ecological anxieties dominated by the climate crisis, especially among the young.[11] Eleven years after the landmark study "The Psychological Impacts of Global Climate Change,"[12] one of their authors summarizes the current situation: "Climate change is described as an existential threat. . . . It undermines people's sense of security in a basic way."[13]

Intensity of anxieties and its combination with other affections matter. Combined with affections such as anger and even rage, even well-founded anxieties can turn into impulsive behavior and panic. Thus, climate policies have become highly emotional affairs. Climate policies are not just an important field of environmental policy reforms but are perceived as a matter of life and death for humanity, of either saving the world or going "worst-ward." Radical politics of "climate emergencies" are demanded by protesters.

To address the troublesome situation, we first have to understand that contemporary Western societies are not just, as many believe, societies being governed by scientific, technological, commercial ("rational") standards; they are as well emotivistic cultures, not in metaethical theory, but in "everyday practice."[14] In her "Monarchy of Fear," Martha Nussbaum confirms MacIntyre's claim that anxieties are a paradigm case of public affections in modern societies.[15] To Nussbaum, anxiety is a primordial feeling that underlies all other feelings. Under the surface of an optimistic culture, as in the United States, anxieties encroach into the minds of many individuals.

Here, we take Nussbaum's analysis some steps further and distinguish between a philosophical and a psychological perspective to propose a proper attitude to anxieties. Given the interdisciplinary background of the authors of this chapter, we begin with a conceptional analysis of affections to propose a conceptual framework. Next, we turn to the biopsychology of anxieties. From there, we adopt a discourse-ethical perspective that allows us to analyze how emotional speech acts might be claimed, adopted, refined, and rejected. Next, we take the new anxiety about the climate crisis as paradigm case and argue that these anxieties spur demands for, as we say, "passionate politics."[16] We conclude with some final words.

Conceptual Analysis: From Feelings to Emotions and From Sorrows to Anxieties

In Hegel's philosophy of human spirit (Geist) there are three modes of spirit: (1) subjective spirit, (2) objective spirit, and (3) absolute spirit. Mental states, including sensual experiences and affections, belong to the mode of subjective spirit, while law, morals, and ethical life (Sittlichkeit) belong to the mode of objective spirit.[17] Objective spirit is about how social life is to be institutionalized. Morality is the sphere of objective spirit that is deeply connected to subjective spirit, including inclinations, imaginations, affections, and feelings. Within morals, affections can become demanding. Hegel, as most philosophers, is critical against the immediacy of (intense) affections in morals because affection may rule at the expense of reason. Such criticism, however, does not suggest that there is a dichotomy between reason and emotions. The either-or model of the relation between reason and emotions is simplistic. Emotions can be perfectly reasonable and adequate, but feelings may also distort and overwhelm. If so, we need a more refined conceptual framework to address affections in general and anxieties in particular.

We start our analysis with the unspecific broad term *affections*, but wish to distinguish between different affective modes, as (a) feelings, (b) passions, (c) sentiments, and (d) emotions. Anxieties are particular affections to which we turn later. If a specific affection is not pure, but mixed with other affections, we speak of "clusters."

At the particular layer of the anxiety cluster, philosophers and psychologists have to analyze the semantic and phenomenological differences between

(a) "fearing," (b) "being afraid," (c) "being concerned," (d) "being worried," (e) "being in sorrow," and (f) "being in panic."

At the general layer of affections, we have to distinguish modes of affections. *Feelings* are an immediate given state of mind. If an individual person P utters a feeling F, she expresses a validity claim of sincerity by way of an expressive speech act: "I feel (un)happy, guilty, ashamed, harassed, uncomfortable, anxious." The expressive speech act can be controlled by others only with respect to the consistency between speech act and behavior. "If you feel so sad, why are you laughing all day long?" Feelings as such have neither truth value nor moral force. Feelings do not guarantee rightness of normative statements. There is no moral duty to respect any feelings as such. If someone feels bad about x, it does not follow that x should be omitted.

Feelings might become more forceful if felt by a prudent person. If an expert says: "I have a bad gut feeling with x," we expect that the expert can add the underlying reason. Generally, we expect that persons can and should warrant their feelings. A warrant of a feeling claims its adequacy within a situation. It can be very reasonable to be afraid about a situation S, as the global climate crisis.

Passions are forceful feelings. Ordinary language often states that a person P is a passionate X. If P is a passionate gardener, chess player, smoker, gambler, P will prima facie avoid stopping his passionate activity. One is, as we say in ordinary language, ruled (or dominated) by passion. For centuries, passions have been regarded as opposite to sober rationality. Passions have overriding motivational force, often get out of control, overwhelm, and may become vicious: greed, revenge, envy, wrath, hatred, jealousy, even addiction. Thus, the destructive powers of passions always have been feared. Norbert Elias argued that the entire process of civilization is a process of discipline against passions. As Elias argues that spontaneous and intense feelings and passions must be tamed, dampened, and restrained if society takes the route to civilization in which physical violence is replaced by economic dependencies and rule of law.[18]

As Hirschman has argued in his "Passions and Interests," philosophers since early modern times argued that a society being dominated by economic interests might be more peaceful, decent, and humane than a society ruled by passions.[19] To political liberalism, politics should not be an arena of passions since passions may turn opponents into enemies. Feelings and passions can become targets of manipulation. Feelings can be manipulated by advertisement. Political passions can be enforced by propaganda. The difference between feelings and passions can, in Hegelian perspective, be stated as follows:

Feelings are the state of immediacy, while *passions* are the state of negativity. On reflection, there are reasons to fear passions.

Sentiments are different from feelings and passions. David Hume (*A Treatise of Human Nature*) believed in moral sentiments that are constituted by the societal way of human life.[20] Moral sentiments belong to our evolutionary legacy as hypersocial beings. Rules cover the impartial side of morals and law, whereas moral sentiments, as sympathy and compassion, cover the partial side, as in care for particular persons. Moral education is learning about adequate moral sentiments. Care-based ethics are mostly based on human ideas.

Moral sentiments, however, can become triggered. Mechanisms of how to trigger sentiments have been made explicit by Mark Johnson in "Moral Imagination," which combines metaethical emotivism and cognitive psychology.[21] Such combination remains open for the strategic use of moral language and all kinds of sentimental moralizing. If so, one must take one further step beyond sentiments toward emotions.

Following Hume, Adam Smith in *The Theory of Moral Sentiments* regards the sentiment of sympathy being crucial.[22] Even if one sees humans as egotistic creatures, Smith argues, one can hardly deny some human dispositions to act in altruistic ways. Compassion is a universal disposition that humans cannot get rid of. To Smith, moral sentiments are correlated to the stylized figure of the impartial spectator. The impartial spectator is a decisive step beyond Hume. According to Smith, the ideal spectator is not detached from sentiments, but (s)he also represents reason. If we take, first, the role of the impartial spectator and, second, keep our moral sentiments and motives alive, then we can approve our behavior hypothetically as the approval being given by the sympathy of the impartial spectator.

Following Smith, we see and define *emotions* as being cultivated and reflected sentiments that have passed the "impartial-spectator" test (or some other ethical device) and can presume adequacy with respect to specific situations. We can overcome the weak side of sentimentalism if we adopt some ethical device that provides a test for sentiments, be it a categorical imperative, an impartial spectator, a Rawlsian veil of ignorance, or a Habermasian discourse. Affections that pass the "test-device" gain the status of proper emotions. Such emotions are, ideally, in reflective equilibrium with reason and moral principles. This approach to emotions is acceptable to Kantians also. To Kant, supreme (categorical) moral principles must be grounded in pure practical reason. If such grounding had been fulfilled, emotions may play a beneficial role in moral perception and motivation.

Emotions presume to be adequate (= appropriate) to given situations. In contrast to feelings, passions, and even sentiments, adequate emotions can and should be shared. In some situations, we are inclined to say: "It would be inappropriate to show no anger (grief, sadness, fear)." The concept of adequacy is key to overcome the false dichotomy between reason and affections. Adequacy refers to situations. Situations have different scales, from imminent danger "here and now" to the long-term global scale, as in the climate crisis. Appropriateness of emotions to global scales is an unprecedented challenge for psychology and ethics in the Anthropocene.[23]

In our conceptual scheme, *Affection* serves as a generic term over four more specific concepts:

1. Feelings: given in immediacy, "just so," arational
2. Passions: the negative side of affective life
3. Sentiments: moral feelings open to manipulation
4. Emotions: cultivated and appropriate (adequate) sentiments.

This conceptual scheme indicates the possibility of learning processes in the realm of affections. It presupposes sincerity at the side of individuals. It is critical against all kinds of manipulation of affections, which remained a weak point in Hume and Johnson. The scheme should work for individuals who may be enabled to describe their own affections more nuanced from a first-person perspective sincerely. It is directed against the anarchic position saying that the world of affections is in constant flux and is nothing but a chaotic display of differences. If our scheme is applied to particular affections, as anxieties, there should be anxieties occurring as feelings, as passions, as sentiments, and as emotions. Our nonexclusive ethical device to transform feelings into emotions is practical discourse.[24]

The Biopsychology of Anxieties: Defining a Corridor for "Good Decisions"

From a purely biological and evolutionary perspective, the paramount question about any trait or behavior is always: Is it beneficial for survival? The *it* in this case refers to emotions (using our terminology here) that are mental experiences of body states.[25] With this question in mind, which emotions are reasonable (or in our terminology, adequate) given a certain situation?

"I want you to panic." Greta Thunberg, the global face of the new wave of environmental anxiety, famously put her concerns into words at the World Economic Forum in 2019.[26] She demands and concludes: "I want you to feel the fear I feel every day. And then I want you to act. I want you to act as you would in a crisis. I want you to act as if our house is on fire. Because it is."

Globally activists and campaigners are now connected under the "for future" movement. On a biopsychological level of risk assessment, they have essentially realized that the climate crisis requires urgent and far-reaching changes to the human way of living, if the species wants to ensure humane living conditions on Earth for the current young as well as future generations. Psychologically they have internalized the three aspects of proximity that makes people act: temporal (it happens now), geographical (it happens here), and social (it affects me or people that matter to me). However, this proximity can be overwhelming and in the case of the climate crisis leading straight from "denial to despair."[27] Related to that, the despair can even be utilized by politics and power structures that transfer clinical concepts into their spheres.

A neuroscientist argues that a brain and body "in panic" is not a reasonable brain, because it is essentially a brain and body that is flooded with hormones and neurotransmitters and is essentially in a condition that maximizes immediate survival. Even more so, the expression "one loses one's head" has a biological truth to it. Panic and the related fear and anxiety puts the body into one of the three F's: fight, flight, or freeze. All three place the evolutionary oldest brain regions into the driver's seat and disable the newer, uniquely human architecture of the brain, that is, higher cognitive functions located in the prefrontal cortex (PFC) as well as access to past experiences located in memory structures are temporally disturbed or completely disabled.[28]

Additionally, a growing body of research shows that the bombardment with negative news we experience in a digital and highly connected world, usually coupled with the overarching message that others (politicians, the economy, or the top brass) make the decisions for us and are responsible for the current situation of the world, not only can lead to a state of so-called learned helplessness[29] but also to long-lasting anxiety. In fact, the concepts of eco- and climate anxiety possibly resulting in depression, paralysis, and the need for therapeutic intervention has been smiled at only a decade ago when the initial paper about it was published,[30] but it is now a growing area of research as well as daily practice for therapists and clinics.[31]

In parallel, much research has been conducted about emotions (and the accompanying brain states) that enable reasonable decision-making aligned to personal values, convictions, and goals. In short, positive emotions are those that empower us to think and act in a goal-directed way and trigger curiosity, all helping to find good, that is, adequate, solutions.[32]

To conclude this short excursion into the biopsychology, the task and challenge to define adequate emotions to face crisis—front and foremost the climate crisis—lies in finding the enabling corridor between not caring (enough; think the three aspects of proximity) and panic disabling long-term thinking. In this corridor of positive excitement, the human brain is able to imagine, envision, and build future-oriented ideas and concepts, that is, humans can become reasonable emotional beings.

Anxieties in Discourse

As our conceptual scheme and neuropsychological science imply, we wish to become reasonable emotional beings. Such "becoming" is intrinsically lingual. We must speak to each other about affections to cultivate them, reflect on them, and control them. Mental states must become speech acts (or narratives). All affections that claim political relevance must be deprivatized. Affections articulated via language may gain the status of emotions. Emotions presume that all reasonable persons should share them. If so, shared emotions should be based on reasons we can share.[33]

According to discourse ethics, the force of the better reasons should guide our individual and collective actions and the choice of norms of actions (rules, institutions).[34] Discourse ethics does not separate reasons from emotions in a dichotomic way. It rather entitles and encourages individual persons to articulate their affective states of mind as precisely as possible. The term *reason* refers to deliberation and arguing. Arguing means to give and to take reasons within a public sphere. The force of argument is different from causal determination.[35] In pure moral discourse, participants ask for impartial norms of actions that are in the common interest. In political debates, however, the pool of reasons enlarges. It includes eudaimonic, economic, legal, cultural, and moral reasons. Such an enlarged pool of reasons often must be matched with risk assessment on different temporal and spatial scales. Discourse ethics may concede that perfect agreement becomes impossible if the affective states and degrees of risk aversion of participants in discourse differ widely. Luhmann has argued against Habermas that there will be no such thing as common risk taking in a value-pluralist society.[36] The unlikeliness of agreement will increase if feelings and passions dominate risk assessment, as in the case of the climate crisis. Within discourse, claims about anxieties must presume to be emotional ones. Such claims must be open for refutation and confirmation. Speech acts about anxieties suppose a basic structure: An individual person P feels an anxiety A about a specific threat (danger, risk) X. This is a threefold relation:

P-A-X. In a standard case, P sincerely utters from a first-person perspective some A-X speech act. If many individual persons share the anxiety, there can be collective A-X speech acts: "We all are afraid about X."

Any A-X statement that presumes to be emotional must be substantiated by reasons R. "We (all) are afraid about X—and rightly so!" The "rightly so" is pragmatically implied in the A-X statement itself. A stylized standard type of the many speech acts expressing anxieties takes the following form: "I (we) are afraid A about X (and rightly so) because of R."

Speech acts refer to validity claims. Validity claims refer either to truth (facts, empirical theories, explanations), to rightness (principles, norms, values), or to sincerity (authenticity).[37] In speech acts about anxieties all three validity claims are present:

1. Anxiety is sincerely felt by an individual person P (or a collective).
2. X and R are both credible in terms of truth and probability. R warrants the "rightly so."
3. We should do something about X (reduce, prohibit, avoid, adapt). This opens debates about Who? How much? When? and How?

Validity claim of sincerity: Speech acts relating to anxieties belong, in the first instance, to the *expressives:* "Hereby I sincerely express my anxiety A."[38] At this point, the distinction between (a) feelings, (b) passions, (c) sentiments, and (d) emotions also holds. The sincerity of the speech act does not logically presume that the speaker claims the status of an emotion. She may just tell her affections as mental fact. If so, the sincerity implies an open question to the, for instance, anxiety-discourse community: "Is my feeling well justified? Is it adequate? How do you think about it?" Quite often, however, the presumption of emotion is made within discourse that goes beyond the sincerity claim.

Truth and probability claim: What is the object X to which an emotional anxiety state of mind refers to? X entails a prospect of loss and/or damage to someone (person, collective, humankind, future generations, life on Earth, etc.). An apocalyptic loss would be "the end of the world as we know it" or the extinction of our species within the sixth mass extinction in the history of planet earth.

Some X are ontologically obscure. In former times, people were afraid of ghosts, demons, devils, witches. If someone states, "I fear witchcraft" or "I am anxious about doomsday, final judgment, and hell," we may feel committed to respect such spiritual beliefs but will not agree. Can one reasonably say "I am deeply afraid of some unknown unknowns"? It might be reasonable to be afraid of earthquakes at one location but not at another one. Thus, we must ask which statements cannot fulfill the requirements inside the "and rightly so."

Warrant: R gives some backing and justification for both the anxiety and X. R underscores the presumptive reason of being afraid about X. R may be a scientific forecast, a historical analogy, an extrapolation, a model run, a simulation, or something similar. R can also take the form of a generic rule such as Murphy's Law: "The worst case will always happen." At the core of discourses on anxieties is contest over the credibility of warrants as they determine the "rightly so." In the case of the climate crisis, R refers to climate science as documented in IPCC reports.[39] Contest over R is epistemic, not moral.

From a media perspective, R can take many forms, starting with rumors, some news from an internet source, headlines in newspapers, documents from NGO's, reports from some state's agencies, personal authorities, and so forth. The distinction between true and false is far too simple to get a proper understanding how R's are composed as warrants for some X. If one does not wish to fall prey to relativism, one should argue that R's have different degrees of scientific credibility. Conspiration theories also can stimulate anxieties and will present some R.[40]

If R is not credible, anxiety A is prima facie not reasonable. Emotional anxieties should be grounded in specific X being backed by credible R. To put it in other words: *Emotional anxieties are discursively dependent on X(R), not the other way around.* If the speech act "A-X-R" can be confirmed, some practical consequences result. We cannot simply ignore or be forgetful about X. Ignorance and forgetfulness are not options if emotions are proper. Given this, the practical side of anxiety discourse opens. Within a discourse-ethical framework, each and any claim can be *denied* (refused, rejected, refined). From a discourse-ethical perspective, we can learn as much (or even more) from denials than from claims. Denials can, in principle, attack each component of the very threefold structure: (a) emotion, (b) X, and (c) R. Within the scope of this chapter, we cannot give a detailed analysis of how denials, warrants, refutations, and confirmations may interplay in discourse. Discourse is the decisive ethical device to turn affections into emotions we all can and should share—especially with regard to the climate crisis.

Climate Change as Paradigm Case for "Passionate Politics"

Climate ethics has become an important field of practical philosophy.[41] Most people have underrated the risks of climate change for a long time, thus allowing it to turn into the climate crisis we now face. If the negative consequences of climate change fall on poor people in the Global South, this constitutes a matter of injustice. Since it has become evident that the fossil fuel industries and the US administration knew about the effects of CO_2 emissions since the 1970s but tried to keep it secret or cast pseudo-skeptical doubts[42] in a very effective way, the emotion of anger seems adequate.[43] There are sound reasons to be deeply concerned and anxious about the climate crisis, and there are reasons to be more demanding with respect to abatement and mitigation policies.[44] Young adults who realize that they and their children will have to live their lives under possibly detrimental conditions are entitled to be emotional and demanding. In full liberal democracies, citizens have rights to engage in civil society to push climate policies forward on the agenda, to demonstrate, and to found new climate parties. They may even perform nonviolent actions of civil disobedience. As Christina Lafont argues, agenda setting is emotional, because it wishes to mobilize the "citizenry with slogans, chants, photos, documentaries, demonstrations, first-personal testimonies," and so forth.[45]

To be afraid about the global climate crisis is, however, unprecedented in human history.[46] We face a new moral situation: planetary anxieties. Humans are not experienced with large-scale anxieties that refer to abstract global measures (as global mean temperature). The world of humans was full of local affairs that gave reasons for fear: predators, warriors, robbers, pest, diseases, bad harvests, to name a few.[47] Since the origins of the species, humans have had to fear many events, but they never had to be anxious about something that happened on a global scale.

Now, we are confronted with planetary anxieties that are warranted by scientific evidence. If so, they are emotional (according to our definition). Because such emotions refer to a global scale, they may become highly intense. Scale may trigger intensity up to a paralyzing and even pathological point.[48] Emotions may eclipse back into sentiments and even passions. There can be eclipse of reason as well as eclipse of emotions.[49] We face both: warranted emotions and a regressive eclipse into depression, despair, and panic. This makes the situation genuinely dialectical. And so is the slogan: "I want you to panic."

In planetary anxieties, emotions and demands refer to ultimate and global objectives of climate policies. More than thirty years ago, Article 2 of the United Nations Framework Convention on Climate Change (UNFCCC) was ratified, which demands to prevent dangerous anthropogenic interference with Earth's climate system. Twenty years ago, the "tolerable window" was defined at 2°C GMT increase (compared to preindustrial temperatures) by the

German Advisory Council on Global Change (WBGU).[50] Then there was the objective "well below 2°C."[51] Now, the objective has been reduced to 1.5°C at the Glasgow summit in 2021. The new social movements take the 1.5°C target for granted. It should be reached with high likelihood. Now, the proper emotions refer to the 1.5°C target. The high likelihood to overshoot the 1.5°C target intensifies the proper emotions and concerns. One may overlook that the targets have become more ambitious over time. It makes a huge difference to be concerned about a 1.8°C, 2.5°C, or 3°C GMT increase.

One can, however, interpret the 1.5°C target as a "first defense line," which might be lost for some time but might be reconquered later.[52] Therefore, we should form a prudent portfolio of means to combat the root causes and the impacts of the climate crisis. We can combine aggressive abatement of emissions (as first-best strategy) at all scales with other strategies. If we can keep the mean global temperature rise "well below 2°C," can launch proper adaptation and resettlement programs, realize carbon sequestration in soils, forests, and mires, and perform some large-scale carbon dioxide removal, the impacts of moderate environmental changes might be severe but will not be catastrophic.

Surpassing the 1.5°C line can, however, be perceived as an apocalyptic event to be avoided by (almost) all means. The affective regression (into despair and panic) spurs "passionate politics." There is a crucial divide between long-term reformist portfolio strategies and passionate politics of climate emergency.

Helge Peukert[53] and Bill McKibben[54] demand a radical shift of the economic system in analogy of war economies in the 1940s. Peukert relies on Randers and Gilding[55] who proposed a "one degree war plan." Such proposals are in line with Latour's ideas that there should be a "people" willing to literally fight for "Gaia,"[56] being based on the political philosophy of Carl Schmitt.[57] To Latour, there should be war between different "people," which are united under beliefs in different higher powers, as "Gaia." Such proposals are not in line with political liberalism and deliberative democracy.

Ironically, most protest is uprising in countries that have successfully reduced roughly 40% of former emissions (1990) and are on a route to further reductions, as in Germany. Some young adults went on hunger strike, others pledged to avoid giving birth to any more children (birth strike). Such protests cannot create much impact on global emissions. Even if Western societies will push forward climate policies on the political agenda (as we dearly hope), all savings at location A can be overcompensated by increased emissions at point

B. Historical responsibility of early industrialized countries for past emissions should not be denied, but 50% of all emissions have been released since the Rio summit in 1992. In the summer of 2021, the BRIICS states (Brazil, Russia, India, Indonesia, China) and some other members of the G20 were reluctant to steepen reduction trajectories toward a 1.5°C target. Many middle-income countries are now carbonizing their economy, emphasizing a right to economic development.[58] Passionate politics in some countries is not an option in the absence of global compliance and cooperation, but emotional politics should point at the many deficiencies of former climate policies, as in the United States, and of course at (multinational) companies that still lack proper commitments as well as plans to meet their own net zero goals.[59]

Conclusion and Recommendations

We live in a peculiar dialectical situation. According to Horkheimer and Adorno, it has been the promise of the project of enlightenment to gain control over nature and to eliminate fear.[60] In the age of the climate crisis, fear and anxiety return without much remaining hope in the capabilities of modern civilization. If safety and security belong to the output legitimacy of a democratic order, many citizens get the impression that the democratic state fails. An anxiety culture may invest false hopes into passionate politics, which may split the citizenry. Fear eclipses, from monarchy (Nussbaum) to despotism, in both mental and political life.

Anxieties as proper emotions being warranted in discourse are like collective warning signals indicating fragilities of ecological systems and human lives. Such a "heuristic of fear"[61] is reasonable. Anxieties, however, should not paralyze but motivate. Many options are available to reduce risks and to increase resilience against impacts of the climate crisis. Western democracies should take forerunner roles in international climate policies.[62]

Humans are "children of sorrow." From a virtue ethical perspective, being full of many sorrows should not occupy our minds completely. Totalizing sorrow strips away joy, trust, and hope from our lives. Moreover, there is a high risk that sorrows, anxieties, and fears might be stimulated strategically by others. Therefore, we should not take anxieties at face value but should take them seriously in their ambivalences. There can be adequate emotions but also affective regressions to passions. If so, there is no alternative to discourse. It remains an open question whether Western democracies can cope well with affections of anxieties in a time of uncontrolled digital media. We should not forget that Aristotle was skeptical against democracy because he was aware of the possibility of demagogy igniting the affections of the "demos." The concept of emotion itself requires that we keep the public sphere of reasoning intact.

NOTES

1. Rachel Carson, *Silent Spring* (San Francisco/Dublin: Houghton Mifflin Harcourt, 1992, 2002).

2. John Paull, *The Rachel Carson Letters and the Making of Silent Spring*, in Sage Open 3(3) (2013), https://doi.org/10.1177/2158244013494861.

3. Donella H. Meadows, Jorgen Randers, and Dennis L. Meadows, *The Limits to Growth. The Future of Nature* (New Haven: Yale University Press, 1972), 101–116.

4. Hans Jonas, *Das Prinzip Verantwortung* (Frankfurt: Insel Verlag, 1979).

5. Hans Rosling, Anna Rosling Rönnlund, Ola Rosling, *Factfulness: Ten Reasons We're Wrong About the World—and Why Things Are Better Than You Think* (New York: Flatiron Books, 2018).

6. Fatih Fuat Tuncer, "The Spread of Fear in the Globalizing World: The Case of COVID-19," *Journal of Public Affairs* 20, no. 4 (2020): e2162.

7. Paul J. Crutzen, "Geology of Mankind," in *A Pioneer on Atmospheric Chemistry and Climate Change in the Anthropocence*, eds. Paul J. Crutzen and H.G. Brauch (Cham: Springer Nature Switzerland AG, 2016), 211–215.

8. Will Steffen et al., "Trajectories of the Earth System in the Anthropocene," *Proceedings of the National Academy of Science*, 115, no. 33 (2018): 8252–8259.

9. Johan Rockström et al., "Planetary Boundaries: Exploring the Safe Operating Space for Humanity," *Ecology and Society* 14, no. 2 (2009): 32.

10. K. Richardson, W. Steffen, W. Lucht, J. Bendtsen, et al., "Earth beyond Six of Nine Planetary Boundaries." *Science Advances* 9, no. 37 (2023): eadh2458. https://doi.org/10.1126/sciadv.adh2458.

11. Caroline Hickman et al., "Climate Anxiety in Children and Young People and Their Beliefs About Government Responses to Climate Change: A Global Survey," *The Lancet Planetary Health*, 5, no. 12 (2021), e863–e873.

12. Thomas J. Doherty and Susan Clayton, "The Psychological Impacts of Global Climate Change," *American Psychologist* 66, no. 4 (2011): 265–276.

13. Ellen Barry, "Climate Chance Enters the Therapy Room," *The New York Times*, February 10, 2022, https://www.nytimes.com/2022/02/06/health/climate-anxiety-therapy.html?unlocked_article.

14. Alasdair Chalmers MacIntyre, *After Virtue. A Study in Moral Theory* (Notre Dame, IN: University of Notre Dame Press, 1984), p. 21.

15. Martha Nussbaum, *Monarchy of Fear* (Oxford: Oxford University Press, 2010).

16. Following Nussbaum, we shall argue that anxiety can be combined either (a) with a cluster of other feelings as rage, nausea, envy, and resentment, or (b) with a cluster of attitudes as precaution, risk assessment, concerns, and prudence.

17. Georg F. W. Hegel, *Grundlinien der Philosophie des Rechts. Werke Bd. 7* (Frankfurt: Suhrkamp, 1979 [original 1821]).

18. Norbert Elias, *Über den Prozeß der Zivilisation* (Frankfurt: Suhrkamp, 1980).

19. Albert O. Hirschman, *The Passions and the Interests* (Princeton: Princeton University Press, 1977).

20. See David Hume, *A Treatise of Human Nature* (Oxford: Oxford University Press, 1978).

21. Mark Johnson, *Moral Imagination. Implications of Cognitive Science for Ethics* (Chicago: University of Chicago Press, 1993).

22. Adam Smith, *The Theory of Moral Sentiments* (New York: Penguin, 2010 [original 1759]).

23. See chapter section, "Climate Change as Paradigm Case for 'Passionate Politics.'"

24. See chapter section, "Anxieties in Discourse."

25. Antonio Damasio and Gil B. Carvalho, "The Nature of Feelings: Evolutionary and Neurobiological Origins," *Nature Review Neuroscience* 14 (2013): 143152.

26. Greta Thunberg, "Our House is On Fire: Greta Thunberg, 16, Urges Leaders to Act on Climate," *The Guardian*, January 25, 2019, https://www.theguardian.com/environment/2019/jan/25/our-house-is-on-fire-greta-thunberg16-urges-leaders-to-act-on-climate.

27. Yuval Noah Hariri, "The Surprisingly Low Price Tag on Preventing Climate Disaster," *Time*, January 18, 2022, https://time.com/6132395/two-percent-climate-solution/.

28. For example, see Junchol Park and Bita Moghaddam, "Impact of Anxiety on Prefrontal Cortex Encoding of Cognitive Flexibility," *Neuroscience* 345 (2017): 193–202.

29. Steven F. Maier and Martin E. P. Seligman, "Learned Helplessness at Fifty: Insights from Neuroscience," *Psychological Review* 123, no. 4 (2016): 349–367.

30. Doherty and Clayton, "Psychological Impacts of Global Climate Change."

31. Barry, "Climate Chance enters the Therapy Room."

32. For example, see Christina M. Armenta, Meagan M. Fritz and Sonja Lyubomirsky, "Functions of Positive Emotions: Gratitude as a Motivator of Self-Improvement and Positive Change," *Emotion Review* 9, no. 3 (2017): 183–190; and Barbara L. Fredrickson, "Chapter 1—Positive Emotions Broaden and Build," *Advances in Experimental Social Psychology* 47 (2013): 1–53.

33. Christine Korsgaard, *Creating the Kingdom of Ends*, Chap. 10 (Cambridge: Cambridge University Press, 1996).

34. See, for example, Karl-Otto Apel, *Transformation der Philosophie*, Vol. 1, Sprachanalytik, Semiotik, Hermeneutik, Vol. 2, Das Apriori der Kommunikationsgemeinschaft (Frankfurt: Suhrkamp Verlag, 1976). (*Toward a Transformation of Philosophy* [London: Routledge, 1980], reprinted by Marquette University Press 1998); and Habermas, *Theorie des kommunikativen Handelns*.

35. Habermas, *Theorie des kommunikativen Handelns*.

36. Niklas Luhmann, *Soziologie des Risikos* (Berlin: de Gruyter, 1991).

37. Habermas, *Theorie des kommunikativen Handelns*.

38. J. L. Austin, *How to Do Things with Words* (Oxford: Oxford University Press, 1975).

39. See chapter section, "Climate Change as Paradigm Case for 'Passionate Politics,'"

40. Michael Butter, *Nichts ist, wie es scheint. Über Verschwörungstheorien* (Berlin: Suhrkamp, 2018).

41. See, for example, the contribution of Stephen M. Gardliner et al., *Climate Ethics: Essential Reading* (Oxford: Oxford University Press, 2010).

42. Nathaniel Rich, *Loosing Earth* (Berlin: Rowohlt, 2019).

43. Nathaniel Oreskes and Erik M. Conway, "Defeating the Merchants of Doubt," *Nature* 465, no. 7299 (2010): 686–687.

44. Kondrad Ott, *Domains of Climate Ethics Revisited*, in *Risks and Regulation of New Technologies*, eds. T. Matsuda, J. Wolff, and T. Yanagawa (Singapore: Springer, Kobe University, 2020), 173–200.

45. Christina Lafont, *Democracy without Shortcuts* (Oxford: University Press, 2020), 30.

46. See the chapter introduction on old and new waves about environmental anxieties.

47. The only planetary anxiety in the Christian tradition was about the apocalyptic period, the return of Christ, and the final judgment. This was a terrific anxiety because one might be doomed eternally by the final judgment.

48. See the chapter section, "The Biopsychology of Anxieties: Defining a Corridor for 'Good Decisions.'"

49. Max Horkheimer, *Eclipse of Reason* (Oxford: University Press, 1947).

50. German Advisory Council on Global Change (WBGU), *Climate Change: Why 2°C?* Berlin: Factsheet No. 2, 2009, https://www.wbgu.de/de/; see also Ask MIT Climate, "Why did the IPCC choose 2° C as the goal for limiting global warming?" June 22, 2021, https://climate.mit.edu /ask-mit/why-did-ipcc-choose-2deg-c-goal-limiting-global-warming#:~:text=In%20the%20 1970s%2C%20William%20Nordhaus,any%20human%20civilization%20had%20experienced.

51. The Paris Agreement on Climate Change, 2015, https://unfccc.int/process-and-meetings /the-paris-agreement/the-paris-agreement.

52. Hans Joachim Schellnhuber, "Wir hätten diese Forschung viel früher beginnen können," *Frankfurter Allgemeine Zeitung*, October 21, 2021.

53. Helge Peukert, *Klimaneutralität Jetzt* (Marburg: Metropolis-Verlag, 2021).

54. Mark McKibben, "A World at War. We're Under Attack from Climate Change—and Our Only Hope is to Mobilize Like We Did in WWII," *The New Republic*, August 15, 2016, https:// newrepublic.com/article/135684/declare-war-climate-change-mobilize-wwii.

55. Jorgen Randers and Paul Gilding, "The One Degree War Plan," *Journal of Global Responsibility* 1, no. 1 (2010): 170–188.

56. Bruno Latour, *Kampf um Gaia* (Berlin: Suhrkamp, 2020).

57. Carl Schmitt, *Der Begriff des Politischen* (Berlin, 1963 [original 1932]).

58. Darell Moellendorf, *The Moral Challenge of Dangerous Climate Change* (Cambridge: Cambridge University Press, 2014).

59. See, for example, Thomas Day et al., *Corporate Climate Responsibility Monitor 2022*, Project no. 221013, New Climate Institute, https://newclimate.org/wp-content/uploads/2022/02/Co rporateClimateResponsibilityMonitor2022.pdf; and Jeff Tolleffson, "Climate Pledges from Top Companies Crumble Under Scrutiny," *Nature* February 9, 2022, https://www.nature.com/articles /d41586-022-00366-2.

60. Horkheimer, *Eclipse of Reason*.

61. Jonas, *Das Prinzip Verantwortung*.

62. Christian Baatz and Konrad Ott, "Why Aggressive Mitigation Must Be Part of Any Pathway," in *Climate Justice and Geoengineering*, ed. Christopher Preston (Lanham, MD: Rowman & Littlefield, 2016), 93–108.

CHAPTER TWENTY-TWO

No Longer Waiting for Messiah

The Antidote for the Tyranny of Happiness in Therapeutic Culture

JULIE RESHE

Mapo Bridge bears the notoriety as the "suicide bridge." Among the 23 suspension bridges in South Korea, Mapo Bridge had the highest number of suicides: from 2007 to 2012, more than 100 people killed themselves by jumping from it. A major suicide prevention campaign to reduce the number of suicides was launched in 2012. It was led by the municipal government and involved cooperation with big enterprises like Samsung Life Insurance. The suicide prevention program aimed to transform Mapo Bridge into a "bridge of life" by turning it into a happy, therapeutic, life-affirming place. To this end, interactive panels with inspirational slogans were installed all along the bridge's guardrails. The panels say things like, "The brightest moments are coming soon," "The sun will surely rise tomorrow," "Worries are nothing." There are also images of babies, smiling people, young lovers, and so on. The selection of phrases and images were carefully chosen by psychiatrists, psychologists, and suicide prevention specialists. The program has won several awards, including a Titanium Lion award at the Cannes Lions International Festival of Creativity.

Ironically enough, the suicide prevention campaign has had the opposite effect, with the number of suicides at Mapo Bridge increasing by more than six times in the two years since the campaign began.[1]

The Triumph of the Therapeutic

The story of Mapo Bridge can serve as an exaggerated illustration of a more general tendency in modern society. We are desperately struggling to turn our society into one big, happy therapeutic community. The myth that humans are built to be happy (alternatively, that the ultimate goal of society is to achieve happiness) is all-pervasive and permeates every aspect of contemporary society: it unites liberal ideology, religious thinking, economics, and scientific and popular takes on psychology. Our happiness-oriented culture can be defined as therapeutic, in which separate individuals and social groups are treated as psychotherapy patients in need of treatment for their emotional suffering—it is what Philip Rieff famously called "the triumph of the therapeutic" in his 1966 book on culture after Freud. The key figure of therapeutic culture, the figure of the therapist, was perceived by Rieff as a corruption of Freud's psychoanalysis, since the therapist substitutes the purpose of psychoanalytic processes with a detrimental messianic attitude. As any reader of *Civilization and its Discontents* will know, Freud was not exactly a messiah who promised psychological health and happiness. Despite the demand for happiness and the massive efforts of therapeutic culture to heal individuals and society from emotional suffering, we are not getting any happier; on the contrary, each year humanity is hitting record levels of depression.[2]

Slavoj Žižek's psychoanalytic framework describes modern society as governed by the repressive ideology of joy and happiness. Deriving his thought from the Frankfurt School critique, Žižek suggests that in post-liberal societies the agency of social repression no longer acts in the guise of an internalized prohibition that requires renunciation and self-control. Instead, "it assumes the form of hypnotic agency . . . , its injunction amounts to a command: 'Enjoy yourself!' "[3] Elsewhere Žižek claims, "Today, . . . , we are bombarded from all sides by different versions of the superego injunction 'Enjoy!', from direct enjoyment of sexual performance to the enjoyment of professional achievement or spiritual awakening."[4] Such enjoyment is dictated by the social environment that most notably includes Anglo-Saxon psychotherapies whose main goal is to render the patient capable of so-called normal, healthy pleasures. Žižek connects the call for happiness, indeed internalized in our culture, with voluntary submission to manipulation, "Truth and happiness don't go together. Truth hurts; it brings instability; it ruins the smooth flow of our daily lives. The choice is ours: do we want to be happily manipulated or expose ourselves to the risks of authentic creativity?"[5]

Even as the COVID-19 pandemic ruined the smooth flow of our daily lives and made us face harsh truths about the uncertainty of our existence, the imposition of happiness has not disappeared. On the contrary, it has been reinforced with renewed vigor. A *Psychiatric Times* entry titled "Life, Liberty, and the Pursuit of Happiness—In Spite of the Pandemic" continues to equate psychological normality with happiness and reminds us that "the functional outcome of successful treatment should help a patient to find more happiness."[6] Perhaps during the crisis it seems even more tempting to succumb to the idea that we are built to be happy since this idea functions like a shield from reality: It implies that the reality we are facing is not a reality at all, but merely a temporary glitch, after whose fixing we will again do as we are supposed to—obtain happiness.

In consonance with Žižek, Alenka Zupančič argues that our present reality is conditioned by a rather repressive ideology of positivity. The demand of happiness and positive affect is what Zupančič, revising Foucauldian terminology, calls the biomorality of our time. The demand of this current biomorality is to turn everything negative into a positive. Zupančič claims,

> In the contemporary ideological climate, it has become imperative that we perceive all the terrible things that happen to us as ultimately something positive—say as a precious experience that will bear fruit in our future life. Negativity, lack, dissatisfaction, unhappiness, are perceived more and more as moral faults—worse, as a corruption at the level of our very being or bare life . . . for who dares to raise her voice and say that as a matter of fact, she is not happy, and that she can't manage to—or, worse, doesn't even care to—transform all the disappointments of her life into a positive experience to be invested in the future?[7]

Happiness and pleasure are presented as normality, while the whole spectrum of activities that do not bring pleasure and happiness are considered deviations and pathologies that must be eliminated. Furthermore, there is evidence that these sad, "bad people" are now discriminated against by employers[8] and rejected by potential romantic partners—they are socially demanded to prepare for work and romantic relationships by going into therapy and changing themselves for the better.[9]

Zupančič goes further to claim that within the framework of today's ideology, we are not only discriminated against by the equation happy = good person (who is ultimately an imaginary entity), but rather have turned ourselves into our own gulag. Not only are we unhappy, but we also torture ourselves for the immorality of our unhappiness, that is, for not corresponding to the main moral demand of our time. Zupančič's insights about the self-gulag of positivity and the demand for happiness have been confirmed by various theoretical research endeavors and empirical findings.[10] This moral demand of happiness transforms our struggles, to which we adequately react with sadness and anxiety, into an unbearable disaster full of apathy, isolated self-pity, and shame. The world is our common Mapo Bridge, where we are bridging to each other by substituting genuine care and solidarity for the repressive demand of positivity.

In therapeutic culture, anxiety and intense sadness, for which *depression* is the current medical term, are the most stigmatized phenomena, considered to be better if fully erased from existence. In their controversial book *The Loss of Sadness*, Allan Horwitz and Jerome Wakefield put the tendency of our culture to consider sadness as a depressive psychiatric disorder that necessarily requires professional treatment under scrutiny. They find this surprising and detrimental, since "sadness is an inherent part of the human condition, not a mental disorder."[11] They acknowledge the need to confront psychiatry's definition of depressive disorder to "consider a painful but important part of our humanity that we have tended to shunt aside in the modern medicalization of human problems."[12] Horwitz and Wakefield acknowledge that, against the current belief, depression is not a modern malaise, it is not a pandemic disease that is specific to our culture and historical moment. Sadness and anxiety have been an omnipresent phenomenon in human history. What has changed is the attitude toward them. The major problem with present medical and cultural pathologization of sadness and anxiety is its decontextualization: Current thinking about depression has lost the idea that mental suffering is not a mental disorder (at least not necessarily) or a moral failure, but first of all it is an adequate though painful reaction to harsh life realities.

Among the key reasons why depression is pathologized, Horwitz and Wakefield list the following:

> All professions strive to broaden the realm of phenomena subject to their control, and whenever the label of disease is attached to a condition, the medical profession has the primary claim to jurisdiction over it. Symptom-based conceptions of mental disorder thus expand the range of conditions that can be the legitimate objects of psychiatric management. Piggybacked on justifiable exercises of psychiatric power aimed at mental disorder, normal human emotions, once they have been classified as disorders, are generally subjected to technologies such as psychotropic medications or psychotherapy.[13]

The COVID-19 pandemic serves as a relevant example of this phenomenon. The magnitude of depressive symptoms during the pandemic is much larger than has been seen in the past. Researchers have claimed that "These rates were higher than what we've seen in the general population after other widespread trauma," referring to depression and anxiety that was observed following the 9/11 terrorist attacks.[14]

If one would de-contextualize this, they would have to assert that half the world's population has gone insane, and the other half is well on its way to joining them! The technical problem is that when the majority suffer symptoms that would qualify for a certain psychiatric disorder, it should no more be considered a disorder but redefined as a normal human condition (normal conditions are by definition the average or typical condition). The present depressed and anxious majority includes psychologists and psychiatrists, because they are also witnessing the same crisis as the rest of us. Perhaps they are even more at risk of being happiness gulag victims because others now increasingly rely on their support as professionals. Recently the World Health Organization (WHO) add to their website a page titled, "Mental Health & COVID-19," stating that "Fear, worry, and stress are normal responses to perceived or real threats, and at times when we are faced with uncertainty or the unknown. So it is normal and understandable that people are experiencing fear in the context of the COVID-19 pandemic."[15] This is a much better measure than the demand for happiness in spite of the pandemic. Following the logic of Mapo Bridge, perhaps it has prevented a substantial number of suicides.

Let us think. What are the roots of our equation of happiness with psychological normality and a societal ideal, and what about the accompanying equation of emotional suffering and anxiety with disorder and deviation? Why does it sit so deep in us that whenever we are trying to overcome it or doubt it, we end up using the same logic we are trying to fight? In our post-Freudian therapeutic culture an answer lies in the history of psychoanalysis, especially its unresolved and ambivalent transition from religion to secularism. If we want to move beyond the traps of what Lauren Berlant has called "cruel optimism,"[16] we need to move beyond a messianic framework and cultivate a less transcendent, more imminent orientation toward our own anxiety and pain.

The Uneven Secularization of Psychoanalysis

One of the basic foundations of our therapeutic culture is the Judeo-Christian inheritance that still largely shapes modern Western morality—an ethic of individual and societal care. Among those who acknowledge the problem of the overvaluation of happiness, Anders Dræby Sørensen suggests that modern secular aspirations to attain happiness and to remove pain and anxiety is at least partly based on a religious idea of deliverance from worldly suffering to a heavenly condition. He writes, "our present understanding of happiness might be characterized as an expression of a secularization of the Christian idea of everlasting salvation from the suffering of sin and the fall of man and salvation for participation in the Reign of God."[17] A Christian understanding of suffering is more complex, but it is hard not to agree that, in its essence, a Christian vision associates suffering with evil. Equating Christian struggle against sin and the current ideology of positivity, Sørensen states, "As the Christians believed that man stands in need of salvation from sin and suffering, for 250 years modern man has been in need of liberation from the negative aspects of worldly existence."[18] This thinking implies that the sin of psychological suffering is today's form of the initial Christian sin of a corrupted soul. Such stigmatization conveys an ideal of an uncorrupted human as the one who overcame suffering and finally came to satisfy the injunction to enjoy. In the secularized world, deprived of the illusion of posthumous life, salvation becomes a task that must be accomplished in our earthly life.

The hope for heaven goes together with waiting for the Messiah who would lead us toward it. Medical-psychological discourse is today's main intermediary of such a messianic attitude. The Foucauldian genealogy of modernity was one of the first to demonstrate inherited similarities between the ethical postulates of Christianity and modern medical discourse. Although the medical models of psychic health and pathology appear largely unquestionable, as did the ethical postulates of Christianity, Foucault shows their conditional nature, socially rooted and for the most part contingent. In Foucault's interpretation from *The Birth of the Clinic*, the medicalization of society was embodied "by way of quasi-religious conversion."[19] With a secularization of Christian salvation, the religious care of souls was transformed into an issue of medicine and common sense. Christian pastors were to save us from the influence of the devil, while today's therapeutic practitioner saves us from the secular sin of suffering from depression and anxiety. What largely goes without questioning in our culture is that there is a need to alleviate all kinds of human emotional suffering, to heal human minds from sorrow, and to establish individual and societal happiness and well-being.

Foucault's theory of medicalization and mental health promotion is typically discussed in the context of "biopower" (or in case of Zupančič, "bio-morality"). However, it is also advantageous to elaborate Foucault's less discussed concept of *pastoral* power. Foucault introduces this concept to explain one of the modes of power that operates in democracies. It functions through an organization of societal care. The figure of the pastor "designates a very special form of power."[20] It refers to the Christian image of the loving shepherd protecting and caring for the flock. The shepherd "goes ahead and shows his people the direction they must follow" and "guides to salvation, prescribes the law, and teaches the truth."[21] The initial religious goal of pastoral care was to deliver the individual to salvation from sin. This process was exclusively tied to the institution of the Church—in accordance with the axiom *extra Ecclesiam nulla salus* (outside the Church there is no salvation). In the eighteenth century the goal of salvation was reshaped into one of health, well-being, and protection.[22] The Church delivering salvation from sin has been transformed into a diagnostic and therapeutic infrastructure bringing salvation in the form of mental health. Likewise, we now believe that there is no salvation outside of the therapeutic domain and normally do not even doubt the very need for such a secular type of salvation.

The attitude of care and sacrifice involves intimacy unknown to the relationship between the sovereign and the individual subject. Such an intimate relationship is not the opposite of repressive power. On the contrary, it is a dispersed, indirect, and therefore more delicate form of it, which enables less noticeable and therefore less deniable, more everyday and therefore more pervasive forms of power. Pastoral power has become a substantial part of governance, directing individuals toward specifically defined psychological health and well-being associated with happiness.

The latest stage of the progress of medicalization and pastoral power is embodied in medical humanism, which "aims to provide health care with honesty, empathy, compassion, altruism, and respect to dignity and beliefs of the patients and their families."[23] One of the principles of medical humanism is the patient-centered approach. Such an approach seeks to establish egalitarian relations between patient and practitioner. It includes the patient into the medical relationship as a way of improving diagnosis and treatment. Diagnosis is supposed to be determined in the process of mutually engaging negotiation and consensus. Pastoral power gets more efficient in such a model since it is not an open manipulation but an implicit web of organization that does not require any control from the outside. Christopher Mayes points out that the doctor in modern patient-centered models of care still clearly resembles a pastoral power as described by Foucault. Even if the purpose of client-centered models is the empowerment of a client to move beyond hierarchical relations, it finds no escape from the trap of its latent hierarchical structure. As Mayes maintains,

> Despite the desire for the patient-centered relationship to be an egalitarian meeting of shared expertise, there is a strong tension between the physician's authoritative knowledge and the patient's experiential knowledge. As the patient approaches the physician, the physician will always be an authority and hold greater expertise in medical matters. This is not to deny the patient's role, but the relationship is always in favour towards the physician's authority and expertise as the patient implicitly recognises the physician as an authority and expert by making an appointment to meet with them. Thus, in the patient-centered approach it can be seen that the physician is an authority, albeit an uncomfortable one, that (to return to Foucault) "requires the confession, prescribes and appreciates it."[24]

The structure of the relationship between patient and practitioner, even if it uses a patient-centered approach, presupposes objectification by reducing the patient to the position of a sick person with a certain diagnosis, problem, or disability. Analyzing the contemporary form of medical power, in which the figure of medical authority is getting eliminated and dispersed by the common practice of self-analysis via the internet, Aisha Kamilah McGriff claims that, here too the principle of medical gaze itself is preserved. The medical gaze becomes internalized while getting more accessible, more dispersed, and therefore more consolidated.

McGriff agrees with the general modern convention that online availability of medical information increases patient autonomy and breaks down the hierarchy between patient and doctor. However, she disagrees that the patient gains full autonomy when they learn to use the medical gaze. She argues that there still remains a reinforcement of the doctor as the final authority, "Thus the patient becomes a type of assistant to the doctor: the patient can self-diagnose for minor ailments and can administer their own care; however, for more complex medical problems, those beyond the medical gaze of the consumer-patient, a doctor is still necessary to use their advanced level medical gaze to identify disease in the body."[25]

Although Foucault is critical of psychoanalysis and medical discourses, he is not trying to imply that there are evil therapeutic messiahs and good oppressed people in need of emancipation from them. The "messiahs" are equally oppressed by the social dynamics that produce them. One should not be misguided that modern pastoral care prevents or oppresses genuine social care and emancipatory self-understanding. Rather, Foucault's concept of pastoral power describes *the only* type of care known to us and therefore *the only* type of care we are currently capable of embodying. There is no other more genuine care outside of this structure. Trying to fight it we end up back in it again, maybe in its more dispersed, less visible manifestations. Discourses of medicine, psychology, and psychoanalysis, with their heritage of Christian ideology, are the only currently possible domains of care. Whenever we practice social care, when we care for our partners and children, when we try to be supportive friends, we end up being mediated by those discourses—perhaps, more or less critically, but never outside of this structure. It is known that Foucault himself, after critically refuting psychoanalysis, nonetheless recommended Freudian psychoanalysis to his young acquaintance.[26] Notwithstanding his pessimism, Foucault asserted a fundamental malleability of power regimes to be reshaped beyond recognition, though still not independently of their historical forms.

Freud's Tragic Psychoanalysis

One might claim that psychoanalysis exists simultaneously in its more conventional version and in a reshaped version of what it initially was. On one hand, Foucault was quite accurate in looking for the roots of psychoanalytic practice in religious morality. Psychoanalysis, being the origin of therapeutic culture, was in a deeply ambiguous relationship with religion, both supplementary and conflicting. Psychoanalysis uses a quasi-religious self-referential jargon and scientifically suspicious techniques. It presents itself both as a care for the soul and a source of truth. Freud himself is known for his messianic attitude, a desire to relieve human suffering, though this is oddly mixed with misanthropic views. For instance, in his early years he wrote to his bride Martha Bernays about his expectations from a travel grant to study under Charcot (not without self-irony): "Oh, how wonderful it will be! I am coming with money . . . and then go on to Paris and become a great scholar and then come back to Vienna with a huge, enormous halo, and then we will soon get married, and I will cure all the incurable nervous cases."[27]

Freud often corresponded with Oskar Pfister, a Protestant minister who was interested in psychoanalysis as an aid to his pastoral work. Despite his openly anti-religious views, Freud seems to have encouraged Pfister's idea of combining a ministry practice and psychoanalysis. At that time, perhaps because he was interested in expanding ways of converting people to the new practice, Freud did not see a contradiction in combining psychoanalysis with religious methods. Freud writes, "Our capacity for expansion in the medical profession is unfortunately very limited and it is important to secure a footing elsewhere where we can."[28] He also recognized that his goals coincided with Pfister's: "We know that by different routes we aspire to the same objectives for poor humanity."[29]

When considering Foucault's attitude toward psychoanalysis, perhaps one should also give credit to another Freud, one with a less messianic and more tragic version of psychoanalysis. Freud was often presented as having two guises; he himself fought what he simultaneously promoted. Freud gradually became more disillusioned, pessimistic, and self-doubting. For the later Freud, the pleasure principle started to seem far from being exhaustive, if not erroneous in describing humans. Because the phenomena associated with mental suffering (such as repetition of traumatic experience, instead of forgetting and avoidance of painful memories) did not fit into the conception of humans as pleasure seekers, in his later works Freud started to look for another principle that governs mental life—the one beyond the pleasure principle. This search would ultimately lead him to consider the concept of the death drive, previously suggested by the psychoanalyst Sabina Spielrein. Thus, contrary to his initial intuition, by using the concept of the death drive, Freud suggested that human beings might also be driven by the repetition of suffering and refraining from pleasure. In relation to this Freud also implied that it is not possible to draw a sharp line between what is called normal or "healthy" and neurotic, or as he put it more directly, "We are all somewhat hysterical."[30]

The problem we now face is that the practice of psychoanalysis, as well as our routine therapeutic strategies, are still based on Freud's early understanding of humans as seekers of happiness. As Freud himself showed, this view is unsustainable upon further scrutiny. Some types of psychotherapy, like existential psychotherapy, while recognizing the semblance of a Freudian death drive, still sees it as a pathological though inevitable part of human nature. Though therapeutic approaches differ in techniques, the goal of a return to the supposedly natural state of pleasure still goes largely unchallenged.

When psychoanalysis was already well established, Freud more openly stated both his anti-religious and anti-medical views. In 1928 he wrote to Pfister, "I do not know if you have detected the secret link between [*The Question of*] *Lay Analysis* and the [*The Future of an*] *Illusion*. In the former I wish to protect analysis from the doctors and in the latter from the priests. I should like to hand it over to a profession which does not yet exist, a profession of lay curers of souls who need not be doctors and should not be priests."[31] In *The*

Question of Lay Analysis Freud claims, "We do not consider it at all desirable for psychoanalysis to be swallowed up by medicine and to find its last resting place in a textbook of psychiatry under the heading of 'Methods of Treatment.'"[32]

Indeed, in America, psychoanalysis became a part of the medical establishment as a result of "assimilation" into the American scene.[33] Turkle explained that Freudianism was brought in line with American beliefs about the virtue and necessity of an optimistic approach. These revisions of Freud focused on adaptation to a reality whose justice was rarely challenged. As Turkle wrote, "in America, medical professionalization contributed to defusing much of what was most radical in [Freud's] vision."[34]

There is a rumor that Freud, on his way to America, said, "they don't realize we are bringing them the plague."[35] A possible interpretation is that Freud was placing psychoanalysis on the side of the plague,[36] as opposed to the goal of health and salvation. It is not the goal of cure, health, or happiness that defines this version of psychoanalysis. One might doubt that it even has any goals or intentions at all, but the sure thing is that, same as the plague, it can painfully disrupt our illusions that secure a semblance of smooth daily and social lives.

Therapy Without Messiahs

This all probably means that the equation of happiness and positive affect with mental health and normality is not the best idea, not only during pandemics but also possibly for eternity until death do us apart. Instead of persecuting ourselves and others with the unsatisfiable demand to be happy and stay positive, perhaps we should rather be more attentive to the devalued voice of psychological suffering like sadness and anxiety. It does not feel good, it does not sound enthusiastic, it will not make anyone happier either, but it could have something important to say. When you think about it, we have nothing else to share, at least nothing more sincere, than our psychological suffering. Happiness always has a tint of a lie and insincerity in it; it disconnects. Everyone's life is hiding sadness and pain behind the veil of positivity. The only way we can truly get in touch with others is first to get in touch with this universally shared collective aspect of our lives. Involvement in togetherness and supporting others comes with acknowledging their suffering. It is tempting to say that the voice of suffering must be heard so that we can do something to eliminate its causes. But there are so many reasons for suffering that we can do nothing about, and there are even more reasons for which we do not know what we should do. Maybe one of the problems is that we rush too fast into the framework of help, solutions, and healing, instead of dwelling in support and understanding—the basics for any possible help and solutions. We should be careful here, understanding that sharing of suffering with an explicit or implicit demand or expectation to completely relieve it does not count as proper sharing. This would be falling into a vicious circle of the pursuit of happiness burden with its oppressiveness.

The possible way out (or rather just "a way," since a way out is normally associated with a single positive outcome and a happy ending) would not be to oppose therapeutic culture but rather to more fully embrace it. Let us say such a culture will remain therapeutic, but this time without messiahs, only with permanently mentally unwell and vulnerable people having (sadly) realized that they have no one to rely on except each other. It would be a therapeutic culture of those who are not relying on an expert's prescriptions but who are persisting together in a state of confusion and shared suffering. This time, we would not be mutually objectifying each other by reducing ourselves and others to their mental disorder diagnosis. None of us is a messiah, no one knows precisely how the psychologically healthy human being or a human collective looks. It is this despair of not knowing that truly unites people—not the hope and reliance on someone as bearer of truth and bringer of happiness to the world. Such a therapeutic culture would not contradict the existence of medicine, psychiatry, and psychology; their development was always associated with their critical self-doubt. This therapeutic society will not be a happy society, but it will be more equal, inclusive, and supportive, which requires the discipline of shared suffering, not the anticipation of joy.

Such a therapeutic culture would be our Mapo Bridge, that will forever remain the bridge of death, the place where we are vanishing from the earth, not toward heaven and salvation but toward nowhere (let us face it, each of us is born to die). It is not the choice between the happy ending and the sad ending. It will not end up well, for sure. The choice is whether we are going through the bridge of suffering together or suffering separately.

NOTES

1. Casey Baseel, "Seoul Anti-Suicide Initiative Backfires, Deaths Increase by More Than Six Times," SoraNews24, February 2014, https://soranews24.com/2014/02/26/seoul-anti-suicide -initiative-backfires-deaths-increase-over-than-six-times/.

2. "What Is Depression?," ADAA.org, 2000. https://adaa.org/understanding-anxiety/ depression.

3. Slavoj Žižek, *The Metastases of Enjoyment: On Women and Causality* (London: Verso, 2005), 16.

4. Slavoj Žižek, *The Parallax View* (Cambridge, MA: MIT Press, 2009), 304.

5. Slavoj Žižek, "Happiness? No, Thanks!" *The Philosophical Salon*, April 2018, http://thephilosophicalsalon.com/happiness-no-thanks/.

6. Steven Moffic, "Life, Liberty, and the Pursuit of Happiness—In Spite of the Pandemic," *Psychiatric Times*, August 4, 2020, https://www.psychiatrictimes.com/view/life-liberty-pursuit-happiness-spite-pandemic.

7. Alenka Zupančič, *The Odd One In: On Comedy* (London: MIT Press, 2008), 5.

8. E. P. M. Brouwers et al., "Discrimination in the Workplace, Reported by People with Major Depressive Disorder: A Cross-Sectional Study in 35 Countries," *BMJ Open* 6, no. 2 (Feb 2016): 1–8.

9. Allen Frances, "The New Somatic Symptom Disorder in DSM-5 Risks Mislabeling Many People as Mentally Ill," *BMJ* 346, no. 3 (March 2013): f1580.

10. Russ Harris, *The Happiness Trap* (London: Robinson, 2008); Jonathan W Schooler, Dan Ariely, and George Loewenstein, "The Pursuit and Assessment of Happiness Can be Self-defeating" in *The Psychology of Economic Decisions*, ed. Isabelle Brocas and Juan D. Carrillo (Oxford: Oxford University Press, 2003); Anders Dræby Sørensen, "The Paradox of Modern Suffering," *The Journal for Research in Sickness and Society* 13, (2010): 131–159.

11. Allan V. Horwitz and Jerome Wakefield, *The Loss of Sadness: How Psychiatry Transformed Normal Sorrow into Depressive Disorder* (New York: Oxford University Press, 2007), 225.

12. Horwitz and Wakefield, *Loss of Sadness*, 225.

13. Horwitz and Wakefield, *Loss of Sadness*, 213.

14. Erin Schumaker, "Depression Rates Tripled During the Pandemic: Study," *ABC News*, September 2, 2020, https://abcnews.go.com/Health/depression-rates-tripled-pandemic-study/story?id=72724832.

15. "Mental Health & COVID-19," World Health Organization, accessed February 4, 2021, https://www.who.int/teams/mental-health-and-substance-use/mental-health-and-covid-19.

16. Lauren Berlant, *Cruel Optimism* (Raleigh, NC: Duke University Press, 2011).

17. Sørensen, "Paradox of Modern Suffering," 142.

18. Sørensen, "Paradox of Modern Suffering," 147.

19. Michel Foucault, *The Birth of The Clinic* (London: Routledge, 2012), 36.

20. Michel Foucault, "The Subject and Power," in *Michel Foucault: Beyond Structuralism and Hermeneutics*, eds. Hubert L. Dreyfus and Paul Rabinow (Chicago: University of Chicago Press, 1983), 214.

21. Michel Foucault, *Security, Territory, Population* (Basingstoke: Palgrave Macmillan, 2009), 224.

22. Foucault, "Subject and Power," 215.

23. Mohey Hulail, "Humanism in Medical Practice: What, Why and How?" *Hospice and Palliative Medicine International Journal* 2, no. 6 (2018): 2336–2339.

24. Christopher Mayes, "Pastoral Power and the Confessing Subject in Patient-Centred Communication," *Bioethical Inquiry* 6 (2009): 490.

25. Aisha McGriff, "Healthy Bodies Matter: Analysis of the Disclosure of Race and Health Care on WebMD.com," PhD Diss. (University of Bowling Green, 2015).

26. James Miller, *The Passion of Michel Foucault* (London: Harper Collins, 1993), 42.

27. Sigmund Freud, "Letter from Sigmund Freud to Martha Bernays, June 20, 1885," in *Letters of Sigmund Freud 1873-1939*, ed. Ernst L. Freud (London: Hogarth, 1961), 154–155.

28. Sigmund Freud, "Letter from Sigmund Freud to Oskar Pfister, May 2, 1912," The International Psycho-Analytical Library, https://www.pep-web.org/document.php?id=ipl.059.0055a.

29. Freud, "Letter from Sigmund Freud to Oskar Pfister, May 2, 1912."

30. Sigmund Freud, *Three Contributions to the Theory of Sex* (New York: Nervous and Mental Disease Publishing Co: 1920), 34.

31. Sigmund Freud, "Letter from Sigmund Freud to Oskar Pfister, November 25, 1928," The International Psycho-Analytical Library, https://www.pep-web.org/document.php?id=ipl.059 .0125a.

32. Cited in Russel Jacoby, "When Freud Came to America," *Chronicle of Higher Education*, September 21, 2009, https://www.chronicle.com/article/when-freud-came-to-america/.

33. Russel Jacoby, *Social Amnesia. A Critique of Conformist Psychology from Adler to Laing* (Boston: Beacon Press, 2018); and Sherry Turkle, *Psychoanalytic Politics: Freud's French Revolution* (New York: Basic Books, 1978).

34. Turkle, *Psychoanalytic Politics*, 150.

35. Cited in Duane Rousselle, "The Truth About Coronavirus" in *Coronavirus, Psychoanalysis, and Philosophy: Conversations on Pandemics, Politics, and Society*, eds. Fernando Castrillón and Thomas Marchevsky (London: Routledge, 2021), 140.

36. Rousselle, "The Truth About Coronavirus," 140.

Afterword

*Time and time again stories are told about the survival strategies
folks use to maintain a sense of hope in desperate life-threatening
situations of oppression, dehumanization, and violence. . . . I first
heard such stories listening to Baba talk about living in slavery and
beyond. She talked about hearing about the hardships, experiencing them as a girl, and she talked about the role of quiltmaking as
both a functional necessity of life . . . , but also she told stories about
the life-sustaining energy of the imagination, the artistry behind the
creation of quilts.*[1]

bell hooks

As this volume attests, there are many paths by which one can approach, discuss, and make sense of anxiety. Citing one of the most horrendous aspects
of human history—slavery—which is intrinsically tied to what facilitated it—
colonialism—might jolt our moral imaginary out of any conceivable proportion. Luckily for us, there were courageous and beautiful souls like bell hooks
who, out of such inconceivable tragedies, managed to retrieve and even build
meaningful bridges which, failing a solution, could at least come close to help
us "speak about it" and try to bring a modicum of human value where one ex-
pects none.

Retracing the experience of slavery and colonialism through expressions of
belonging sounds "safe" enough to argue that even when, as in quiltmaking,
we begin to piece the fragments of a historic contingency together,[2] we also
realize that in such an understanding we are bound to *curate* the anxiety that
marks this fragmentary recognition. Quiltmaking, particularly that which
hooks refers to, embraces (by articulating) the fragmentary. Since the quilts of
the Gee's Bend made it to the official space of the art world,[3] many have realized that far from just making blankets for a loved one, quiltmaking was an act
of resistance in the face of the horror of slavery.

While it is inconceivable to think that any sense of belonging could be
recouped from such horror (let alone anxiety), quiltmakers like hooks's
grandma Baba did find a way out of slavery's attempt to annihilate her human

dignity. Not without paradox, the subsequent curation of these quilts as works of art became symbolic of another form of coping with history's anxiety—this time, in the act of curation itself.

To curate is to arrange and edit, to put together by way of making sense of contingent events and random situations that were never meant, or allowed, to make a coherent whole. Baba made a coherent sense of her life through quiltmaking, but she never meant to curate her life of strife and suffering. Like art, history presents us with such forms of curation. Yet under the pretext of teaching and understanding, history's curation has a habit of papering the cracks and gaps of historic contingency with the aim of presenting knowledge as a form of certainty.

As Abdulrazak Gurnah has noted, "[T]hey left too many spaces unattended to, could not in the nature of things do anything about them, so in time gaping holes began to appear in the story. It began to fray and unravel under assault, and a grumbling retreat was unavoidable. Though that was not the end of stories. There was still Suez to come, and the inhumanities of the Congo and Uganda, and other bitter bloodlettings in small places."[4]

In *By the Sea*, Gurnah recalls his history lessons back in his childhood home in Zanzibar. Through his novel's character, he describes how history was curated in its schooled imaginary. Such forms of historical curation recall one's own colonial experience as a subject of someone else's history that is imposed on one's own personal story. Even when not enslaved and reduced to become someone else's property, history was never made one's own. It belonged to the colonialist. Schooled by the colonialist, this was a history that *curated* anxiety by a curricular covering of "too many spaces [left] unattended to."

"Then it would seem that the British had been doing us nothing but good compared to the brutalities we could visit on ourselves. Their good, though, was steeped in irony. They told us about the nobility of resisting tyranny in the classroom and then applied a curfew after sunset, or sent pamphleteers for independence to prison for sedition. Never mind, they did drain the creeks, and improve the sewage system and bring vaccines and the radio. Their departure seemed so sudden in the end, precipitate and somehow petulant."[5]

In contemporary scholarship, the word *archive* often comes to mind as scholars from several disciplines seek to compensate for the lagging conversations by which we helplessly try to make sense of a world afflicted by internalized forms of anxiety. Opening his long discussion of the archive, Derrida reminds us that archives are forms of *domiciliation*.[6] Gathering an archive is a *homed* event, and those who keep the archive are the holders of its interpre-

tation. The archive extends to a horizon of phenomena in whose manifestation we curate the disparate by embracing the paradoxical—what Gurnah
identifies in the colonialist's "good . . . steeped in irony." However, while the
notion of a curated anxiety culture might offer some ironic solace, beyond
such a desideratum of domestication, the rise of anti-politics, populist nationalism, and authoritarianism reveals once more a series of gaps that come
back to haunt us.

In Gurnah's history lessons the colonial narrative was aimed to cover the
gaps and normalize the irony. Those who grew up learning such stories would
recognize how they were embedded in the sense of the familiar through faith,
country, and tradition.[7] The familiar *evens out* all the gaps and history's curation of what is odd and foreign becomes complete. The colonialist's aim was
always intent on justifying the curfew after sunset and legitimizing the sedi-
tionist's arrest.

To reveal the gaps over which anxiety has become gradually socially and
culturally normalized, one seeks a way out of an existential impasse through
acts of estrangement. Curating, just like archiving, implies an outside. "There
is no archive without a place of consignation, without a technique of repetition, and without a certain exteriority."[8] However, to the educator's mind, what
remains out—what is *estranged*—presents an opportunity. The same happens
in art, where a body of work previously considered as "outsider art," like the
quilts of Gee's Bend, opened a world of unexpected perspectives.

To embrace the unexpected is to become a stranger in neighborhoods that
were hitherto closer to home. This comes akin to what Maxine Greene, after
Jean Paul Sartre, regards as the realm of the imagination. As Sartre used to say,
we cannot imagine something that is already in front of us.[9] Pedagogically
speaking, Greene turns this on its head.[10] "To take a stranger's vantage point
on everyday reality," she argued, "is to look inquiringly and wonderingly on
the world in which one lives. It is like returning home from a long stay in some
other place. The homecomer notices details and patterns in his environment
he never saw before. (. . .) To make it meaningful again, he must interpret and
reorder what he sees in the light of his changed experience. He must consciously engage in inquiry."[11]

Becoming strangers to our curated anxieties becomes key to how we can
counter the curation of anxiety by forfeiting the comforts of certainty. To become a stranger is to embrace uncertainty and make of it a method of counter-
curation, and in Baba's case, an act of resistance. Only the estranged would
occasion us with an opportunity to embrace the paradox of certainty itself,

which is to say that only as willed strangers could we recognize the pitfalls of a curated anxiety culture by identifying history's gaps and fragments.

As willed strangers we remain open to the unexpected by seeking the error—just as Socrates suggests in the *Meno*[12] when he demonstrates how learning comes from that moment of aporia where nothing seems to make sense anymore. Some think this causes anxiety, but Kierkegaard sees this as an *occasion* for learning. "If the Teacher serves as an occasion by means of which the learner is reminded, he cannot help the learner to recall that he really knows the Truth; for the learner is in a state of Error. What the Teacher can give him occasion to remember is, that he is in Error."[13] The occasion of error suggests a *practice*—a form of knowing, doing, and making—that hosts an occasion that prompts our imagination, and by which one moves out of a curated anxiety. Just like Baba's quilting, this practice will piece it all together.[14]

Kierkegaard invites us to "consider the dialectical determinations of anxiety." "Anxiety," he argues, "is a sympathetic antipathy and an antipathetic sympathy."[15] Moving this away from "inordinate desire" (*concupiscentia*), he argues that we can speak of a "pleasing anxiety, a pleasing anxiousness [*Beængstelse*], and of a strange anxiety, a bashful anxiety, etc." The take on original sin (which out of its theological contexts, one could rearticulate as a source of existential anxiety), one could see how the dialectical determinations of which Kierkegaard speaks come close to a curated state where what is sympathetic merges into the antipathetic by dint of what is normalized. Here, anxiety and anxiety culture become implicit to our existence as its inherent *practice*.

In the process of the imagination, we are prompted to *represent*—that is, present twice over—what we expect to be presented with. This warrants a different order and place for the *practice* of anxiety outside its curated state. As a site of gaps, anxiety culture is turned into a practice that hosts the spaces left behind by the certainties and histories which have hitherto colonized our imagination. This is where I see this compelling volume as an opportunity by which we engage with what elsewhere I have called the *uncolonial*,[16] that is, a space that moves beyond the declared locations of a post- and precolonial narrative (both of which, incidentally, have conveniently curated the anxieties of historical contingency), and where, as willed strangers, we reaffirm a sense of belonging that becomes akin to Baba and her quiltmaking.

John Baldacchino

NOTES

1. bell hooks, *Belonging. A Culture of Place* (New York: Routledge, 2009), 163.
2. Agnes Heller, *A Philosophy of History in Fragments* (Oxford: Blackwell, 1993).
3. William Arnett et al., *The Quilts of Gee's Bend* (Atlanta, GA: Tinwood Books, 2002).
4. Abdulrazak Gurnah, *By the Sea* (London: Bloomsbury, 2001), 18.
5. Gurnah, *By the Sea*, 19.
6. Jacques Derrida, *Archive Fever. A Freudian Impression* (Chicago: University of Chicago Press, 1996), 2ff.
7. See John Baldacchino and Faisal Abdu'Allah, "Doing Art, (Un)Colonized Bodies. Immersing Curricula in Our Acts of Living," in *Expanding Inclusive Learning in Primary Classrooms and Schools*, eds. Kristine Black-Hawkins and Ashley Grinham-Smith (London: Routledge, 2022).
8. Derrida, *Archive Fever*, 11.
9. Jean Paul Sartre, *The Psychology of Imagination* (New York: Philosophical Library, 1948).
10. Maxine Greene, *Teacher as Stranger: Educational Philosophy for the Modern Age* (Belmont, CA: Wadsworth Publishing, 1973).
11. Greene, *Teacher as Stranger*, 267–268.
12. Plato, *Five Dialogues. Euthyphro, Apology, Crito, Meno, Phaedo* (Indianapolis, IN: Hackett, 2002).
13. Soren Kierkegaard, *Philosophical Fragments, or A Fragment of Philosophy by Johannes Climacus* (Princeton: Princeton University Press, 1974), 17.
14. hooks, *Belonging*, 162–168.
15. Soren Kierkegaard, *The Concept of Anxiety* (Princeton: Princeton University Press, 1980), 42.
16. John Baldacchino, "Resemblance, Choice and the Hidden: Mediterranean Aesthetics and the Political 'Logics' of an Uncolonial Subjective Economy," in *Critically Mediterranean: Aesthetics, Theory, Hermeneutics, Culture*, eds. Yasser Elhariry and Edwige Tamalet Talbayev (Cham, Switzerland: Palgrave Macmillan, 2018)

History of Meetings of the Anxiety Culture Project

June 2015	Christian Albrechts University of Kiel, IPN Leibniz Institute for Science and Mathematics Education at Kiel University, and Teachers College, Columbia University "Come-Into-Touch" Conference at Kiel University
June 2016	Kieler Woche (Kiel Week) Symposium at Kiel University
August 2017	Hamburg Foundation Lubeck Conference at Gut Siggen on "The Perception of Social Threats and Crisis in Public Life and Education"
February 2018	International Workshop on "Anxiety Culture" at Columbia University
November 2018	International Workshop on "Living and Learning in a World of Anxieties" at Kiel University
May 2019	German Conference on "Anxiety Culture—Beyond Fear" at Gut Siggen
June 2019	Council for European Studies International Conference of Europeanists Panel on "Euro-Anxiety? Anxiety

	Discourses in European Education, Literature, Politics, and Public Health" at Madrid
November 2019	"Night of the Profs" Symposium on "Angst Macht Kultur" (Anxiety Power Culture) at Kiel University
December 2019	International Workshop on "Varieties of Anxiety—A Global Perspective" at New York University
September 2020	Digital Theme Day "Everyday Racism—Solidarity and Creativity Against Everyday Discrimination of Different Social Groups" at Kiel University
October 2022	Expert Talk on "Anxiety Index 2025: Understanding Citizens—Protecting People" at the Representation of Schleswig-Holstein, Berlin

The Editors

DR. JOHN ALLEGRANTE is the inaugural Charles Irwin Lambert professor of
health behavior and education at Teachers College, Columbia University, where
he has been a member of the faculty since 1979 and has served as department
chair, deputy provost, and associate vice president for international affairs.
He has held appointments in sociomedical sciences at the Mailman School of
Public Health and in the Graduate School of Arts and Sciences at Columbia,
and has been a visiting professor at several universities in Europe and Asia.

An applied behavioral scientist, Dr. Allegrante's research has focused on investigating new approaches to understanding, predicting, and intervening on
the barriers and facilitators of behavioral self-management of chronic diseases.
He also has written extensively about epistemological, theoretical, and methodological issues, as well as research-to-practice translation in the science of
health promotion. He began collaborating with Icelandic behavioral and social
scientists at Reykjavik University in the early 2000s on research that has investigated risks and protective factors for substance use, including the impact of
COVID-19 on mental health, among children and adolescents. He is a cofounder of the Anxiety Culture research project.

Allegrante was a W. K. Kellogg Foundation national fellow and postdoctoral
Pew policy career development fellow in health policy at the RAND Corporation. A past president of the Society for Public Health Education and an editor emeritus of *Health Education & Behavior*, he has been a fellow of the New
York Academy of Medicine, the Academy of Behavioral Medicine Research,
and the Society of Behavioral Medicine. Dr. Allegrante is the recipient of numerous awards, including Fulbright and Erasmus awards, an honorary doctorate from the State University of New York, and the 2017 CDC Foundation

Elizabeth Fries Health Education Award for his contributions to the fields of behavioral science and health education as a researcher, academician, and ambassador.

DR. ULRICH HOINKES is a professor of Romance studies and teacher education at the Christian Albrechts University of Kiel, Germany. He has made numerous research contributions during his academic career as a Romance philologist (French, Spanish, Italian, Catalan, and Occitan) and as a linguist specializing in semantics, history of linguistic thought, variety linguistics, language sociology, and minority languages.

After studying Romance philology, German philology, and general linguistics at the University of Münster, he received his doctorate in 1990 with a thesis on philosophy and grammar in the French Enlightenment, which was awarded the Doctoral Thesis Prize of the University of Münster and the Strasbourg Prize of the F.V.S. Foundation of Hamburg. He subsequently habilitated in 1999 with an empirically based thesis on bilingualism and technical language use in regionally relevant fields of work that was funded by the German Research Foundation (revised online edition, 2018). During his studies and between academic promotions, he spent extended periods in Spain, France, and Belgium, where he did extensive empirical field research on social multilingualism and was a visiting professor at the Multilingualism Research Centre of the Katholieke Universiteit Brussel (1998–1999).

Since his appointment at Kiel University, he has turned attention to education and foreign language didactics, becoming director of the Centre on Humanities in Education at Kiel University in cooperation with the IPN Leibniz Institute for Science and Mathematics Education in Kiel. As a university teacher, Hoinkes built long-term projects on student filmmaking, international exchange in teacher education, the social responsibility of professional education, and the creation of artistic performances (jazz, spoken word) with students. Since 2015, he has been energetically dedicated to building the international and interdisciplinary Anxiety Culture research project in collaboration with Teachers College, Columbia University, where he was a visiting scholar during the 2017–2018 academic year.

DR. MICHAEL SCHAPIRA, an independent scholar, is an adjunct professor of philosophy at Saint Joseph's University in Philadelphia, Pennsylvania. He has taught at a number of institutions of higher education, including Hofstra University, Rutgers University, Columbia University, Ursinus College, and the School of Advanced Studies in Tyumen, Russia. He also has a keen interest in teaching philosophy at the pre-college level, which he has done at the Brooklyn Free School and for the Johns Hopkins University's Center for Talented Youth.

Dr. Schapira's research interests fall into three fields of inquiry. As a philosopher of education with an interest in history, he has written on the intellectual and institutional foundations of the modern research university, which emanated out of Germany in the early 19th century. A central part of this story is the prevalence of "crisis of the university" narratives that mark key periods of institutional transformation. This has led to a secondary interest in the interplay between narrative conventions and policy debates, with a particular focus on the relationship between crisis and theories of tragedy. His third field of inquiry, represented in this volume, has been developed in collaboration with linguists, behavioral scientists, education scholars, and anthropologists in the Anxiety Culture research project. His scholarly work has been published in the *Journal of Philosophy of Education*, the *Oxford Research Encyclopedia of Education*, the *Journal of Educational Controversy*, the *Philosophy of Education Yearbook*, and *Europe Now*.

He is the author of *University in Crisis: From the Middle Ages to the University of Excellence* (Rowman & Littlefield, 2023). In addition to his scholarly work, Dr. Schapira is an editor of *Full Stop*, a Whiting Award-winning journal of literature and culture.

DR. KAREN STRUVE holds the professorship in Franco-Romance and literary studies at Bremen University in Germany. She has also taught at the Christian Albrechts University of Kiel, where she has worked as the research manager for the Anxiety Culture research project, and at the Technical University of Dresden, where she held the professorship in Francophone Literature and cultural studies. Dr. Struve's research and scholarship focuses on Francophone Literature (18th to 21st century) and French theory.

In the field of cultural theory, her main research interests lie in the field of postcolonial, transcultural and poststructuralist literary and cultural theory, in epistemology, and in the cultural theories of anxiety. She is the cofounder of research projects dealing with New Approaches to Reception and Transmission of Literature (Literaturvermittlung hoch[3]), and with Imaginations of the North in Francophone and Italian Literature. Her scholarly works have been published in both German and French volumes. These include the monographs, *Écriture Transculturelle Beur. Die Beur-Literatur als Laboratorium Transkultureller Identitätsfiktionen* (*Cross-Cultural Writing Beur. Beur-Literature as Laboratory of Transcultural Fictions of Identity*, 2009); *Zur Aktualität von*

Homi K. Bhabha. Einleitung in sein Werk (Introduction to the Work of Homi K. Bhabha, 2013); and *Wildes Wissen in der Encyclopédie. Koloniale Alterität, Wissen und Narration in der Französischen Aufklärung (Wild Knowledge in the Encylcopédie. Colonial Alterity, Knowledge and Narration in French Enlightenment,* 2020).

Dr. Struve was a research fellow on the Mare Balticum Fellowship of the University of Rostock. In recognition of her scholarly work, she was awarded the Germaine de Staël Prize from the Association of French Studies (Frankoromanistenverband) in 2008 and the Elise Richter Prize from the Association of Romance Studies Scholars in 2019.

The Contributors

KRISTINA ALLGOEWER, a molecular biologist and public health scientist, is a scientific project manager in the Institute of Legal Medicine at the University Medical Center Hamburg-Eppendorf.

BRYNDIS BJORK ASGEIRSDOTTIR, a psychologist whose research has focused on sexually abusive youth, victimization, and adolescent substance use, is professor and dean of the School of Social Sciences at Reykjavik University.

JOHN BALDACCHINO, a philosopher of education and the author of 14 books, the most recent being *Educing Ivan Illich: Reform, Contingency and Disestablishment* (Peter Lang, 2020), is professor of art and education at the University of Wisconsin-Madison.

CHRISTINE BLAETTLER is a professor of philosophy specializing in the history and philosophy of science and technology at the Christian Albrects University of Kiel. She is the author of books and articles on the tradition of cultural science around 1900.

MICHEL BOURBAN is assistant professor of environmental ethics at the University of Twente. His research focuses on sustainability ethics, eco-anxiety, climate justice, and ecological and cosmopolitan citizenship.

DOMINIC BOYER, a cultural anthropologist, writer, and filmmaker whose work focuses on relationships between energy and environment, media and politics, teaches at Rice University.

EVA J. DAUSSÀ is a senior lecturer at the University of Amsterdam whose scholarly interests include linguistic phenomena associated with multilingualism and the dynamics of the social, political, and psychological realities of complex linguistic ecologies.

NICHOLAS FREUDENBERG, the author of *At What Cost: Modern Capitalism and the Future of Health* (Oxford University Press, 2021), is distinguished professor of public health at the City University of New York Graduate School of Public Health and Health Policy.

MONICA VAN DER HAAGEN-WULFF, a social and literary theorist with interests in communication and media, is a lecturer in the Institute for Educational Research and Social Science at the University of Cologne.

KELSEY HUDSON chairs the Youth Subcommittee and serves on the Steering Committee through the Climate Psychology Alliance—North America. She is a practicing child/adolescent clinical psychologist whose work focuses on the mental health impacts of climate change on young people.

KARENA KALMBACH, a specialist in social and cultural history of technology and the environment, is the author of *The Meanings of a Disaster: Chernobyl and its Afterlives in Britain and France* (Berghahn Books, 2021). She is head of strategy and content at the FUTURIUM in Berlin.

EMMANUEL KATTAN, a Canadian philosopher and the author of four novels in French and an essay on the politics of memory, is the director of the Alliance Program at Columbia University.

MARKUS LEMMENS, an editor, publisher, and founder and CEO of three companies (media, software, energy), currently manages a deep technology consortium that is bringing growth-critical topics into application through scientific knowledge and technology transfer.

ERIC LEWANDOWSKI is a clinical associate professor in child and adolescent psychiatry at New York University. He is a coauthor of *The Lancet* report, "Young People's Voices on Climate Anxiety, Government Betrayal and Moral Injury: A Global Phenomenon."

RAPHAËL LIOGIER is a professor of sociology and philosophy at the Institut d'études politiques d'Aix-en-Provence and a research scholar at the University of Paris 10.

ROMAN MAREK, the former scientific coordinator for the Future of Medicine interdisciplinary research group at the Berlin-Brandenburg Academy of Sciences and Humanities, is the director of the charitable German Sepsis Foundation.

CHRISTIAN MARTIN, a professor of comparative politics at the Christian Albrechts University of Kiel, German, held the Max Weber Visiting Chair in German and European Studies at New York University from 2016 to 2021.

PAUL MECHERIL, formerly director of the Centre for Migration, Education and Cultural Studies at Carl von Ossietzky University, where he developed his interest in migration and education, is professor of education at Bielefeld University.

ANGELIKA MESSNER, a sinologist specializing in the history of medicine, is professor and head of the China Centre at the Christian Albrechts University of Kiel and is an author and editor of *Civilizing Emotions: Concepts in Nineteenth Century Asia and Europe* (Oxford University Press, 2015).

CAINE C. A. MEYERS, an instructor and undergraduate thesis supervisor at Reykjavik University, has held various alternative-academic positions. His research has focused on adolescent health and well-being.

JULIE MOSTOV, whose scholarship focuses on national identity, sovereignty, and citizenship, is professor and dean of Liberal Studies at New York University and author of the book, *Soft Borders: Rethinking Sovereignty and Democracy* (Palgrave Macmillan, 2008).

DIRK NABERS is professor of international political sociology at the Christian Albrechts University of Kiel and the author of *A Poststructuralist Discourse Theory of Global Politics* (Palgrave Macmillan, 2015).

FRAUKE NEES, a professor of psychology at the Christian Albrechts University of Kiel, is director of the Institute of Medical Psychology and Medical Sociology at the University Medical Center Schleswig-Holstein.

KONRAD OTT, a philosopher whose scholarly interests in discourse analysis and ethical theory of sustainable environments and climate change, is professor of philosophy at the Christian Albrechts University of Kiel.

SONALI RAJAN, a professor of health education at Teachers College, Columbia University, and founding president of the Research Society for the Prevention of Firearm-Related Harms, is a school violence prevention researcher.

JULIE RESHE, a philosopher and psychoanalyst, is currently a visiting professor at the University College Cork and University College Dublin director of the Institute of Psychoanalysis at the Global Center for Advanced Studies.

BÀRBARA ROVIRÓ is a lecturer in the Department of Languages and Literatures at the University of Bremen and works as a teacher educator in the field of Romance languages. Her research focuses on sociolinguistic issues in multilingual society and particularly in educational institutions.

RENATA SALECL, a Slovene philosopher, sociologist and legal theorist, is a senior researcher at the Institute of Criminology, Faculty of Law, at the University of Ljubljana, and holds a professorship at Birkbeck College, University of London. She is the author of *A Passion for Ignorance: What We Choose Not to Know and Why* (Princeton University Press, 2020).

INGA DORA SIGFUSDOTTIR is scientific director of the Icelandic Centre for Social Research and Analysis, a professor at Reykjavik University, and an honorary research professor at Teachers College, Columbia University. She studies healthy adolescent development.

FRANK A. STENGEL is a research fellow with the Research Group on International Political Sociology at the Christian Albrechts University of Kiel and author of *The Politics of Military Force: Antimilitarism, Ideational Change and Post-Cold War German Security Discourse* (University of Michigan Press, 2020).

INGIBJORG EVA THORISDOTTIR is the chief analytics and advisory officer for Planet Youth and teaches at Reykjavik University. Her research focuses on adolescent mental health, substance use, and the impact of social media and technology in the lives of young people.

MAREN URNER is a neuroscientist and professor of media psychology at the Media University of Applied Sciences in Cologne. She has written three bestselling books and focuses on effective communication, especially in the field of sustainability and transformation.

IRIS WIECZOREK is a senior research fellow at the German Institute for Global and Area Studies (GIGA) in Hamburg and GIGA Representative in Japan. Her research focuses on comparative assessment of the Japanese research and innovation system.

ZHAO XUDONG is professor for psychology and psychiatry and managing director of the Division of Humanities in Medicine and Behavioural Science at Tongji University, Shanghai.

LIYA YU, a political scientist and freelance writer based in Taipei and Berlin, is the author of *Vulnerable Minds: The Neuropolitics of Divided Societies* (Columbia University Press, 2022) and co-editor of the forthcoming *Routledge Handbook on Neuropolitics*.

illiberalism: and cognition, 13, 15, 17, 22; Illich, Ivan, 2; and immigration, 245, 249; rise of, 46, 245, 249, 321–22. *See also* right-wing parties
imaginaries, 284
immigration: and belonging, 186, 190, 192–93, 195, 197–205, 243; deaths, 193, 195, 203, 205; dehumanization of immigrants, 20, 201–2; democracy and migration crisis, 186–87, 243–51; economic refugees, 192–93, 244; and fantasy discourse and Trumpism, 330–31; fears of migrants, 185–87, 189–206, 215–16; immigrants' support for Trump, 17; indifference to suffering of, 200; and integration, 227–29; and labor, 193–94, 246; and language, 186–87, 226–39; and media, 186, 190–96, 202–3, 330–31; and mental health, 185, 186; motivations for, 185, 237; narrative anxiety and Francophone literature, 186–87, 211–23; numbers of people migrating, 185, 191–92; and the Other, 200–206, 244–50; overview, 185–86; political hostility to, 185, 186–87, 190–96, 244–50; and political legitimacy, 186, 189–206; and political orientation, 104, 105–8, 110; selectivity in, 194–95
incels, 272–73
Indigenous peoples, 67n17, 75, 76, 89, 95–96
industrialism, 254, 257–74
Industry 4.0, 306, 312, 314, 316
inequities: in climate change effects, 79, 89, 92; and fundamental causes in public health, 127, 133–34
Inglehart, Ronald, 102
inhibition, 36
interdependence hypothesis, 233
ISIS/Daech, 271–72
Islam: and British fantasy discourse, 328; and Muslim immigrants, 194–95, 202–3, 204, 249; and terrorism, 271–72

Jabareen, Yosef, 124
January 6 insurrection, 324, 332–33
Japan: dehumanization of Japanese, 20; technology policy, 255, 305–6, 311–17
Jasanoff, Sheila, 284
jetztzeit, 217, 221
Johnson, Mark, 343
Johnston, Adrian, 327
jouissance, 324, 326–28
joy. *See* happiness
Judeo-Christian origins of morality, 359–63
Jünger, Friedrich Georg, 297

Kalmbach, Karena, 254
Karazsia, Bryan, 86
Kierkegaard, Søren, 2, 3, 11, 12, 42, 281, 372
Kim, Sang-Hyun, 284
Kittler, Friedrich, 298–99
Klein, Melanie, 73
Kleinginna, Anne, 197
Kleinginna, Paul, 197
Kleyn, Tatyana, 233, 239
knowledge transfer, 309–10, 316
Koch, Lars, 285
Koopmans, Ruud, 237–38
Korea, anti-suicide campaigns, 355
Koselleck, Reinhart, 196, 283–84, 285
Kvaløy, Berit, 103

labor and immigration, 193–94, 246
Lacan, Jacques: and anxiety, 80, 81, 261, 263; and fantasy discourse and Trumpism, 324, 326–29, 334; and nihilism, 260; and the Other, xii
Laclau, Ernesto, 208n31, 326, 329, 330
Lafont, Christina, 349
Laguna de la Vera, Rafael, 309
language: anxiety terms in languages other than English, 41, 171–72; heritage languages, 186–87, 226–39; L2 languages, 235; and linguistic diversity, 227
Lanz, Tilman, 229
Latour, Bruno, 350
learning: anxiety's role in, 3, 12, 372; and collective effort, 9; fear *vs.* anxiety, 26–27; and gun violence, 141–42, 149; and heritage languages, 233, 235; machine learning, 54, 105–6, 109–15; and managing anxiety, 12, 27, 31, 37; and reflection, 3; strategies and culture, 32
Ledoux, Joseph, 50
Lee, Crystal, 18
Lee, Jin Sook, 233
Lefranc, Sandrine, 220
leisure habits and youth mental health, 155, 157, 158, 161–62, 163, 166, 167
Le Mammouth (Samson), 222–23
LeMenager, Stephanie, 70, 71, 81
Le pays des autres (Slimani), 216–17
Le silence des esprits (N'Sondé), 216
Levi, Primo, 220
liberalism and cognition, 13–19, 22–23
"The Limits to Growth" (Club of Rome report), 71, 102, 339
Link, Bruce G., 127